FETAL HEART RATE MONITORING

THIRD EDITION

FETAL HEART RATE MONITORING

THIRD EDITION

ROGER K. FREEMAN, M.D.

Professor
Department of Obstetrics and Gynecology
University of California, Irvine
Orange, California
Director of Obstetrics & Gynecology, Newborn Careline
Women's Hospital
Long Beach Memorial Medical Center
Long Beach, California

THOMAS J. GARITE, M.D.

E. J. Quilligan Professor and Chairman
Department of Obstetrics and Gynecology
University of California, Irvine
Orange, California

MICHAEL P. NAGEOTTE, M.D.

Professor
Department of Obstetrics and Gynecology
University of California, Irvine
Orange, California
Executive Careline Director
Women's Hospital
Long Beach Memorial Medical Center
Long Beach, California

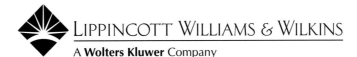

LIPPINCOTT WILLIAMS & WILKINS
A **Wolters Kluwer** Company
Philadelphia • Baltimore • New York • London
Buenos Aires • Hong Kong • Sydney • Tokyo

Acquisitions Editor: Lisa McAllister
Developmental Editor: Kerry Barrett
Production Editor: Elaine Verriest McClusky
Manufacturing Manager: Colin Warnock
Cover Designer: Christine Jenny
Compositor: Lippincott Williams & Wilkins Desktop Division
Printer: Maple Press

Printed in the USA

Library of Congress Cataloging-in-Publication Data

Freeman, Roger K., 1935–
    Fetal heart rate monitoring / Roger K. Freeman, Thomas J. Garite, Michael P. Nageotte.—3rd ed.
        p. ; cm.
    Includes bibliographical references and index.
    ISBN 0-7817-3524-6
      1. Fetal heart rate monitoring. I. Garite, Thomas J. II. Nageotte, Michael P.
    III. Title.
    [DNLM: 1. Fetal Monitoring. 2. Heart Rate, Fetal. 3. Fetal Heart.
    WQ 210.5 F855f2003]
    RG628.3.H42F73 2003
    618.3′20754—dc21

                                                                    2002043363

Care has been taken to confirm the accuracy of the information presented and to describe generally accepted practices. However, the authors and publisher are not responsible for errors or omissions or for any consequences from application of the information in this book and make no warranty, expressed or implied, with respect to the currency, completeness, or accuracy of the contents of the publication. Application of this information in a particular situation remains the professional responsibility of the practitioner.

The authors and publisher have exerted every effort to ensure that drug selection and dosage set forth in this text are in accordance with current recommendations and practice at the time of publication. However, in view of ongoing research, changes in government regulations, and the constant flow of information relating to drug therapy and drug reactions, the reader is urged to check the package insert for each drug for any change in indications and dosage and for added warnings and precautions. This is particularly important when the recommended agent is a new or infrequently employed drug.

Some drugs and medical devices presented in this publication have Food and Drug Administration (FDA) clearance for limited use in restricted research settings. It is the responsibility of the health care provider to ascertain the FDA status of each drug or device planned for use in their clinical practice.

10 9 8 7 6 5 4 3 2 1

The authors dedicate this book in the hope that an in-depth, physiologically oriented understanding of electronic fetal heart rate monitoring (EFM) will result not only in the best possible outcome for babies and mothers, but also an understanding of the limits of this technology. Fetal heart rate (FHR) monitoring is after all, a diagnostic, not a therapeutic device; and no thermometer, EKG, or other diagnostic tool can do more than give us better information and help us make better decisions. It cannot in and of itself improve outcome. The unrealistic expectations that EFM has created and the frequency of abnormal FHR patterns have together led to a labor and delivery environment that is one of high anxiety, both for patients and their caregivers. We hope that with a better understanding of EFM, we are not only able to optimize outcome and understand the limits of this technology, but also to react more appropriately—minimizing interventions and making the labor and delivery unit the happy, fulfilling environment it should be.

CONTENTS

PREFACE

The first edition of this book was published in 1981 when electronic fetal heart rate monitoring was becoming the preferred modality in most hospitals for intrapartum fetal surveillance. The retrospective and non-controlled prospective trials comparing electronic fetal monitoring to non-intensive auscultation were encouraging. The second edition was published in 1991. At that time questions about the validity of the modality and its potential impact on outcomes were emerging. Through randomized controlled trials, it was discovered that intensive auscultation appeared to give equivalent outcomes to electronic fetal heart rate monitoring. Electronic fetal heart rate monitoring was associated with increased operative delivery rates in some studies. It became apparent that the incidence of cerebral palsy had not changed with the introduction of electronic fetal heart rate monitoring. It was clear, however, that when comparing outcomes before electronic fetal heart rate monitoring and intensive auscultation, to those outcomes after its advent, the incidence of intrapartum stillbirth in term pregnancies had declined by a factor of three. This would suggest that the window may have moved, resulting in some previously stillborn infants surviving but with damage and some previously damaged infants surviving intact with a net result of no decrease in cerebral palsy.

Nevertheless, electronic fetal heart rate monitoring offers a more cost effective means of surveillance than does intensive intermittent auscultation. Presently, most hospitals in the United States offer electronic fetal heart rate monitoring as the primary means of fetal surveillance. It therefore becomes incumbent on providers of obstetric care to have a good understanding of the technique and the interpretation of the data produced. This third edition provides the obstetrical clinician a framework within which to interpret and understand fetal heart rate tracings and their implications.

Since the last edition, the use of the term "fetal distress" has fallen into disfavor because it assigns a significance to fetal heart rate patterns that exceeds the scientific information available. It is clear that most fetal heart rate patterns are reassuring with respect to adequacy of fetal oxygenation. Patterns that are not reassuring of adequate fetal oxygenation are better termed "nonreassuring" rather than fetal distress because a large percentage of such tracings ultimately do not have evidence of significant fetal hypoxia. Further-more, there are tracings that may suggest fetal central nervous system abnormalities that are not associated with hypoxia or any ongoing "distress." They would also be considered nonreassuring, but not necessarily associated with any condition that may benefit from intervention.

Another factor that has been introduced since the last edition is the National Institutes of Health consensus workshop on intrapartum fetal heart rate monitoring interpretation. The result of this workshop was that only completely reassuring patterns, and those patterns that were of such concern that imminent risk of death or damage was present could be agreed upon. This leaves a large area of "nonreassuring" patterns for which there was no real consensus, but still concern. This magnifies the need for other methods of evaluation of such patterns including fetal scalp blood sampling, fetal scalp stimulation, and fetal pulse oximetry.

The third edition has added a chapter on fetal pulse oximetry which offers a means by which the clinician can continuously clarify the significance of fetal heart rate patterns that are nonreassuring. While this new technique appears to offer a great advantage in such situations, further clinical experience and research with the technique will serve to clarify its roll for the obstetrical clinician faced with problematic tracings.

Finally, since the last edition, the role of infection resulting in a fetal inflammatory response that is mediated through inflammatory cytokines has been identified as a major causative factor in the later development of cerebral palsy, especially in pre-term infants. It is not clear what fetal heart rate patterns may be associated with such conditions or if there are any strategies that we may employ to avoid the damage resulting from this fetal inflammatory response. It is clear, however, that the neonatal encephalopathy resulting from this fetal inflammatory response may be indistinguishable from hypoxic ischemic encephalopathy. The authors have attempted to review this new area of concern.

We hope the third edition will provide obstetrical care providers with assistance in the management of their patients using fetal heart rate monitoring as a means of primary surveillance.

Roger K. Freeman, M.D.
Thomas J. Garite, M.D.
Michael P. Nageotte, M.D.

ACKNOWLEDGMENT

The authors wish to acknowledge and express our appreciation to Kimberly Peters-Phair, M.N., R.N., who found many new cases, provided organization and editing skills, and kept us on schedule. Without her dedication and skill it is hard to imagine that this edition would have ever been completed.

1

HISTORY OF FETAL MONITORING

It is somewhat surprising that something as potentially accessible as the fetal heart was neither heard nor described until the 17th century when Phillipe LeGaust first depicted fetal heart tones in his poetry in an ancient French dialect. LeGaust was a colleague of Marsac, a physician of the province of Limousin, who is credited with first having heard the fetal heart.

Marsac's observation apparently went unnoticed until 1818, when Swiss surgeon Francois Mayor reported the presence of fetal heart sounds when he placed his ear on the maternal abdomen in an attempt to hear the fetus splash about in the liquor amnii. Three years later, French nobleman Lejumeau Kergaradec, apparently unaware of Mayor's report, described both the fetal heart tones and the uterine souffle. He suggested auscultation to be of value in the diagnosis of pregnancy and twins, and in determining fetal lie and presentation.

As with many discoveries, the obstetricians of the time were slow to respond to Kergaradec's observations and recommendations. To convince clinicians of the value of Kergaradec's findings, Evory Kennedy of Dublin published an extensive book in 1833, *Observations on Obstetric Auscultation* (1). The text contains many anecdotal examples of cases in which auscultation was clearly beneficial. In addition, Kennedy described the funic souffle for the first time.

THE FETOSCOPE

Before the development of the fetoscope, much attention was paid to whether mediate (stethoscopic) auscultation using Laennec's instrument, or immediate auscultation, with direct application of the ear to the gravid maternal abdomen, was the more appropriate choice. Rauth and Verardini (2) suggested vaginal stethoscopy as more valuable in the early detection of fetal life. The development of the head stethoscope (fetoscope) is a story of controversy and

professional jealousy. It was first reported, in 1917, in *The Journal of the American Medical Association* (Fig. 1.1), by David Hillis (3), an obstetrician then working in Chicago Lying-In Hospital. In 1922, J.B. DeLee, who was chief of staff at the same institution, and who became a legend in American obstetrics for many contributions, published his report of a similar instrument (4). Although the order of publications is clear, DeLee claimed that he openly talked of this idea for many years preceding the Hillis publication. The instrument, which subsequently came to be known as the DeLee-Hillis stethoscope, has changed little since its early development.

DIAGNOSIS OF FETAL DISTRESS

Thirty years after Mayor first described heart sounds, Killian (5) first proposed that changes in the fetal heart rate might be used to diagnose fetal distress and to indicate when the clinician should intervene on behalf of the fetus. He formulated what is sometimes called "the stethoscopal indication for forceps delivery," and suggested that heart rates below 100 or above 180 beats per minute (BPM), and those with loss of purity of tone or distinct intermission, or in which only one tone could be heard, were indications for forceps application without delay. In 1893, Von Winckel (6) described the criteria of fetal distress that were to remain essentially unchanged until the arrival of fetal scalp sampling and electronic heart rate monitoring: tachycardia (heart rate more than 160 BPM), bradycardia (less than 100 BPM), irregular heart rate, passage of meconium, and gross alteration of fetal movement. Few studies either challenged or supported the validity of these auscultative and clinical criteria for fetal distress. It was not until 1968, when Benson et al. (7) published the results of the Collaborative Project, commissioned by the National Institute of Neurologic Diseases and Blindness, that these criteria came under serious scrutiny. The Benson study reviewed the

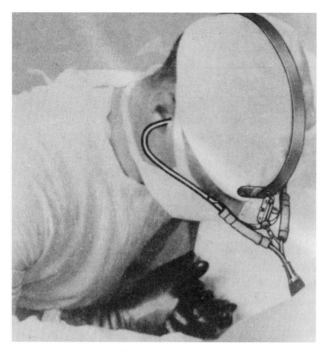

FIGURE 1.1. Original illustration of the head stethoscope or fetoscope. (From Hillis DS: Attachment for the stethoscope. *JAMA* 68:910, 1917.)

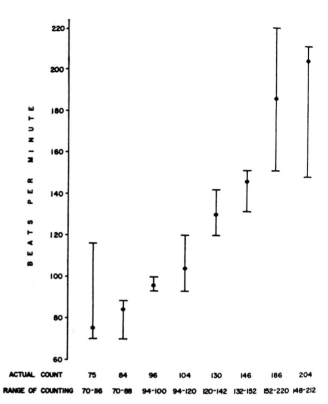

FIGURE 1.2. Range of error in auscultative counting of fetal heart rate (FHR) by 15 obstetricians asked to count from recorded FHR. Count as reported by obstetrician on vertical scale vs. actual count on horizontal scale. (From Hon EH: The electronic evaluation of the fetal heart rate. *Am J Obstet Gynecol* 75:1215, 1958.)

benefits of fetal heart rate auscultation in the management of intrapartum fetal distress in 24,863 deliveries. Benson concluded that there was "no reliable indicator of fetal distress in terms of fetal heart rate save in extreme degree." Ten years earlier, Hon (8) asked 15 obstetricians to count several rates from audiotape. He found a wide divergence in counting and pointed out the unreliability of human computation of the fetal heart rate (FHR) (Fig. 1.2).

As new information has emerged, the term fetal distress has been determined as an inappropriate term to describe FHR patterns that may be associated with decreases in fetal oxygenation. Because a large proportion of such patterns do not result in neonates with signs of fetal hypoxia and/or acidosis, the term nonreassuring FHR pattern has been adopted to refer to such tracings. In addition, the original recommendations for intervention based on periodic FHR patterns alone is undergoing an evolution in which the presence of spontaneous or evoked accelerations, FHR variability, fetal pH, and fetal pulse oximetry allow the clinician to sometimes avoid intervention for nonreassuring patterns. These approaches will be discussed in later chapters.

With these serious doubts, and with the age of electronic technology fast making its impact on modern medicine, it was inevitable that obstetric research would turn to more sophisticated methods of fetal evaluation.

THE FETAL ELECTROCARDIOGRAPH

Cremer (9) recorded the FHR electronically for the first time in 1906, by means of abdominal and intravaginal leads. For the first half of the century, the application of fetal electrocardiography was used primarily for the diagnosis of fetal life. It was Southern (10) who, in 1957, suggested that certain fetal electrocardiograph (ECG) changes might correlate with fetal hypoxia. Shortly thereafter, Hon and Hess (11) reviewed all the applications of fetal electrocardiography, including fetal presentation, diagnosis of twins, antenatal diagnosis of congenital heart disease, diagnosis of fetal maturity, and fetal distress. They concluded that the ECG waveform was not of consistent value in any of these situations and, specifically, that in 75 cases of fetal distress "no consistent fetal ECG changes could be detected." Subsequently, Pardi et al. (12) used group averaging techniques to demonstrate ST segment depression with fetal hypoxia (Fig. 1.3). Unfortunately, this technique has not been developed to the point where it has become clinically applicable.

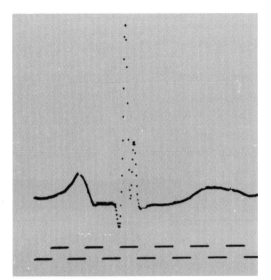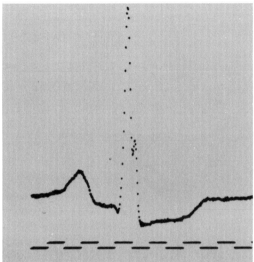

FIGURE 1.3. Left: Average of 25 electrocardiograph (ECG) complexes performed before the onset of a contraction: baseline 160 beats/min. **Right:** Average of 25 ECG complexes performed immediately after the end of the same contraction, during a late deceleration. Notice the depression of the ST segment. Scalp capillary blood pH 7.34, Apgar score 4/9, umbilical artery pH 7.25. (From Crosignani PG, Pardi G: *Fetal evaluation during pregnancy and labor.* Academic Press, New York, 1971, p 235.)

The history of the development of electronic FHR monitoring, or cardiotachometry, is a complex merger of technologic development with empirical observations of those heart rate patterns associated with various causes of fetal distress.

The earliest preliminary report of FHR monitoring came in 1958 from Edward Hon, MD, (8) then at the Yale University School of Medicine. He reported on the continuous instantaneous recording of FHR via fetal ECG monitor on the maternal abdomen. He began to elucidate causes of fetal bradycardia and, more specifically, defined when bradycardia was indicative of fetal distress. In the years that followed, Hon, Caldeyro-Barcia in Uruguay, Hammacher in Germany, and their many coworkers reported their observations on the various heart rate patterns associated with fetal distress. Bradycardia and tachycardia were well-known signs of fetal compromise. In 1959, Hon (13) defined the type of variable deceleration associated with umbilical cord compression and proposed a mechanism for the hypoxic uteroplacental causes of delayed decelerations. In 1963, Caldeyro-Barcia et al. (14) reported their observations on the "prognostic significance" of similar heart rate decelerations, which they called type III and II. In addition, long- and short-term FHR variability was defined for the first time. Hammacher (15) subsequently described this parameter's significance in terms of loss of heart rate variability in association with fetal distress.

With many investigators throughout the world making similar observations, FHR terminology became extremely confusing. Hon, Caldeyro-Barcia, and many of their colleagues met at an international conference on monitoring of the fetal heart in December 1971 in New Jersey and in March 1972 in Amsterdam to discuss nomenclature and develop standards for FHR monitoring. They developed and agreed upon a common nomenclature. Efforts were made to agree upon universal scales and paper speed for fetal monitors, but these remained variable. Much of the subsequent history has been one of technologic development for the clinical application of electronic FHR monitoring. The first practical commercially available fetal monitor to be of clinical use was produced by Hammacher and Hewlett-Packard in 1968 using external tocography and phonocardiography (Fig. 1.4). Before this time, monitors were bulky and generally limited to research, although attempts were made to market some equipment for general use (Fig. 1.5). Technologic advances since that first generation of fetal monitors have allowed further and more accurate definition of FHR patterns and have provided the clinician with a practical tool. Direct ECG monitoring was realized with Hon's introduction of an electrode that could be applied directly to the fetal scalp (16). This was originally a modification of a surgical skin clip (Fig. 1.6). Subsequently, Hon developed a more convenient disposable spiral electrode (Fig. 1.7) that is widely used in this country today. Doppler ultrasound and exter-

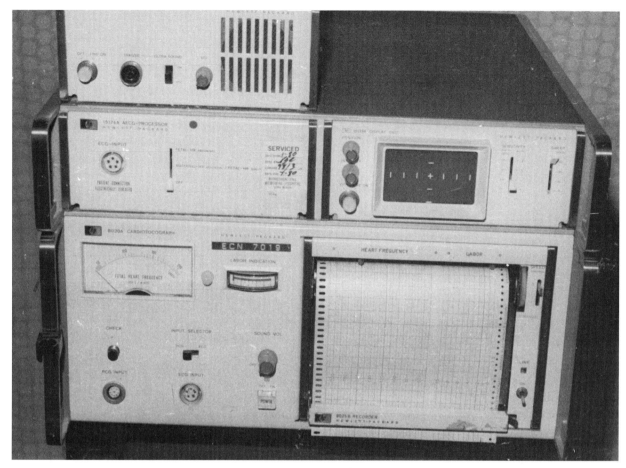

FIGURE 1.4. First generation of practical commercially available fetal monitors. The original model used external monitoring with phonocardiography only. The upper two modules were subsequently added, allowing the addition of external ultrasound and internal fetal electrocardiographic monitoring (Hewlett-Packard Model 8020A).

nal ECG and logic systems that provide adequate approximations of the real beat-to-beat heart rate have been more recent developments.

ERA OF QUESTIONING

Benson's report on the data collected by the Collaborative Project set the stage for rejection of auscultation and the boom in electronic cardiotachometry. By 1978, it was estimated that fetal monitoring was in routine use in over half of labors (18). Enthusiasm for its use, however, came without clear documentation of its efficacy and safety. There were many retrospective analyses of fetal monitoring and nearly all agreed to a beneficial effect, including reduction of intrapartum stillbirth rate and perinatal mortality, as well as improved Apgar scores (19). Randomized controlled trials have now been reported (20–23). While mixed, they do not uniformly show electronic monitoring as beneficial and, indeed, suggest that such monitoring may substantially increase the rate of cesarean sections. Details of all these studies and an analysis of the risks and benefits of fetal monitoring are reviewed in Chapter 3. The era of consumer demand in obstetrics in particular, coupled with a period of heightened government intervention into cost, risks, and benefits of medical care, have provided further impetus for questioning electronic fetal monitoring.

Electronic fetal monitoring has become common practice for patients during labor, and antepartum electronic fetal heart rate monitoring is one of the best means currently available to assess the fetus at high risk for antenatal uteroplacental insufficiency. Further applications will depend on continuing evaluation and adjustment of current methodologies as well as the development of new technology. It is clear, however, that assessment of the human fetus for hypoxia is one end result of the development of electronic fetal heart rate monitoring.

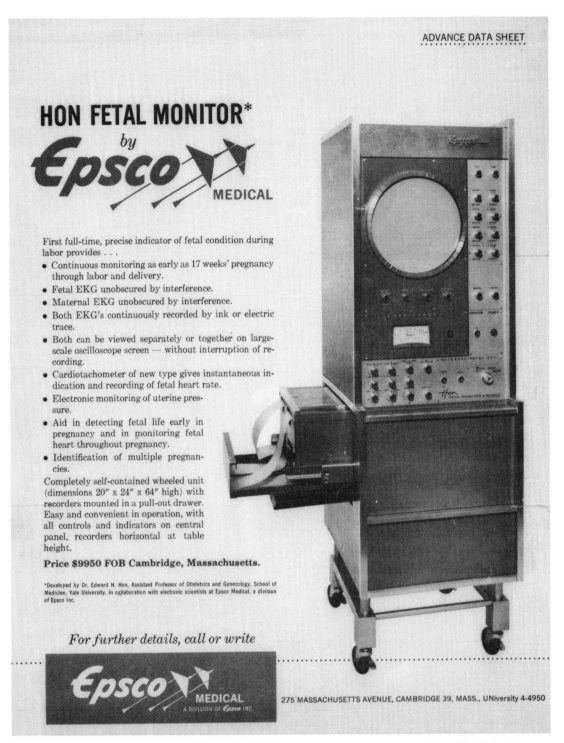

FIGURE 1.5. This bulky machine was the first attempt at making a commercially available fetal monitor. (Courtesy of Epsco, Inc.)

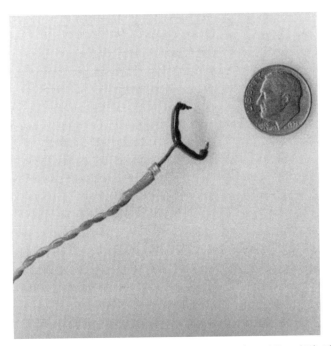

FIGURE 1.6. Vaginal fetal scalp electrode as described by Dr. Edward Hon (16). This is a modification of a Michelle surgical skin clip. A specially made long forceps and a vaginal speculum are necessary for application.

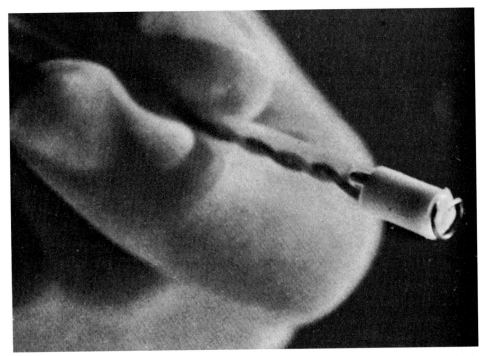

FIGURE 1.7. Spiral silver–silver chloride fetal scalp electrode described by Hon (17) in 1972. This is packaged within a plastic sheath which allows direct application without the aid of a speculum.

REFERENCES

1. Kennedy E: *Observations on Obstetric Auscultation.* Hodges and Smith, Dublin, 1833.
2. Rauth, Verardini: quoted in: Hirst BC: *An American System of Obstetrics.* Lea Brothers Co, Philadelphia, 1888.
3. Hillis DS: Attachment for the stethoscope. *JAMA* 68:910, 1917.
4. DeLee JB: Ein nues stethoskop für die Geburtshilfe besonders geeignet. *Zentralbl Gynaekol* 46:1688, 1922.
5. Kilian: quoted in: Goodlin R: History of fetal monitoring. *Am J Obstet Gynecol* 133:325, 1979.
6. Von Winckel F: *Lehrbuch der Geburtshilfe,* Weisbaden, 1893, p 634.
7. Benson RC, Shubeck F, Deutschberger J, et al.: Fetal heart rate as a predictor of fetal distress: a report from the Collaborative Project. *Obstet Gynecol* 32:529, 1968.
8. Hon EH: The electronic evaluation of the fetal heart rate. *Am J Obstet Gynecol* 75:1215, 1958.
9. Cremer M: *Munch Med Wochenschr* 53:811, 1906.
10. Southern EM: Fetal anoxia and its possible relation to changes in the prenatal fetal electrocardiogram. *Am J Obstet Gynecol* 73:233, 1957.
11. Hon EH, Hess OW: The clinical value of fetal electrocardiography. *Am J Obstet Gynecol* 79:1012, 1960.
12. Pardi G, Brambati B, Dubini S, et al.: Analysis of the fetal electrocardiogram by the group averaging technique. Presented at the Proceedings of the 2nd European Congress of Perinatal Medicine, London, 1970.
13. Hon EH: Observations on "pathologic" fetal bradycardia. *Am J Obstet Gynecol* 77:1084, 1959.
14. Caldeyro-Barcia R, Mendez-Bauer C, Poseiro JJ, et al.: Control of human fetal heart rate during labor. In: Cassels D, ed. *The Heart and Circulation in the Newborn Infant.* Grune & Stratton, Inc., New York, 1966.
15. Hammacher K: In: Kaser O, Friedberg V, Oberk K, eds. *Gynakologie v Gerburtshilfe BD II.* Georg Thieme Verlag, Stuttgard, 1967.
16. Hon EH: Instrumentation of fetal heart rate and electrocardiography. II. A vaginal electrode. *Am J Obstet Gynecol* 86:772, 1963.
17. Hon EH, Paul RH, Hon RW: Electronic evaluation of fetal heart rate. XI. Description of a spiral electrode. *Obstet Gynecol* 40:362, 1972.
18. Williams RL, Hawes WE: Cesarean section, fetal monitoring and perinatal mortality in California. *Am J Public Health* 69:864, 1979.
19. Task Force on Predictors of Fetal Distress, NICHD Consensus Development Committee on Antenatal Diagnosis, NIH Publication no 79-1973, 1979.
20. Haverkamp AD, Thompson HE, McFee JG, et al.: The evaluation of continuous fetal heart rate monitoring in high risk pregnancy. *Am J Obstet Gynecol* 125:310, 1976.
21. Renou P, Chang A, Anderson I, et al.: Controlled trial of fetal intensive care. *Am J Obstet Gynecol* 126:470, 1976.
22. Kelso IM, Parsons RJ, Lawrence GF, et al.: An assessment of continuous fetal heart rate monitoring in labor: a randomized trial. *Am J Obstet Gynecol* 131:526, 1978.
23. Haverkamp AD, Orleans M, Langendoerfer S, et al.: A controlled trial of the differential effects of intrapartum fetal monitoring. *Am J Obstet Gynecol* 134:399, 1979.

2

PHYSIOLOGIC BASIS
OF FETAL MONITORING

Clinical fetal heart rate (FHR) monitoring is an ongoing observation of human fetal physiology. The question being asked by the clinician is: What is the adequacy of fetal oxygenation? Because the FHR pattern appears to assume certain characteristics under the influence of various hypoxic and nonhypoxic stresses, it becomes important for the clinician to have a basic understanding of the physiology of fetal respiratory exchange and the physiologic control of the FHR. In this chapter, an attempt will be made to outline the principle factors involved in fetal oxygenation and carbon dioxide transfer as well as the basis for our current understanding of FHR responses to changes in fetal respiratory status.

THE ANATOMY OF MATERNAL-FETAL EXCHANGE

The placenta is an organ that functions as the fetus' extracorporeal life-support system. The placenta serves as the fetal lung (respiration), kidney (excretion), gastrointestinal tract (nutrition), and skin (heat exchange), and as a barrier against certain substances dangerous to the fetus. In addition, it is an endocrine organ that produces steroid (estrogen, progesterone) and protein (human chorionic gonadotropin, human placental lactogen) hormones. Very early in gestation, the blastocyst implants in the decidualized endometrium and the trophoblast cells invade the maternal circulation, creating a lake of maternal blood that bathes the trophoblast and developing embryo. As the gestation grows, a number of spiral arteries that supply blood to the endometrium are penetrated and provide the basic architecture as the placenta develops, with villi forming cotyledons arranged around these spiral arteries. The fetal chorionic villi develop many convolutions and float in the maternal blood supplied from the previously invaded spiral arteries. This maternal blood occupies an area referred to as the intervillous space, and it is between this space and the fetal capillary (contained within the chorionic villus) that mater-

nal-fetal and fetal-maternal exchange occurs. The human placenta is thus referred to as a hemochorial type because the mother's blood comes into direct contact with the fetal chorionic villus (1). Oxygen, carbon dioxide, nutrients, waste products, water, and heat are exchanged at this level and must cross two layers of fetal trophoblast, the fetal connective tissue within the villus, and the fetal capillary wall (Fig. 2.1).

The uterine blood flow is supplied principally from the uterine arteries, but anastomoses occur between these vessels, other branches of the hypogastric arteries, and ovarian arteries. Significantly, the spiral arteries must traverse the full thickness of the myometrium to reach the intervillous space. Anything that affects maternal cardiac output will, of course, affect the flow through the spiral arteries. Additionally, as the uterus contracts, the intramyometrial pressure

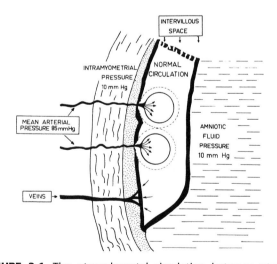

FIGURE 2.1. The uteroplacental circulation between uterine contractions is shown. Note that the intramyometrial pressure is less than the arterial pressure, allowing the arteries to remain open and provide a supply of blood to the intervillous space. (From Poseiro JJ, Mendez-Bauer C, Pose SV, et al.: Effect of uterine contractions on maternal blood flow through the placenta. In: *Perinatal factors affecting human development.* Pan American Health Organization, Scientific Publication no 185, Washington, DC, 1969:161–171, with permission.)

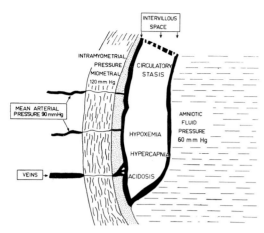

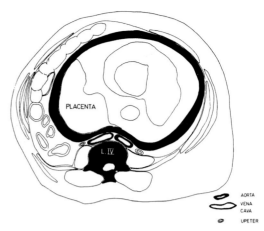

FIGURE 2.2. The uteroplacental circulation during a uterine contraction is shown. Note that the intramyometrial pressure exceeds the arterial pressure, causing circulatory stasis in the intervillous space. (From Poseiro JJ, Mendez-Bauer C, Pose SV, et al.: Effect of uterine contractions on maternal blood flow through the placenta. In: *Perinatal factors affecting human development.* Pan American Health Organization, Scientific Publication no 185, Washington, DC, 1969:161–171, with permission.)

FIGURE 2.3. A cross-section of a pregnant uterus lying on the maternal vertebral column with the interposed great vessels, which are subject to occlusion when the mother is supine. (From Poseiro JJ, Mendez-Bauer C, Pose SV, et al.: Effect of uterine contractions on maternal blood flow through the placenta. In: *Perinatal factors affecting human development.* Pan American Health Organization, Scientific Publication no 185, Washington, DC, 1969:161–171, with permission.)

may exceed the intraarterial pressure, causing occlusion of these vessels and resulting in cessation of blood flow to the intervillous space (Fig. 2.2) (2).

Most authorities agree that approximately 85% of the total uterine blood flow goes to supply the placental (intervillous) circulation and approximately 15% supplies the extraplacental uterine musculature (3). The intervillous space blood supplies the vascular support to the placenta itself and, if the blood flow to any area is sufficiently compromised, an infarction of the placenta may occur (4,5).

For clinical purposes, the intervillous space circulation is probably maximal when the mother is at rest, in the lateral position. Although estrogen administration to the pregnant ewe will increase uterine blood flow, it is not certain that this results in increased intervillous space flow (5). Therefore, although we know of nothing that will increase effective uterine blood flow above that found in the resting lateral position, there are many things that will decrease uterine blood flow.

FACTORS THAT DECREASE UTERINE BLOOD FLOW

Position

Changes in the mother's position may decrease blood flow to the uterus by at least two mechanisms. The supine position is characterized by an exaggeration of the lumbar lordotic curve, resulting in uterine compression of the vena cava, the aortoiliac vessels, or both. With vena caval occlusion, the return of blood to the heart is decreased, and this

may result in a fall in maternal cardiac output, maternal hypotension, and decreased uterine blood flow (7,8). Compression of the aorta against the spine or iliac vessels as they cross the pelvic brim may result in decreases in uterine blood flow without maternal hypotension (Fig. 2.3). Abitbol et al. (9) showed that patients in the supine position had an increased incidence of late decelerations during labor and this correlated with a fall in femoral arterial pressure, a decrease in the amplitude of the big toe capillary pulse, and a drop in the fetal scalp blood pH, all of which were reversible when patients were returned to the lateral position.

Exercise

Maternal exercise may serve to divert blood away from the uterus to supply somatic muscle groups, resulting in decreased uterine blood flow. Clapp (10) has shown that baseline FHR increases consistently following exercise in pregnant women. The tachycardia following exercise is not believed to be due to hyperthermia or increased fetal activity but rather is a sympathetic response to a period of reduced fetal oxygen. Artal et al. (11) have described three cases of fetal bradycardia occurring during postexercise fetal tachycardia, suggesting that in those cases there was more profound hypoxia. These studies in humans tend to support the caution originally suggested in Emmanouilides et al.'s research into exercising pregnant sheep (12). Although there is evidence that exercise is not detrimental to the fetus where there is normal uteroplacental function (13), it is possible that some fetuses could be adversely affected by excessive maternal exercise.

Uterine Contractions

The spiral arteries that traverse the myometrium are subject to collapse as the uterus contracts and the intramyometrial pressure exceeds the spiral arterial pressure. During normal pregnancy, the uterus has certain inherent contractility (Braxton-Hicks contractions), and as labor begins, the contractions increase in intensity. If the uteroplacental reserve is normal, the Braxton-Hicks contractions and labor contractions do not appear to significantly compromise the total intervillous space blood flow. However, a normal fetoplacental unit may have its uteroplacental reserve exceeded if uterine activity is excessive, as with spontaneous or oxytocin-induced uterine hypertonus and/or tetanic contractions (14,15). Patients with abruptio placenta may have hypertonus and polysystole, resulting in decreased intervillous space perfusion producing fetal hypoxia. Orgasmic coitus has been reported to be associated with increased uterine activity and prolonged FHR deceleration in three patients studied with simultaneous FHR and uterine contraction monitoring (16).

Surface Area

Anything that will decrease the effective surface area of the placenta will clearly increase the potential for fetal hypoxia. Abruptio placenta is a classic example of reduced placental surface area available for exchange. Patients with multiple placental infarcts, as may be seen in hypertensive disorders and prolonged pregnancy, are also subject to having the fetus suffer from uteroplacental insufficiency. There is recent evidence that hypercoagulable states in the fetus may result in thromboses of the fetal vessels in the placenta that may lead to growth restriction and decreased available oxygen to the fetus (17).

Anesthesia

The administration of conduction anesthetics carries the potential for reduced intervillous space blood flow secondary to maternal hypotension, resulting from the sympathetic blockade that may occur to a greater or lesser degree in all such patients. The pharmacologic correction of such hypotension with α-adrenergic agents may not restore uterine blood flow because the α-adrenergic agents will increase uterine circulatory resistance along with the other somatic components of total peripheral resistance that are responsible for the increase in blood pressure. For this reason, it is recommended that an agent such as ephedrine (a mixed α- and β-adrenergic stimulator) be used to restore maternal blood pressure after hypotension induced by the sympathectomy of conduction anesthesia (18). Usually, however, the uterine blood flow is easily restored in such situations by correcting positional factors and expanding maternal blood volume, thus obviating the need for any pressor agents.

Using isotope techniques, reports of increased uterine blood flow following epidural anesthesia have given rise to some questions regarding the classic understanding of sympathectomy caused by conduction anesthesia, resulting in diversion of blood from the uterus (19). Recent data using Doppler flow techniques have shown that diastolic flow in the arcuate arteries may actually increase in prehydrated patients following epidural anesthesia (20). The proposed mechanism involves a decrease in sympathetic tone in the uterine circulation, resulting in decreased resistance. It is not clear, however, whether this finding actually represents increased placental flow or merely opening of the nonplacental portion of the uterine circulation. The reason one must question data suggesting that epidural anesthesia increases uteroplacental blood flow is related to the frequent finding of late deceleration following epidural activation. Further research in this area is needed to clarify the exact relation of conduction anesthesia to uteroplacental blood flow.

Hypertension

Maternal hypertensive syndromes may result in decreased intervillous space blood flow as a result of either acute vasospastic or chronic atheromatous changes in the uterine arterial blood supply. If one lowers blood pressure in the hypertensive patient either intentionally with antihypertensive agents or unintentionally as a result of administering a conduction anesthetic, one runs the risk of diverting blood away from the intervillous space if the caliber of the uterine arterial circulation remains diminished as other vascular beds are dilated.

Diffusion Distance

The thickness of the placental membrane between the intervillous space and the fetal capillary may also decrease the transfer of oxygen. An example of a clinical entity demonstrating this phenomenon can probably be found in fetal erythroblastosis with placental edema. Perhaps this is also a factor in certain conditions of fetal dysmaturity where there is an increase in fibrin deposition between the intervillous space and the fetal capillary. Villous hemorrhage and edema in diabetics may also play a role in increasing the thickness of the placental membrane.

THE FETAL CIRCULATION

The anatomy and physiology of the fetal circulation are very complex. For the purposes of this chapter, we will focus on the umbilical circulation and factors that affect placental exchange (Fig. 2.4).

The umbilical vessels are contained within the umbilical cord and are protected with an abundance of a substance

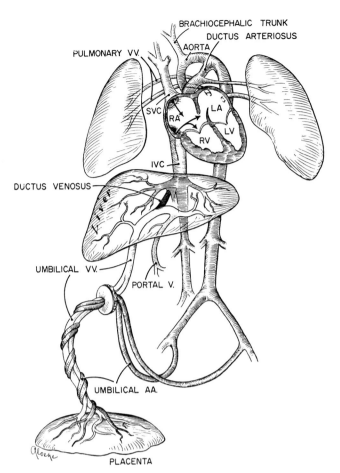

FIGURE 2.4. Schematic representation of the fetal circulation in the lamb. Note that the well-oxygenated blood returning from the placenta via the inferior vena cava *(IVC)* crosses into the left atrium *(LA)* while the superior vena cava *(SVC)* blood tends to run into the right ventricle *(RV)*. (From Assali NS: Fetal and neonatal circulation. In: *Biology of gestation. II.* Academic Press, New York, 1968:254, with permission.)

called Wharton's jelly. Normally, there are two umbilical arteries that arise from the terminal ends of the hypogastric arteries and a single umbilical vein that returns blood to the fetus from the placenta, channeling it partly through the liver and partly to the inferior vena cava via the ductus venosus. This well-oxygenated blood enters the right atrium and follows a course directing it mainly to the cephalic circulation, while blood returning from the upper body via the superior vena cava is channeled principally through the ductus arteriosus to the lower body and the placenta. Approximately 30% of the fetal cardiac output goes to the placenta, which comprises a low resistance vascular bed. The oxygen content of the umbilical venous blood closely approximates that of the uterine venous drainage, which suggests that the pattern of umbilical and uterine flows functionally follows a concurrent relationship, although the flow relationships are clearly much more complex and authorities in the field are not in total agreement concerning this fact (21).

One must ask how the fetus can exist at a maximum pO_2 below that of the uterine vein (about 35 mm Hg), whereas the adult would be unable to survive under similar circumstances. The fetus has a number of unique characteristics that allow it to do well with such a low pO_2.

First, the fetal hemoglobin concentration is higher than that in the adult, allowing for a much greater oxygen-carrying capacity. Second, the fetal cardiac output far exceeds that of the adult on a volume per unit body weight basis. Third, the fetal hemoglobin dissociation curve favors a higher saturation at a given pO_2 (Fig. 2.5). So, although the fetal pO_2 is lower, the fetus is able to compensate by having an increased oxygen content, due to the high hemoglobin concentration and the characteristic of the fetal hemoglobin dissociation curve. The more rapid circulation then increases the amount of oxygen that can be delivered to the fetal tissue per unit time (22).

Oxygen crosses the placenta by simple diffusion. If the relative flows on the two sides of the placenta are held constant, the differential pO_2 between the intervillous space and the fetal capillary determines the rate of maternal-fetal oxygen transfer. Thus, administration of high concentrations of oxygen to the mother may increase her pO_2 several hundred millimeters of mercury and the maternal fetal oxygen gradient may be markedly increased by this maneuver (23). Moreover, if the fetal pO_2 is increased by only a few millimeters of mercury, the fetal blood oxygen

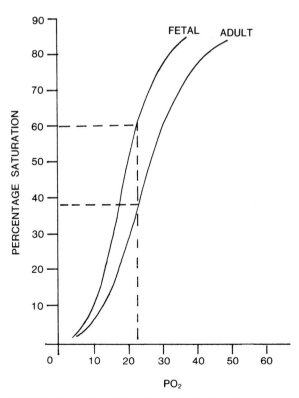

FIGURE 2.5. Adult and fetal hemoglobin dissociation curves.

content may increase significantly because, in either the physiologic or hypoxic range, the fetal hemoglobin saturation curve is quite steep (Fig. 2.5) (24).

Clinically, however, even though maternal hyperoxia may be of some help, most causes of fetal hypoxia are related to restriction of umbilical or intervillous space blood flow. Under conditions of diminished flow on either side of the placenta, changing the pO_2 gradient will not be of as much help as restoring the blood flow. It is still reasonable to administer oxygen to the mother (25) in such situations, but one must remember that restoration of flow is usually more important.

Fetal Circulatory Response to Hypoxia

Fetal circulatory responses to hypoxia involve redistribution of blood flow.

These include:

A redistribution of cardiac output resulting in preservation of blood flow to certain vital organs, including brain, myocardium, and adrenal glands, at the expense of flow to certain less vital organs including the parathyroid glands, lungs, liver, kidneys, intestines, bone marrow, and somatic muscles.

A loss of cerebral vascular autoregulation resulting in a pressure-passive cerebral circulation.

An eventual decrease in cardiac output resulting in hypotension and ultimately a decrease in cerebral blood flow (26–28). Fetal cerebral vascular resistance can decrease by at least 50% and maintain cerebral blood flow allowing for only a minimal decrease in oxygen delivery. With persistent hypoxemia leading to arterial hypotension, cerebral vascular resistance cannot maintain flow by decreasing, leading to a marked reduction in cerebral blood flow. This can then lead to neuronal necrosis in the fetal brain.

There are also noncirculatory responses to hypoxia that are important in preserving neuronal integrity under hypoxic conditions. These include:

A slower depletion of high-energy compounds during hypoxia-ischemia in the fetus compared with the term infant or adult.

The use of alternate energy substrate, the neonatal brain having the capacity to use lactate and ketone bodies for energy production.

The relative resistance of the fetal and neonatal myocardium to hypoxia-ischemia.

The potential protective role of fetal hemoglobin.

Because of these circulatory and noncirculatory responses to hypoxia, the fetus has considerable protection from neuronal damage, and even with severe hypoxic insults, most fetuses that survive have little or no central nervous system damage.

CONTROL OF THE FETAL HEART RATE

The FHR, under physiologic conditions, represents the final product of intrinsic and extrinsic rate-determining or modifying factors. Technically, the FHR represents the reciprocal of the interval between two successive beats, or more simply stated, the interval between beats is inversely related to the instantaneous rate. Most data on FHR use an electrical marker (specifically the peak of the fetal electrocardiogram [ECG] R wave) to signify the time of the beat. Unless otherwise stated, we will refer to the rate calculated from intervals between fetal ECG R waves. FHR changes constitute the basis for electronic fetal monitoring, and for this reason, one must look carefully at the factors that determine or modify the rate.

Schifferli and Caldeyro-Barcia (29) pointed to the fact that the baseline heart rate decreases with gestational age. At 15 weeks' gestation, the average baseline rate is approximately 160 beats per minute (BPM) (Fig. 2.6). Although premature fetuses may have a slightly increased rate over that found at term, within the limits of fetal viability (from 28 weeks to term), the average baseline FHR difference is only approximately 10 BPM. One must, therefore, be careful not to attribute a baseline tachycardia to prematurity when it may well be a sign of fetal compromise. Surely, any baseline FHR above 160 BPM must be explained on some basis other than fetal prematurity.

Schifferli and Caldeyro-Barcia (29) further noted that if one administers atropine to a fetus, the resulting increase in heart rate is of greater magnitude as one approaches term, and that the postatropine heart rate is usually in the range of 160 BPM. Because atropine is a parasympathetic blocking agent, it would appear that the gradual decrease in FHR

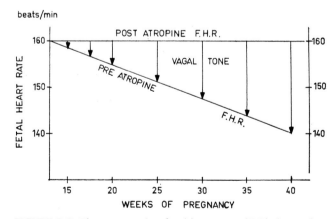

FIGURE 2.6. The preatropine fetal heart rate (FHR) shows that the average FHR decreases as gestational age increases. The postatropine FHR shows that the FHR after atropine administration rises to approximately 160 beats per minute, regardless of gestational age, indicating increasing vagal tone as gestational age increases. (From Schifferli P, Caldeyro-Barcia R: Effects of atropine and beta adrenergic drugs on the heart rate of the human fetus. In: Boreus L, ed. *Fetal pharmacology.* Raven Press, New York, 1973:264, with permission.)

that occurs with increasing gestational age can be explained as an increase in parasympathetic tone (Fig. 2.6).

Renou et al. (30) have shown that upon administering atropine directly to a human fetus during labor, three phenomena are observed. First, there is a modest increase in the baseline FHR, presumably due to blocking of the tonic parasympathetic effect described by Schifferli and Caldeyro-Barcia (29). Second, Renou et al. noted a loss of the variability of the FHR, suggesting that a continuous balance between the parasympathetic slowing effect and the sympathetic accelerating effect may have been disturbed. Third, they noted that a majority of patients demonstrated the appearance of FHR accelerations during uterine contraction. This suggests that, before release of parasympathetic tone by atropine, the accelerating forces were present but suppressed. Renou and co-workers then added a β-adrenergic blocking agent (propranolol) to these atropinized fetuses and noted abolition of the accelerations and a decrease in the baseline FHR (Fig. 2.7). It

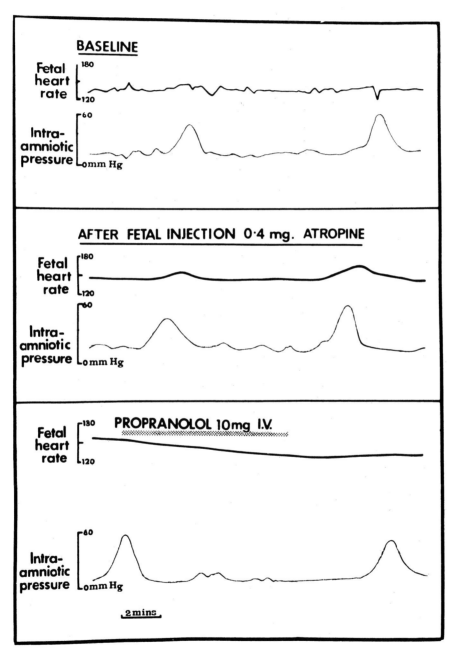

FIGURE 2.7. The **upper panel** shows a normal fetal heart rate (FHR)-uterine contraction tracing. The **middle panel** shows that after atropine administration to a human fetus the FHR rises, the FHR variability decreases, and accelerations appear with contractions. The **lower panel** shows that after maternal propranolol administration, the FHR decreased and the FHR accelerations disappeared. (From Renou P, Newman W, Wood C: *Am J Obstet Gynecol* 105:953, 1969, with permission.)

would thus appear that the accelerating forces unmasked by atropine blockade were of β-sympathomimetic origin. With this information, it is then possible to think of the baseline FHR as a product of the modulated influences of the parasympathetic and sympathetic nervous systems. Furthermore, the baseline FHR variability probably represents an instantaneous product of these two forces that are constantly working in a push-pull relationship; the presence of good FHR variability probably requires the integrity of these two modulating forces.

Under normal circumstances at term, the rate determined by the atrial pacemaker and modulated by parasympathetic and sympathetic factors usually ranges between 120 and 160 BPM. In a fetus with heart block, the rate is usually in the range of about 60 BPM, which represents the intrinsic ventricular or nodal rate.

Parasympathetic impulses originate in the brain stem and are carried over the vagus nerve to the heart. Sympathetic impulses also originate in the brain stem and are carried via the cervical sympathetic fibers to the fetal heart. Sympathetic influences on the fetal heart may also come from humoral stimulation of the cardiac β-receptors via release of epinephrine from the adrenal medulla. In clinical practice, conditions such as fetal anencephaly, marked hydrocephaly, and anoxic brain damage may all be associated with an absence of FHR variability and a very "blunted" FHR response to stress. In the adult who experienced cerebral death, the heart rate, when recorded instantaneously, has no variability. These clinical examples support the notion that heart rate variability is largely under central nervous system (CNS) influence. These examples further suggest that higher centers in the brain also play a role. Although these mechanisms of CNS control of FHR cannot be completely understood with current available data, clinically it is important to recognize that the FHR pattern does depend on certain CNS controls and that factors influencing the CNS such as drugs, anatomic brain damage, or cerebral hypoxia may also affect the FHR pattern. The FHR patterns associated with CNS dysfunction are discussed in more detail in Chapter 14.

FETAL STATE

The normal fetus has certain FHR changes that are related to the fetal state. It is well-established that, after about 32 weeks' gestation, virtually all normal fetuses demonstrate episodes of FHR acceleration associated with fetal movement. This has been called fetal reactivity and has been found to have a high association with fetal well-being. Before 24 weeks, fetal reactivity is rare, and it would seem that the appearance of FHR reactivity is related to the CNS maturation that is occurring at the beginning of the third trimester (31,32). Normal fetuses exhibit episodes of reactivity that last 20 to 40 minutes or longer (33). When the FHR accelerates, there is virtually always fetal movement, but the converse is not true (34). There are intermittent periods of low reactivity that correlate with fetal electroencephalogram (EEG) signs of deep sleep. During the periods of reactivity, fetal EEG measurements are suggestive of rapid eye movement (REM) sleep. Fetal state has a circadian rhythm with maximal reactivity occurring late at night (35). There is also a relation between fetal baseline heart rate and maternal heart rate that varies in a diurnal fashion. Brown and Patrick (36) have shown that normal fetuses rarely go more than 80 minutes without reactivity; when they do, they are very likely severely compromised. Drugs such as phenobarbital (37) and propranolol (38) will decrease reactivity. Also, fetuses with primary CNS abnormalities will have decreased reactivity. The loss of reactivity appears to be a change that occurs later than the appearance of late decelerations in fetuses undergoing progressive hypoxia (39).

The Effect of Uterine Contractions on the Fetal Heart Rate

FHR monitoring consists of a series of observed changes in instantaneous heart rate with and without uterine contractions. Uterine contractions subject the fetus to an intermittent hyperbaric state. They also cause intermittent decreases in intervillous space blood flow, may influence cerebral blood flow under certain circumstances, and, depending on the location of the umbilical cord, may cause intermittent umbilical cord occlusion. These situations may all influence the FHR by giving rise to contraction-related or "periodic" FHR changes. The physiologic bases for these periodic changes are discussed below.

Early Deceleration

Pressure on the fetal head causes slowing of the heart rate. It is believed that this is due to local changes in cerebral blood flow (40), resulting in stimulation of the vagal centers. While the fetal head undoubtedly undergoes compression of a greater or lesser degree in all vaginal deliveries, the typical gradual onset, gradual offset FHR deceleration described as characteristic of fetal head compression is rather uncommon. Certainly during the second stage of labor, when pronounced variable FHR decelerations are commonly seen, it is not possible to say for sure that these decelerations may not be partially or entirely due to compression of the fetal head as it passes through the birth canal. Hon (41) studied neonates, using different sized doughnut pessaries, and found that placing the circular pessary over the fetal vertex, when the center was 4 to 6 cm in diameter, usually resulted in point pressure from the edge of the pessary over the anterior fontanelle, and that this was associated with an FHR deceleration. This seemed to fit clinically with the fact that the FHR deceleration pattern

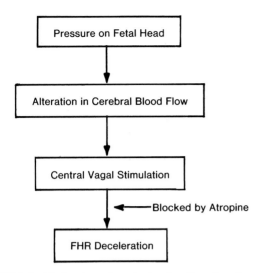

FIGURE 2.8. Mechanism of early deceleration (head compression).

that reflected the uterine pressure curve as a mirror image is usually found when patients are between 4 and 6 cm of cervical dilatation. The symmetric deceleration pattern resulting from fetal head compression is called early deceleration and will be described in more detail in Chapter 6. Further studies have shown that early deceleration may be abolished or markedly altered by the administration of atropine, thus confirming the theory that this is a vagal reflex (42). Although all authorities do not agree, there is good evidence that this deceleration pattern does not carry asphyctic implications (Fig. 2.8) (43).

Variable Deceleration

The umbilical cord is easily compressed as the fetus moves in relation to the uterine contents. Uterine contractions are the usual cause of intermittent umbilical cord occlusion, especially if the cord is around the fetal neck or fixed in another location, resulting in its impingement during contractions.

Our understanding of the mechanism of FHR changes in association with umbilical cord occlusion began with the work of Barcroft (44). He studied exteriorized fetal goats and showed that there was an almost instantaneous rapid and profound decrease in the FHR when the umbilical cords of these fetal goats were occluded. Because the response was so rapid, he reasoned that it may be due to a neurologic reflex. He then repeated the experiment after interrupting the vagus nerves of these fetal goats and found that there was a delay in the onset of the FHR deceleration. This then suggested that indeed the initial rapid deceleration associated with cord occlusion in the animal with intact vagi did appear to be caused by a vagal reflex, but the fact that a delayed deceleration was observed even with

interruption of the vagal nerves suggested a second mechanism for the delayed portion of the deceleration (Fig. 2.9).

If one examines the hemodynamic effects of umbilical cord occlusion, some clues concerning the mechanism for the early component of the FHR deceleration emerge. When the umbilical arteries are occluded, there is a sudden increase in total fetal peripheral resistance resulting from a cutoff of the low resistance fetal placental circulation. This increase in peripheral resistance in the fetal circulation causes sudden fetal hypertension (45,46). Stimulation of fetal baroreceptors occurs instantly, sending reflexes up the afferent limb of the neural reflex. The baroreceptor impulses affect the central vagal nuclei and result in a parasympathetic outflow that produces a sudden slowing effect on the fetal atrial pacemaker. Fetal ECG changes during cord occlusion show a gradual shortening of the P-R interval and, with profound cord occlusion, the P wave disappears, resulting in a ventricular rate of about 60 BPM (47). With release of the cord occlusion, the atrial pacemaker returns with a gradual lengthening of the P-R interval back to predeceleration values. Hon et al. (42) have shown that atropine administered to the human will greatly alter, if not abolish, this profound deceleration associated

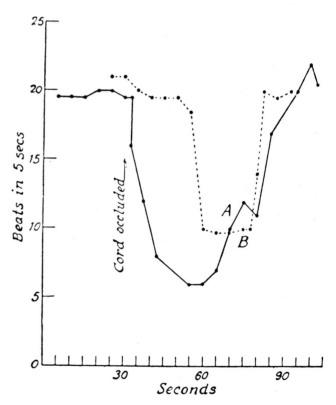

FIGURE 2.9. The solid line represents the fetal heart rate (FHR) after total umbilical cord occlusion in the intact exteriorized fetal goat. The broken line represents the FHR after total umbilical cord occlusion in the vagectomized exteriorized fetal goat. (From Barcroft J: *Researches on prenatal life*. Blackwell Scientific Publications, Oxford, 1946, with permission.)

with umbilical cord occlusion. This tends to support Barcroft's hypothesis about the vagal reflex nature of at least one component of the FHR deceleration associated with umbilical cord compression.

This FHR deceleration pattern may bear no consistent temporal relationship to the contraction, presumably because the location of the umbilical cord may vary from one contraction to another. The pattern of cord occlusion has therefore been referred to as variable deceleration. Further description of the pattern will appear in Chapter 6.

Siassi et al. (48) have made suggestions, based on observations in neonates, that the afferent limb of this reflex bradycardia, due to umbilical cord compression, may result from changes in arterial pO_2. They noted that neonates on continuous heart rate monitors had heart rate changes similar to variable deceleration after apneic episodes. Because the deceleration seemed to follow the apnea, it appeared that one might explain this phenomenon by a decrease in the neonatal arterial pO_2 (paO_2), causing a chemoreceptor initiation of the afferent limb to the vagal reflex. Next, they looked at neonates on respirators and noted that the delay in the onset of deceleration after cessation of respiratory assistance was related to the level of the paO_2 before the cessation of breathing. The onset of the deceleration indeed appeared to occur at a critical paO_2. This observation would support Barcroft's theory and suggest that the delayed deceleration was possibly due to hypoxia.

Siassi expanded these studies by returning to exteriorized fetal sheep. By connecting the fetal umbilical circulation to a membrane oxygenator, he was able to show that the onset of variable deceleration after umbilical cord occlusion could be delayed by first raising the paO_2 of the fetus via the membrane oxygenator. Because these sheep were anesthetized, however, one cannot say that the baroreceptor afferent limb does not play a role in variable deceleration. However, these experiments clearly point to the presence of a hypoxemic stimulus as at least having a role in variable deceleration. Certainly, the paO_2 decreases rapidly with total umbilical cord occlusion, but, fortunately, the paO_2 also increases rapidly with release of the occluded cord, accounting for the apparent clinical benignity of variable deceleration patterns in their mild-to-moderate forms.

Itskovitz et al. (49) showed that FHR responses in fetal lambs resembling variable decelerations did not occur until flow was reduced by at least 50%. With partial cord occlusion, there was no significant change in blood pressure and the variable decelerations were abolished by atropine. With partial cord occlusion, the deceleration was of chemoreceptor origin and was mediated via the vagus nerve. Only with total cord occlusion did they see an increase in fetal blood pressure, and they determined that, under those circumstances, the deceleration was of combined chemoreceptor and baroreceptor origin.

Along with the sudden increase in pressure and the sudden decrease in paO_2, there is an acute increase in the pCO_2

during umbilical cord occlusion. This may result in varying degrees of respiratory acidosis, and it is not clear what role this plays in the physiologic mechanism involved in the development of variable deceleration. It is not until cord occlusion is prolonged that a significant oxygen debt develops, resulting in fetal hypoxemia of a more than transient nature as evidenced by the development of metabolic acidosis reflecting significant anaerobic metabolism. When variable deceleration is severe, the late component of Barcroft comes into play. It is believed that this component is due to myocardial depression and represents significant hypoxemia and fetal metabolic acidosis (see the discussion of late deceleration below).

It has been suggested that lesser degrees of umbilical cord compression may result in only occlusion of the low-resistance venous return from the placenta. James et al. (50) and Lee et al. (51) have stated that this venous occlusion may result in a decreased return of blood to the fetal heart, decreased fetal cardiac output, and a compensatory FHR acceleration (Figs. 2.10 and 2.11). Clinical evidence to support this concept comes from the observation that periodic FHR acceleration associated with uterine contractions often leads to variable deceleration as labor progresses.

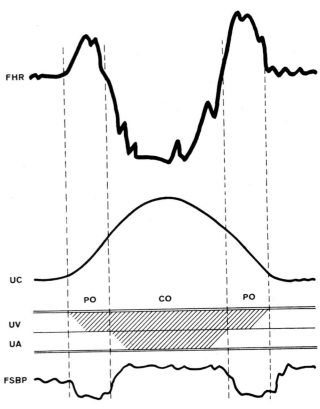

FIGURE 2.10. This figure represents fetal heart rate *(FHR)* and fetal systemic blood pressure *(FSBP)* occurring during compression of the umbilical vein *(UV)* and the umbilical artery *(UA)*. UC, uterine contraction. (From Lee CV, Di Loreto PC, O'Lane JM: A study of fetal heart rate acceleration patterns. *Obstet Gynecol* 45:142, 1975, with permission.)

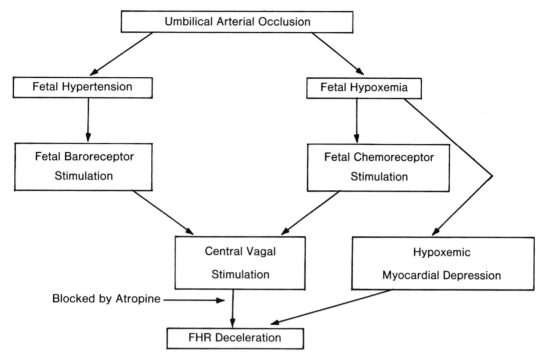

FIGURE 2.11. Mechanism of variable deceleration.

Indeed, often there are accelerations before and after variable decelerations.

Oligohydramnios may be associated with variable decelerations even before the onset of labor. The protective nature of amniotic fluid is suggested by the fact that it is less common to see evidence of umbilical cord occlusion in antepartum patients when there are adequate amounts of amniotic fluid present. Gabbe et al. (52) showed that one was able to induce variable decelerations in laboring monkeys by removing amniotic fluid and to relieve them by restoring the amniotic fluid volume. More recently, Miyazaki and Nevarez (53) showed that saline amnioinfusion via a transcervical catheter to patients having variable deceleration in labor decreased the variable decelerations, and Nageotte et al. (54) showed, in a randomized prospective study on patients with preterm premature rupture of membranes, that prophylactic amnioinfusion decreased the incidence and severity of variable decelerations and resulted in improved umbilical arterial pH. This technique will be discussed in more detail in Chapter 9.

In summary, the variable deceleration reflex appears to have both baroreceptor (hypertensive) and chemoreceptor (hypoxia) afferent limbs with the efferent limb being vagal. With severe hypoxemia and fetal metabolic acidosis, there may be a delayed deceleration component due to hypoxic fetal myocardial depression. With mild forms of umbilical cord compression, only the vein may be occluded, resulting in FHR acceleration (Fig. 2.10).

Late Deceleration

Earlier in this chapter, it was pointed out that intervillous space blood flow may be diminished by a number of causes. When intervillous space blood flow is decreased to a point that the fetus becomes hypoxemic, uteroplacental insufficiency (UPI) is said to exist. Clinical UPI may manifest itself in the chronic form with intrauterine growth retardation, antepartum fetal death, or both; or, in the acute form, with the onset of fetal distress during labor, asphyxia neonatorum; or, in the extreme, intrapartum fetal death.

Before electronic FHR monitoring, there was little known by practitioners of the art of obstetrics about characteristic FHR patterns that are associated with UPI. Among the first to describe FHR changes associated with UPI were Hon (55) and Caldeyro-Barcia et al. (56). They pointed to a slowing of the FHR that was related to uterine contractions with a gradual onset, usually after the peak of the contraction and a delayed return to baseline, usually after the end of the contraction. This was referred to as late deceleration by Hon and a type II dip by Caldeyro-Barcia. This late deceleration pattern is believed to have both a reflex component and a hypoxic component somewhat similar to the mechanisms described in variable deceleration, but because of the nature and timing of the stimulus, the FHR pattern has different characteristics.

Work by Martin et al. (57) clarifies our understanding of the physiologic mechanisms involved in hypoxemic FHR changes. Martin devised a sheep model with an inflatable cuff that could be used to occlude the maternal sheep's common hypogastric artery and was able to measure blood pressure, heart rate, and blood gases in this chronic fetal sheep preparation. Inflation of the implanted cuff around the common hypogastric artery resulted in cessation of blood flow through the uterine arteries. Intermittent compression could then simulate the changes in uterine blood flow that result from uterine contractions. The FHR changes noted with intermittent hypoxia in this model were a delayed FHR deceleration associated with transient fetal hypertension.

Treatment with phentolamine (α-adrenergic blockade) resulted in a loss of the hypertensive response and a decrease in the late decelerations. Fetal atropine administration (parasympathetic blockade) resulted in periodic FHR accelerations in response to intermittent hypoxia. These accelerations were blocked by propranolol (β-adrenergic blockade). With combined blockade (α-adrenergic, parasympathetic, and β-adrenergic), there was no change in FHR with intermittent hypoxia in the nonacidemic fetus. When the hypoxia was prolonged enough to produce acidemia, the initial hypertensive response was lost and the

FHR deceleration occurred even in the presence of triple blockade, indicating that, with hypoxia and acidemia, the FHR deceleration is presumably due to myocardial depression.

With the knowledge of this work by Martin and coworkers, it would appear that late deceleration is primarily a reflex change with nonacidemic hypoxia, but when hypoxia is severe enough to result in acidemia, the mechanism of late deceleration appears to be nonreflex myocardial depression. Clinically, the use of fetal scalp blood sampling or fetal scalp stimulation may be of value to determine whether late deceleration is occurring in association with acidemia (Fig. 2.12).

Variability of the Fetal Heart Rate

The interval between successive heartbeats in the intact fetus is characterized by its nonuniformity. This beat-to-beat variability is known as short-term variability. Average interval differences are usually in the magnitude of 20 to 30 msec or 2 to 3 BPM when converted to rate. When variability is diminished, the usual beat-to-beat interval differences average about 1 BPM or less.

The long-term fluctuations in FHR have a cyclicity of 3 to 5 per minute, and the amplitude is usually from 5 to 20 BPM. A long-term variability of less than 5 BPM is considered to be reduced (Fig. 2.13).

Parasympathetic influences tend to have a short time constant, resulting in more rapid decelerations than the longer time constant sympathetic influences that cause slower and more sustained accelerations. Druzen et al. (58) have shown that the parasympathetic system is more responsible for short-term variability, whereas the sympathetic effect appears to be strongest on long-term variability. Dalton and coworkers found that, even after double blockade with atropine and β-sympathetic blockade, 35% to 40% of FHR variability remained in fetal sheep. They interpreted this as suggesting some nonneural component to FHR variability (59). However, it is possible that there are some nonautonomic efferent neural components to variability that are operable in the presence of double autonomic blockade. With absent CNS function, as seen in some anencephalics, variability may be completely absent (60). Studies by Modanlou et al. (61) suggested that short-term variability appeared to be reduced early in the course of neonatal hypoxemia, with loss of long-term variability being a later change. Interestingly, with neonatal recovery, long-term variability reappeared first, and the return of short-term variability was delayed.

According to our understanding of the control of FHR, these changes in variability are probably related to changes in CNS status. Generally, the intact fetus has good short- and long-term variability. Drugs that depress the CNS or interfere with autonomic reflexes will tend to decrease FHR variability. There also appears to be a gradual increase in

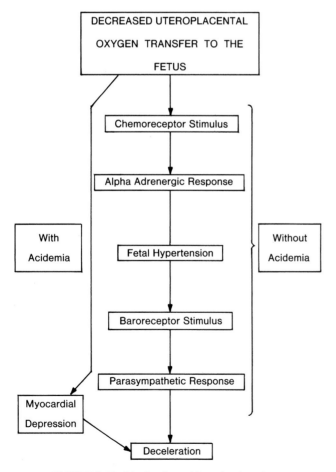

FIGURE 2.12. Mechanism of late deceleration.

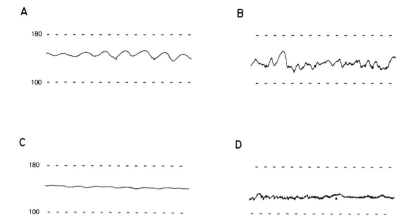

FIGURE 2.13. Components of fetal heart rate (FHR) variability for fetal ECG-derived FHR. **A:** Long-term without short-term variability. **B:** Long-term and short-term variability. **C:** No long-term and no short-term variability. **D:** Short-term without long-term variability. (From Zanini B, Paul RH, Huey JR: *Am J Obstet Gynecol* 136:43, 1980, with permission.)

FHR variability as gestational age progresses. However, in the viable fetus of more than 28 weeks' gestation, one should not attribute loss of variability to prematurity alone, because most fetuses in the 28- to 32-week range will have reasonably good FHR variability but perhaps slightly less than the term fetus will have.

Although much attention has focused on the difference between short- and long-term variability, they usually go hand in hand—when one is reduced, so is the other. One exception to this is the sinusoidal pattern where there is absent short-term variability and very uniform long-term variability. With the newer monitors, a much closer representation of short-term variability can be appreciated on external systems even though technically true short-term variability is defined as differences in R-waves from the fetal ECG.

The major significance of FHR variability is that it may be affected by hypoxemia. Druzen et al. (58) showed that the earliest effect of fetal hypoxemia on FHR variability appears to be an increase in both long- and short-term variability. These investigators showed that mild hypoxia resulted in adrenergic discharge and fetal hypertension, causing stimulation of the fetal baroreceptors and a reflex vagal discharge. Thus, a general increase in autonomic tone during early fetal hypoxia results in an increase in both short- and long-term variability. Prolonged and severe fetal hypoxia with acidemia will reduce FHR variability, presumably due to the CNS effects of hypoxia and acidosis.

A very curious pattern known as a sinusoidal FHR pattern is exceedingly rare. It is characterized by an absence of short-term variability and a very uniform long-term variability pattern in the shape of a sine wave. It has been seen with chronic fetal anemia associated with erythroblastosis (62). It has also been reported with acute intrapartum fetal asphyxia (63), after alphaprodine administration (64), and with fetal-maternal hemorrhage (65). The physiologic basis for this pattern is not clear, but a report by Elliott et al. (66) showed that the pattern observed in the fetus with erythroblastosis was also seen in the neonate and did not respond

to adequate neonatal oxygenation but disappeared after neonatal blood transfusion. They suggested that tissue hypoxia may have been relieved by increasing the hemoglobin concentration.

Recent work by Murata et al. (67) in fetal lambs indicates that anemic fetuses had increased levels of arginine vasopressin but that one could not produce a sinusoidal pattern simply by the infusion of this substance. However, with high doses of atropine or with fetal vagectomy, sinusoidal patterns were produced with high-dose arginine vasopressin infusion. Because cerebral ischemia may result in phasic vasomotor activity, perhaps through alteration in central parasympathetic function, these data suggest that the sinusoidal pattern may involve cerebral ischemia as well as increased arginine vasopressin levels. Certainly, this work suggests that the sinusoidal pattern is related to a change in the CNS control of FHR and implies cerebral ischemia. It is not clear, however, why the pattern is so rare and is usually associated with fetal anemia but can also be seen in hypoxemic fetuses with no anemia.

The FHR is believed to be under the direct control of the fetal autonomic nervous system. We are beginning to understand the reflex mechanisms involved with hypoxic changes in FHR patterns and variability. With early hypoxia, whether caused by cord compression or uteroplacental insufficiency, the FHR patterns are primarily of neural reflex origin, whereas with severe hypoxia and fetal acidosis, the periodic FHR changes are probably primarily due to myocardial depression. The correlation between physiologic studies and clinical observations remains incomplete, but, clearly, as we learn more about physiologic mechanisms involved in the control of the FHR, the clinical observations become more and more meaningful.

REFERENCES

1. Ramsey EM, Martin CB Jr, et al.: Fetal and maternal placental circulation. *Am J Obstet Gynecol* 98:419, 1967.
2. Poseiro JJ, Mendez-Bauer C, Pose SV, et al.: Effect of uterine

contractions on maternal blood flow through the placenta. In: *Perinatal factors affecting human development.* Pan American World Health Organization, Scientific Publication no 185, Washington, DC, 1969, p 161–171.

3. Greiss FC Jr: Concepts of uterine blood flow. In: Wynn RM, ed. *Obstetrics gynecology annual.* Appleton-Century-Crofts, New York, 1973, vol. 2, p 55-83.

4. Wallenburg HS, Stolte LAM, Janassens J: The pathogenesis of placental infarction. I. A morphologic study in the human placenta. *Am J Obstet Gynecol* 116:835, 1973.

5. Wallenburg HC, Hutchinson DL, Schuler HM, et al.: The pathogenesis of placental infarction. II. An experimental study in the rhesus monkey placenta. *Am J Obstet Gynecol* 116:841, 1973.

6. Greiss F, Marston E: The uterine vascular bed: effect of estrogens during ovine pregnancy. *Am J Obstet Gynecol* 93:720, 1965.

7. Howard BK, Goodson JM, Mengert WIT: Supine hypotensive syndrome in late pregnancy. *Obstet Gynecol* 1:371, 1953.

8. Kerr NG: The mechanical effects of the gravid uterus in late pregnancy. *J Obstet Gynaecol Br Commonw* 72:513, 1965.

9. Abitbol M: Supine position in labor and associated fetal heart rate changes. *Obstet Gynecol* 65:481, 1985.

10. Clapp JF 3d: Fetal heart rate response to running in midpregnancy and late pregnancy. *Am J Obstet Gynecol* 153:251, 1985.

11. Artal R, Romem Y, Paul RH, et al.: Fetal bradycardia induced by maternal exercise. *Lancet* 2(8397):258, 1984.

12. Emmanouilides GC, Hobel CJ, Yashiro K, et al.: Fetal response to maternal exercise in the sheep. *Am J Obstet Gynecol* 112:130, 1972.

13. Collings C, Curet LB: Fetal heart rate response to maternal exercise. *Am J Obstet Gynecol* 151:498, 1985.

14. Lees MH, Hill JD, Ochsner AJ 3d, et al.: Maternal and placental myometrial blood flow of the rhesus monkey during uterine contractions. *Am J Obstet Gynecol* 110:68, 1971.

15. Greiss FC Jr: Pressure flow relationship in the gravid uterine vascular bed. *Am J Obstet Gynecol* 96:41, 1966.

16. Chayen B, Tejani N, Verma UL, et al.: Fetal heart rate changes and uterine activity during coitus. *Acta Obstet Gynecol Scand* 65:853, 1986.

17. Kraus FT, Acheen VI. Fetal thrombotic vasculopathy in the placenta: cerebral thrombi and infarcts, coagulopathies, and cerebral palsy. *Hum Pathol* 30:759–769. 1999.

18. Greiss FC Jr, Crandell DL: Therapy for hypotension induced by spinal anesthesia during pregnancy. *JAMA* 191:793, 1965.

19. Hollmen A, Jouppila R, Jouppila P, et al.: Effect of extradural analgesia using bupivacaine and 2-chloroprocaine on intervillous blood flow during normal labour. *Br J Anaesth* 54:837, 1982.

20. Giles WB, Lah FX, Trudinger BJ: The effect of epidural anaesthesia for cesarean section on maternal uterine and fetal umbilical artery blood flow velocity waveforms. *Br J Obstet Gynaecol* 94:55, 1987.

21. Dawes GS: Foetal and neonatal physiology. In: *The foetal circulation.* Year Book Medical Publishers, Chicago, 1968:91–105.

22. Dawes GS: Foetal and neonatal physiology. In: *Foetal blood gas tensions and pH.* Year Book Medical Publishers, Chicago, 1968:106–116.

23. Longo LD: Placental transfer mechanisms. An overview. In: Wynn RM, ed. *Obstetrics gynecology annual 1972.* Appleton-Century-Crofts, New York, 1973.

24. Khazin AF, Hon EH, Hehre FW: Effects of maternal hyperoxia on the foetus. *Am J Obstet Gynecol* 109:628, 1971.

25. Edelstone DI, Peticca BB, Goldblum LJ: Effects of maternal oxygen administration on fetal oxygenation during reductions in umbilical blood flow in fetal lambs. *Am J Obstet Gynecol* 152:351, 1985.

26. Behrman RE, Lees MH, Petersen EN, et al.: Distribution of circulation in the normal and asphyxiated fetal primate. *Am J Obstet Gynecol* 108:956–969, 1970.

27. Cohn EH, Sacks EJ, Heyman MA, et al.: Cardiovascular responses to hypoxemia and acidemia in fetal lambs. *Am J Obstet Gynecol* 1974;120:817–824.

28. Peeters L, Sheldon R, Jones M, et al.: Blood flow to fetal organs as a function of arterial oxygen content. *Am J Obstet Gynecol* 1979;135:637–646.

29. Schifferli P, Caldeyro-Barcia R: Effects of atropine and beta adrenergic drugs on the heart rate of the human fetus. In: Boreus L, ed. *Fetal pharmacology.* Raven Press, New York, 1973: 259–279.

30. Renou P, Warwick N, Wood C: Autonomic control of fetal heart rate. *Am J Obstet Gynecol* 105:949, 1969.

31. Smith CV, Phelan JP, Paul RH: A prospective analysis of the influence of gestational age on the baseline fetal heart rate and reactivity in a low-risk population. *Am J Obstet Gynecol* 153:780, 1985.

32. Druzin ML, Fox A, Kogut E, et al.: The relationship of the nonstress test to gestational age. *Am J Obstet Gynecol* 153:386, 1985.

33. Patrick J, Campbell K, Carmichael L, et al.: Influence of maternal heart rate and gross fetal body movements on the daily pattern of fetal heart rate near term. *Am J Obstet Gynecol* 144:533, 1982.

34. Navot D, Yaffe H, Sadovsky E: The ratio of fetal heart rate accelerations to fetal movements according to gestational age. *Am J Obstet Gynecol* 149:92, 1984.

35. Patrick J, Campbell K, Carmichael L, et al.: Patterns of gross fetal body movements over 24-hour observation intervals during the last 10 weeks of pregnancy. *Am J Obstet Gynecol* 142:363, 1982.

36. Brown R, Patrick J: The nonstress test: how long is enough? *Am J Obstet Gynecol* 141:646, 1981.

37. Keegan KA, Paul RH, Broussard PM, et al.: Antepartum fetal heart testing. III. The effect of phenobarbital on the nonstress test. *Am J Obstet Gynecol* 133:579, 1979.

38. Margulis E, Binder D, Cohen AW: The effect of propranolol on the nonstress test. *Am J Obstet Gynecol* 148:340, 1984.

39. Murata Y, Martin CB Jr, Ikenoue T, et al.: Fetal heart rate accelerations and late decelerations during the course of intrauterine death in chronically catheterized rhesus monkeys. *Am J Obstet Gynecol* 144:218, 1982.

40. Paul WM, Quilligan EJ, MacLachlan T: Cardiovascular phenomenon associated with fetal head compression. *Am J Obstet Gynecol* 90:824, 1964.

41. Hon EH: Personal communication, 1974, Los Angeles.

42. Hon EH, Bradfield AH, Hess OW: The electronic evaluation of the fetal heart rate. V. The vagal factor in fetal bradycardia. *Am J Obstet Gynecol* 82:291, 1961.

43. Kubli FW, Hon EH, Khazin AF, et al.: Observations on heart rate and pH in the human fetus during labor. *Am J Obstet Gynecol* 104:1190, 1969.

44. Barcroft J: *Researches on prenatal life.* Blackwell Scientific Publications, Oxford, 1946.

45. Lee ST, Hon EH: Fetal hemodynamic response to umbilical cord compression. *Obstet Gynecol* 22:554, 1963.

46. Towell ME, Salvador HS: Compression of the umbilical cord. In: Crasignoni P, Pardi G, eds. *An experimental model in the fetal goat, fetal evaluation during pregnancy and labor.* Academic Press, New York, 1971:143–156.

47. Yeh MN, Morishima HO, Niemann WE, et al.: Myocardial conduction defects in association with compression of the umbilical cord. Experimental observations on fetal baboons. *Am J Obstet Gynecol* 121:951, 1975.

48. Siassi B, et al.: Effect of arterial pO2 in the cardiovascular response to umbilical cord compression. Presented at the 20th

Annual Meeting of the Society for Gynecological Investigation, Atlanta, Georgia, March 28-30, 1973.

49. Itskovitz J, LaGamma EF, Rudolph AM: Heart rate and blood pressure responses to umbilical cord compression in fetal lambs with special reference to the mechanism of variable deceleration. *Am J Obstet Gynecol* 147:451, 1983.

50. James LS, Yeh MN, Morishima HO, et al.: Umbilical vein occlusion and transient acceleration of the fetal heart rate. Experimental observations in subhuman primates. *Am J Obstet Gynecol* 126:276, 1976.

51. Lee CV, Di Loreto PC, O'Lane JM: A study of fetal heart rate acceleration patterns. *Obstet Gynecol* 45:142, 1975.

52. Gabbe SG, Ettinger BB, Freeman RK, et al.: Umbilical cord compression associated with amniotomy: laboratory observations. *Am J Obstet Gynecol* 126:353, 1976.

53. Miyazaki FS, Nevarez F: Saline amnioinfusion for relief of repetitive variable decelerations: a prospective randomized study. *Am J Obstet Gynecol* 153:301, 1985.

54. Nageotte MP, Freeman RK, Garite TJ, et al.: Prophylactic intrapartum amnioinfusion in patients with preterm premature rupture of the membranes. *Am J Obstet Gynecol* 15 3:5 57, 1988.

55. Hon EH: Observations on "pathologic" fetal bradycardia. *Am J Obstet Gynecol* 77:1084, 1959.

56. Caldeyro-Barcia R, Casacuberta C, Bustos R, et al.: Correlation of intrapartum changes in fetal heart rate with fetal blood oxygen and acid base state. In: Adamsons K, ed. *Diagnosis and treatment of fetal disorders.* Springer-Verlag, New York, 1968:205–225.

57. Martin CB Jr, de Haan J, van der Wildt B, et al.: Mechanisms of late deceleration in the fetal heart rate. A study with autonomic blocking agents in fetal lambs. *Eur J Obstet Gynecol Reprod Biol* 9:361, 1979.

58. Druzen M, Ikenoue T, Murata Y, et al.: A possible mechanism for the increase in FHR variability following hypoxemia. Presented at the 26th Annual Meeting of Society for Gynecological Investigation, San Diego, California, March 23, 1979.

59. Dalton KJ, Dawes GS, Patrick JE: The autonomic nervous system and fetal heart rate variability. *Am J Obstet Gynecol* 146:456, 1983.

60. Terao T, Kawashima Y, Noto H, et al.: Neurologic control of fetal heart rate in 20 cases of anencephalic fetuses. *Am J Obstet Gynecol* 149:201, 1984.

61. Modanlou HD, Freeman RK, Braly P: A simple method of fetal and neonatal heart rate beat-to-beat variability quantitation: preliminary report. *Am J Obstet Gynecol* 127:861, 1977.

62. Manseau P, Vaquier J, Chavinie J, et al.: Le rythme cardiaque foetal sinusoidal aspect evocateur de souffrance foetale au cours de la grossesse. [Sinusoidal fetal cardiac rhythm. An aspect evocative of fetal distress during pregnancy.] *J Gynecol Obstet Biol Reprod (Paris)* 1:343, 1972.

63. Gal D, Jacobson LM, Ser H, et al.: Sinusoidal pattern: an alarming sign of fetal distress. *Am J Obstet Gynecol* 132:903, 1978.

64. Gray JH, Cudmore DW, Luther ER, et al.: Sinusoidal fetal heart rate pattern associated with alphaprodine administration. *Obstet Gynecol* 52:678, 1978.

65. Modanlou HD, Freeman RK, Ortiz O, et al.: Sinusoidal fetal heart rate pattern and severe fetal anemia. *Obstet Gynecol* 49:537, 1977.

66. Elliott JP, Modanlou HD, O'Keeffe DF, et al.: The significance of fetal and neonatal sinusoidal heart rate pattern: further clinical observations in Rh incompatibility. *Am J Obstet Gynecol* 138:227, 1980.

67. Murata Y, Miyake Y, Yamamoto T, et al.: Experimentally produced sinusoidal fetal heart rate pattern in the chronically instrumented fetal lamb. *Am J Obstet Gynecol* 153:693, 1985.

3

INTRAUTERINE HYPOXIA AND OTHER CAUSES OF NEONATAL ENCEPHALOPATHY AND CEREBRAL PALSY

Electronic fetal heart rate (FHR) monitoring has been extensively studied with respect to the effects of hypoxia on the FHR. The relationship between uteroplacental insufficiency, umbilical cord compression, and FHR changes are useful in studying the mechanism of FHR change with respect to intrauterine fetal hypoxia. FHR changes also occur when the fetal central nervous system (CNS) control of FHR is impaired. This impairment may or may not have a hypoxic cause. The concept of CNS damage caused by intrauterine fetal conditions is no longer believed to be limited to hypoxia and trauma. Myriad associations have been described and even though a substantial percentage of children with neurologic problems never have a precise etiology assigned, recent research has pointed to mechanisms other than hypoxia, including infection, hypercoagulable states, maternal thyroid disease, and a family history of neurologic abnormalities. It is generally agreed that intrauterine hypoxia in a term fetus, proximate to birth, sufficient to result in later CNS damage, will always be associated with neonatal encephalopathy (1). Recent studies have also pointed to the fact that a substantial portion of cases of neonatal encephalopathy are not caused by intrauterine global fetal hypoxia. Furthermore, ischemia due to cerebral infarcts without global hypoxia may cause neonatal encephalopathy and later neurologic damage. Finally, while prematurity has the largest association with later cerebral palsy, the patterns of neurologic deficits differ from those of children who sustained intrauterine damage at or near term.

INTRAUTERINE FETAL HYPOXIA

When the fetus is exposed to insufficient oxygen to allow the complete metabolism of glucose, lactic acid accumulates and results in metabolic acidosis. Acute impairment of the umbilical circulation will result in hypercarbia and respiratory acidosis due to decreased exchange of CO_2, but utero-placental insufficiency may or may not be associated with hypercarbia because exchange of CO_2 at the placenta is more efficient than is exchange of oxygen. The term fetal asphyxia is overused and should be limited to fetal hypoxia accompanied by metabolic acidosis. Although it has become a popular legal theory, there remains no scientific basis for the notion that cerebral ischemia caused by the pressures of labor and in the absence of fetal hypoxia is a cause of cerebral palsy.

Fetal circulatory responses to hypoxia include redistribution of blood flow to the more vital organs resulting in preservation of circulation to the brain, myocardium, and adrenal glands. There is a resulting decrease in blood flow to the kidney, intestine, and muscle. Another consequence of hypoxia is a loss of cerebral vascular autoregulation resulting in a pressure-passive circulation. When the level of hypoxemia is near lethal, there is a decrease in fetal cardiac output resulting in hypotension and decreased cerebral blood flow (2–4). It appears that when fetal cardiac output declines, resulting in a decrease in cerebral blood flow below a critical level, neuronal necrosis results. Subsequent development of cerebral edema in the neonate further compromises cerebral blood flow aggravating the degree of neuronal necrosis.

When fetal hypoxia occurs at sublethal levels, permanent damage to the fetus may result; however, the frequency with which this occurs in the intrapartum period and the ability of the clinician using fetal monitoring to prevent it is a subject of intense debate. References to perinatal brain damage can be found earlier, but the English orthopedic surgeon, William John Little (5), is credited with the first specific hypothesis suggesting adverse perinatal events as the main etiologic factors in infantile spastic palsies. He reviewed the histories of more than 200 cases of spasticity of congenital origin and presented his paper entitled "On the influence of abnormal parturition, difficult labours, premature birth and asphyxia neonatorum, on the mental and physical condition of the child, especially in relation to deformities" to the Obstetrical Society of London. He concluded that these 200 cases had one thing in common, that is, some abnormal characteristic of parturition. The form of cerebral palsy (CP) that he described has often been called "Little's disease." Little later went so far as to conclude that virtually nothing other than abnormalities of birth could cause the clinical picture he described (5). Subsequently, other neurologic problems including mental retardation, epilepsy, and behavioral and learning disorders have been attributed to various intrapartum problems.

Animal data corroborating the concept that perinatal asphyxia may cause profound sublethal neurologic damage can be found in the classic papers of William F. Windle (6). Between 1943 and 1963, Windle (7) performed experimental asphyxiation of rhesus monkeys and evaluated the immediate, long-term, and neuropathologic effects. The monkeys were asphyxiated in one of two ways, both involving hysterotomy. Either the placenta and membranes were delivered with the fetus within the intact amniotic sac, or the fetal head was covered by a fluid-filled sac and the umbilical cord was completely occluded. The fetal oxygen supply was completely interrupted for 5 to 20 minutes. Monkeys allowed to breathe in 6 minutes or less showed no neurologic deficits and no pathologic brain changes. Asphyxiation for more than 7 minutes produced at least transient motor and behavioral changes and relatively consistent brain pathology, along with necrosis of brain-stem cells in the inferior colliculi and ventrolateral thalamic nuclei with secondary glial proliferative scarring. The most profound changes were found in monkeys left anoxic for 12 to 17 minutes. Resuscitation was invariably necessary. More severe brain-stem lesions were created. Initially, the monkeys were hypoactive and hypotonic. Seizures, ataxia, and athetosis were often seen. The monkeys were observed for 8 years and, as they matured, most deficits gradually improved, leaving residual hypoactivity and clumsiness. Although this model indeed supported the hypothesis that perinatal asphyxia is associated with permanent neurologic damage, the pattern of damage did not seem to correspond with the mental retardation and spasticity seen most commonly in the human. In later experiments, Windle (7) subjected monkeys to prolonged labor with oxytocin and the asphyxiated neonates did not show the midbrain and brain-stem lesions of acute total asphyxia but rather primarily cortical damage.

Ronald Myers (8) suggested that total asphyxia may not be the usual case in humans, and that prolonged partial asphyxia is more likely. Myers was able to produce partial asphyxia in the rhesus monkey by various techniques including uterine hyperstimulation with oxytocin, compression of the maternal abdominal aorta, maternal infusion of catecholamines, and inspiration by the pregnant monkey of reduced oxygen concentrations. These were controlled by maintaining fetal pO_2 at 5 to 9 mm Hg. Myers et al. (9) later demonstrated that late decelerations of the FHR were caused by this hypoxia. Fetuses were maintained in such partially asphyctic states for at least 1 hour, then delivered and resuscitated. The immediate effect on the newborn was flaccidity, which evolved after several hours into generalized hypertonus and decerebrate posturing, at which time the newborns began to have periodic generalized seizures. Many fetuses developed ileus and cardiogenic shock, and then died. A minority of fetuses survived. Extensive histopathologic examination of the brain led Myers to conclude that such prolonged partial hypoxia led to a vicious cycle of brain swelling, which caused decreased cerebral blood flow that further aggravated the brain swelling. In extreme degrees, such diminished blood flow led to total hemispheric cortical necrosis. In lesser degrees, cortical damage was seen in the middle third of the paracentral cerebral cortex and in the basal ganglia. Such lesions correspond closely with the intellectual deficits and spastic motor defects seen in humans in whom prolonged intermittent asphyxia is more common than acute total asphyxia as described by Windle.

ETIOLOGIC FACTORS IN CEREBRAL PALSY

Many authors have reviewed obstetric histories of children with congenital neurologic damage. Early in his career, Sigmund Freud became interested in the etiology of cerebral palsy. In his 1897 monograph, *Die Infantile Cerebrallahmung* (10), Freud concluded that one third of the cases were the result of traumatic birth, one sixth consequent to prematurity, one sixth were of prenatal or postnatal cause, and one third unknown. Interestingly, Freud questioned whether the real etiology of the damage was the birth process or if abnormalities seen at birth were a reflection of a previously existing abnormality. For example, Nelson and Ellenberg (11) found that a third of breech deliveries had major malformations; hence, a conclusion that abnormal development was caused by breech delivery rather than the reality that existing fetal abnormalities contribute to the incidence of breech presentation. Torfs et al. found a 3.8-fold increase in cerebral palsy for breech-delivered children over those presenting as a vertex (12). Lilienfeld and Pasamanick (13) reviewed birth certificates of 561 congenitally spastic children and found a very high incidence of abruptio and placenta previa. Eastman and DeLeon (14) reported an analysis of 96 obstetric records of infants in whom CP developed. Only 18 of these births were uncomplicated; 34 babies were premature. Of the 96 infants, 30% had apnea of more than 30 seconds at birth. Compared with controls, there was a doubling of third-trimester hemorrhage, a threefold increase in breech delivery, a fourfold increase in both anesthetic complications and fetal distress by auscultation, and a tenfold increase in shoulder dystocia among affected infants. Eastman's findings in a subsequent,

TABLE 3.1. OBSTETRIC BACKGROUND OF 753 CASES OF CP 16

Background	CP (%)	Control (%)
Postnatally acquired	8.5	
Premature (less than 2,500 g)	29.0	8.0
Twins (rate twin A = rate twin B)	7.0	1.0
Mid/high forceps	8.0	5.0
Breech	9.0	3.5
Resuscitated at birth	27.0	3.0
Hypoxia	11.0	4.0
Cord prolapse	3.0	0.3
Abruptio placentae	4.0	1.3
Toxemia	5.0	2.0
Prolonged labor	2.4	1.6
Hemolytic disease	6.0	0.3
Congenital anomalies	5.0	1.3

CP, cerebral palsy.

more extensive review (15) of 753 cases are summarized in Table 3.1.

Finally, Steer and Bonney (16) in 1962 reviewed 317 patients with CP and concluded that 5% were a result of kernicterus, 8% were caused by congenital defects and neurologic infections, and 87% were cases "with possible obstetric causes."

Thus, for many years, it has been the impression that CP was primarily caused by perinatal events. Fetal monitoring was developed with the hope that, by identifying fetal hypoxia early enough and with prompt and appropriate intervention, death and damage could be prevented (17).

Contrary to the classic theory of intrapartum hypoxia as the major cause of CP, epidemiologic studies have shown that only a small percentage of CP is attributable solely to intrapartum events, and that most cases of CP with intrapartum factors also have antepartum risk factors. In a 1998 case-controlled review by Badawi and colleagues, involving 164 term infants with moderate or severe neonatal encephalopathy compared with 400 term control infants without neona-

tal encephalopathy, antepartum and intrapartum risk factors for the development of CP were categorized. When adjusting for antepartum risk factors, they concluded that only maternal pyrexia during labor, occipital posterior presentation, an acute intrapartum event, instrumental vaginal delivery, emergency cesarean section, and general anesthesia were significant intrapartum risk factors for neonatal encephalopathy (Table 3.2). Such things as general anesthesia and emergency cesarean section are not believed to be causative in themselves but by association with the reasons for these interventions. They concluded that 70% of term or near-term neonates with neonatal encephalopathy had only antepartum risk factors with no evidence of adverse intrapartum events, 25% had evidence of antepartum risk factors and intrapartum hypoxia, and only 4% had only intrapartum hypoxia as a risk factor (18). This small contribution of intrapartum asphyxia as a cause of cerebral palsy probably accounts largely for the fact that intrapartum FHR monitoring has been disappointing as a preventative strategy (19,20).

FORMS OF CONGENITAL NEUROLOGIC DAMAGE RELATED TO FETAL HYPOXIA

Cerebral Palsy

Cerebral palsy caused by intrapartum fetal hypoxia will always have evidence of encephalopathy in the neonatal period and will be of the spastic quadriparetic or dyskinetic type. Unilateral brain lesions are not likely to be due to global hypoxia as is seen in intrapartum asphyxia (21,22). A recent large population-based survey placed the incidence of neonatal encephalopathy at 3.8 per 1,000 term infants and the incidence of hypoxic ischemic encephalopathy at 1.9 per 1,000 term infants (23). In the collaborative project, the incidence of neonatal encephalopathy was 5.4 per 1,000 births weighing more than 2,500 g. Cerebral palsy, defined as "a persistent but not changing disorder of movement and posture, appearing in the early years of life and due to a non-

TABLE 3.2. RISK FACTORS FOR NEONATAL ENCEPHALOPATHY

Preconceptional Factors	Antepartum Factors	Intrapartum Factors	Decreased Risk
Increasing maternal age	Maternal thyroid disease	Intrapartum fever	Elective C/S
Unemployed, unskilled worker, or housewife	Severe preeclampsia	Prolonged rupture of membranes	
No private health insurance	Bleeding in pregnancy	Thick meconium	
Family history of seizures	Viral illness during pregnancy	Malpresentation and malposition	
Family history of neurologic disorders	Postdate pregnancy	Intrapartum hypoxia	
Infertility treatment	Growth restriction in the fetus	Acute intrapartum events	
	Placental abnormalities	Forceps delivery or emergency C/S	

C/S, cesarean section.
Indicates risk factors that are significant by multiple logistic regression analysis of term infants with neonatal encephalopathy compared with term infants without neonatal encephalopathy.
Adapted from Manning FA, Bondaji N, Harman CR, et al: Fetal assessment based on fetal biophysical profile scoring. VIII. The incidence of cerebral palsy in tested and untested perinates. *Am J Obstet Gynecol* 178:696–706, 1998.

progressive disorder of the brain" (15), will develop in approximately five infants per 1,000 births, with a prevalence of one to two per 1,000 school-age children. As a result, CP affects 350,000 children in the United States today (14,24,25). Approximately 50% have mild intellectual retardation (IQ less than 70), and one fourth are severely affected (IQ less than 50). One fourth of children with CP have a seizure disorder (24). Cerebral palsy is classified according to the distribution of extremities involved (diplegia, paraplegia, tetraplegia, hemiplegia) and the type of movement disorder. Diplegia, a commonly used term, implies bilateral lower extremity involvement. Motor symptom classification describes the dominant movement disorder and includes spasticity, dyskinesia (athetosis), and ataxia.

Spastic diplegia is the abnormality most commonly associated with prematurity (26). Infants born prematurely are also more likely to have periventricular white matter damage (periventricular leukomalacia [PVL]) than infants born at or near term. PVL is frequently associated with intraventricular hemorrhage and ventriculomegaly (27). One study showed that abnormalities of the umbilical cord and frequent moderate variable decelerations seen in premature infants were more common in infants that were shown to have PVL (28). There is no evidence that intervention for moderate variable decelerations in a premature fetus is indicated in that PVL did not develop in more than one fourth of premature fetuses that also had frequent moderate variable decelerations.

Mental Retardation

Estimates of severe mental retardation are surprisingly uniform from country to country at about 3.5 per 1,000 population (29). Mild retardation is somewhat more variable, occurring in 23 to 31 per 1,000, probably because of testing inaccuracy and the effect of environment in this group (29). Mental retardation is a much less specific result of perinatal asphyxia than is CP. Perinatal causes are estimated to be responsible for approximately 10% of cases of mental retardation (30,31); chromosome abnormalities and various hereditary disorders, 65%; infection, 5%; prenatal causes such as toxins and maternal disease, 10%; and the rest are unknown (32). Many studies, including the Collaborative Perinatal Project (33), have conducted prospective analyses of children determined to be asphyctic at birth, examining several criteria including Apgar score, neonatal apnea, shock, or acidosis. The vast majority (generally greater than 90%) have normal IQs, and the mean IQ is usually only 5 to 10 points below average. Mental retardation without associated CP is not believed to be caused by fetal asphyxia (34).

Epilepsy

Although the potential for hypoxia to cause seizures in both newborns and adults is acutely clear, there is not a strong relationship between perinatal events and epilepsy. The Collaborative Perinatal Project did not demonstrate an increase in epilepsy in low birthweight infants or in depressed infants (35); however, epilepsy is found more commonly in infants with CP and mental retardation. Epilepsy without CP is not attributable to fetal asphyxia (34).

Behavioral and Learning Disorders

Because most depressed neonates do not have demonstrable intellectual impairment, many have questioned whether indeed such infants do eventually reach their full intellectual potential. The data suggest the opposite, because many children born hypoxic, with demonstrated intellectual impairment in infancy and preschool periods, will test in normal ranges later on. Whether this implies dissipation of the effects of hypoxia with catch-up intellectual growth or limitations of testing is open to question. Some of Windle's severely asphyxiated monkeys had structural brain defects despite apparent normal behavior. The subtleties of behavioral difficulties and learning disorders make the problem very difficult to analyze. Nichols and Chen (36) found that hyperactivity and learning disorders correlated weakly and inconsistently with perinatal asphyxia. Thus, current knowledge does not link isolated behavioral or learning disorders to fetal hypoxia.

OTHER FACTORS ASSOCIATED WITH NEONATAL ENCEPHALOPATHY AND CEREBRAL PALSY

Asphyxia is one cause of prenatal and perinatal neurologic damage. Other factors may be causative or contributive, or indeed, as pointed out by Freud (10), in babies apparently distressed and hypoxic at birth, there may have been precedent damage or anomaly unrelated to hypoxia.

Prematurity

The association of prematurity and perinatal neurologic insults and their sequelae have long been recognized. Shakespeare's King Richard III, then Duke of Gloucester, proclaimed:

> "I that am curtailed of this fair proportion,
> Cheated of feature by this dissembling nature,
> Deformed, unfinished, sent before my time
> Into this breathing world, scarce half made up—
> And that so lamely and unfashionable
> That dogs bark at me as I halt by them— . . ."

Little pointed out this passage in presenting his paper and documented a high association between spastic rigidity and prematurity.

Of all perinatal factors that are identifiable as being related to CP, prematurity has the highest correlation (11). Many of these data, however, come from 30 or more years ago. Improvements in neonatal care have decreased the incidence of neurologic damage in very low birthweight babies, but survival rates have increased so much that the contribution of prematurity to CP rates becomes very difficult to analyze.

Prolonged Pregnancy

The risk for neonatal encephalopathy increases progressively after 39 weeks' gestational age at birth. Badawi (18) showed the risk at 40 weeks was increased 1.41 times; at 41 weeks, 3.34 times; and at 42 weeks, 13.2 times. Postterm birth had less impact when controlled for small for gestational age and maternal age (37).

Intrauterine Growth Retardation

Intrauterine growth retardation (IUGR) may be caused by perinatal infections, teratogens, congenital anomalies, inadequate nutrition, or uteroplacental insufficiency in which a high incidence is associated with birth asphyxia. Fitzhardinge and Steven (38) observed 96 full-term growth-retarded infants (excluding anomalies and congenital infections) up to 8 years of age. CP occurred in 1% and epilepsy in 6%; however, "minimal cerebral dysfunction (learning difficulties, hyperactivity, and poor coordination) were found in 25%." Of these infants, 30% had speech problems and 40% poor school performance. In a case-controlled review, Badawi found IUGR to be the most significant antepartum risk factor for the development of neonatal encephalopathy with an odds ratio of 4.37 between the third and ninth percentiles and 38.23 for IUGR below the third percentile (39). Because this group of fetuses/newborns is known to have a high incidence of perinatal asphyxia, it is difficult to determine whether an antepartum respiratory and/or nutritional deficiency, intrapartum asphyctic insult, or some combination is responsible for such neurologic damage.

Traumatic Birth

The relatively high incidence of midforceps, high forceps, and breech deliveries in retrospective studies of neurologically damaged babies (14,15) suggests that birth trauma may have played a contributing role. In breech births, further evidence is provided by the reduced incidence of these problems with elective cesarean section (40). Because difficult operative vaginal deliveries have decreased, they are probably a less frequent cause of neurologic damage.

Prolonged Labor

Friedman et al. (41–43), in their series of studies concerning the effects of prolonged labor on adverse developmental

outcome, have demonstrated that this also may have contributed to sublethal CNS damage but that this may not be as important as the means of delivery (i.e., midforceps). Because Friedman's work was largely done before electronic fetal monitoring, it is difficult to know if the association with prolonged labor was due to fetal hypoxia or other causes such as infection.

Anesthesia and Analgesia

Drugs and anesthesia may contribute to neurologic damage in one of two ways. Regional anesthesias may cause maternal hypotension with resultant fetal hypoxia from decreased uterine perfusion. Depressants, whether anesthetic agents or narcotics, may cause neonatal apnea. In a setting with availability of good neonatal resuscitation, this should contribute little to hypoxic damage.

Genetic Factors

Congenital anomalies are associated with high incidences of CP, mental retardation, epilepsy, and developmental disabilities. Generally, researchers evaluating mental retardation report higher incidences of associated congenital defects than those studying CP. In a series of 1,410 autopsies from three hospitals for the mentally retarded, Malamud reports a 61% incidence of anomalies, with Down syndrome the most frequent single cause (44). Fetuses with a family history of neurologic disease or seizures had a twofold to threefold increase in neonatal encephalopathy (34) and CP (11). This suggests a relation to genetic or early developmental causes. Some inherited metabolic abnormalities also are causes of neonatal encephalopathy and cerebral palsy (45).

Fetal Infections

Congenital infections can be associated with CNS damage with or without microcephaly or hydrocephaly. Rubella, cytomegalovirus, syphilis, and toxoplasmosis (TORCH infections) are among well-known causes. As in anomalies, congenital TORCH infections are more likely to contribute to mental retardation and somatic growth retardation than to cerebral palsy. They are estimated to account for 10% of mentally retarded children in developed countries (29).

The fetal inflammatory response associated with maternal fever during labor, chorioamnionitis, and funisitis has been implicated as a cause of later cerebral palsy (46–48). It is believed that inflammatory cytokines can cause cerebral ischemia resulting in damage to the paraventricular area of premature fetal brains (49–53). These lesions appear as periventricular leukomalacia and intraventricular hemorrhage. The relation between chorioamnionitis and cerebral palsy in term fetuses has been demonstrated by Grether and Nelson (54,55). Cytokines have also been implicated in term fetuses (56). As our knowledge of infectious causes of cerebral palsy increases, it may account for some of the large percentage of cerebral palsy with unknown cause and strategies for intervention may become evident.

Coagulation and Autoimmune Disorders

Infants whose blood contains indicators of coagulation or autoimmune disorders have a higher incidence of neonatal encephalopathy, stroke, and, later, cerebral palsy, especially of the hemiparetic subtype (54,57,58). One study looking at placentas of children in whom CP developed showed that thromboses were the most frequent finding (59). This study also showed that some of these mothers had a history of pregnancy loss and some had histories of autoimmune disorders. Thyroid disorders in mothers are a potent risk factor for neonatal encephalopathy and may be related to autoimmune mechanisms (60). Neonatal encephalopathy resulting from cerebral infarcts due to coagulation disorders may closely resemble hypoxic ischemic encephalopathy. Neonates with encephalopathy should be evaluated for thrombophilias and autoimmune disease.

Toxins

Fetal neurotoxins may be the least understood causative factors in neurologic congenital diseases. Certainly, there are examples of environmental toxins (methyl mercury), drugs (folic acid antagonists such as methotrexate), and food and drink substances (alcohol) that are known to affect fetal neurologic development and cause serious mental retardation and even spasticity. Other environmental toxins may be responsible for a portion of the large group of cases of CP and mental retardation of unknown cause.

Antenatal Insults

The contributing role of antenatal factors is perhaps the most controversial and difficult to analyze of the factors involved in neurologic damage. Antenatal insult probably contributes to IUGR, and when one observes the high incidence of antepartum bleeding and toxemia in the histories of children with neurological damage, the contribution of prepartum damage becomes apparent. These babies often appear depressed at birth and have intrapartum fetal distress, but the damage may have occurred before the onset of labor.

Factors other than intrapartum hypoxia do seem very important in the pathogenesis of congenitally acquired neurologic damage. In assessing what contribution one may make with intrapartum assessment techniques, consideration must be given to such insults that may have occurred before the onset of labor. Approximately 75% of cases of CP have no history of neonatal depression or perinatal insults. Furthermore, a large percentage of neonates with encephalopathy and CP have causes other than global hypoxia. Therefore, the abnormally developing child with

features consistent with CP should not be assumed to have suffered antenatal or perinatal asphyxia.

OTHER ORGANS AFFECTED BY HYPOXIC/ASPHYXIC DAMAGE

Redistribution of blood flow in response to fetal hypoxia affects non-CNS organs acutely. Neurological damage is not the only sublethal result of perinatal hypoxia. It is well known that the lungs, kidney, and gastrointestinal tract are also sensitive to ischemia and hypoxia, and that newborn sequelae may result; however, nonneurologic damage usually repairs itself (61).

Respiratory Distress Syndrome

Respiratory distress syndrome (RDS) is the leading cause of neonatal death and serious morbidity in prematurity. The primary etiologic factor is generally thought to be inadequate pulmonary surfactant. The synthesis of pulmonary lecithin (the major component of surfactant) is significantly diminished by hypoxia and acidosis (62). Even in infants with mature ratios of lecithin to sphingomyelin, depressed and acidotic babies are more likely to have RDS (63–65). Hobel et al. and Martin et al. have pointed out that premature newborns, acidotic babies, and those with abnormal heart rate patterns suggesting hypoxia had both higher incidences of and higher mortalities from RDS. Furthermore, Martin found ominous FHR patterns to be even more predictive of RDS than Apgar scores.

Renal Damage

The association between asphyxia and renal damage, that is, anuria and renal failure similar to that in the adult, has been known since 1920. Animal data suggest such ischemic damage may be the result of the decreased renal blood flow after blood redistribution with hypoxia (66–68). Premature fetuses seem more susceptible to renal damage from ischemia.

Gastrointestinal Damage

Similarly, when blood flow is redistributed during periods of fetal hypoxia, blood flow to the fetal gastrointestinal tract is particularly diminished. Alward et al. (69) have shown that in animal fetuses, asphyxia could lead to decreased blood flow to the gastrointestinal tract, thus resulting in dilation of segments of the large and small bowel and scattered mucosal necrosis. Towbin and Turner (70), in looking at autopsies with other hypoxic damage, found intestinal injuries due to venous stasis and infarction with lesions ranging from focal mucosal necrosis to massive gross intestinal infarction. Necrotizing enterocolitis (NEC), seen most frequently in premature infants, may at least in part be the result of such damage. Preliminary data suggest ominous FHR patterns are often seen in fetuses destined to develop NEC (71).

EVIDENCE THAT ABNORMAL FETAL HEART RATE PATTERNS CORRELATE WITH HYPOXIA/ASPHYXIA

Knowing the correlation of hypoxia, asphyxia, and other intrapartum events with sublethal neurologic damage, one must demonstrate the relationship of abnormal FHR patterns with hypoxia and acidosis. If Apgar scores are used to measure neonatal depression, one must show the association of neonatal depression with hypoxia and acidosis. The latter was well demonstrated by Modanlou et al. (72). Biochemical changes, especially pH and base deficit, have a statistically significant correlation with depressed newborns (73).

While it is not within the realm of this chapter to discuss the mechanisms responsible for the genesis of FHR patterns, it has been established that these changes are caused by fetal hypoxemia and acidemia and are correlated with fetal distress and neonatal depression. Barcroft first demonstrated the typical variable-type deceleration caused by umbilical cord occlusion in the fetal goat (74). Subsequently, Lee and Hon (75) were able to reproduce this in the human fetus. Myers et al. (9) were able to reproduce late decelerations in the rhesus monkey by precipitating uterine artery hypotension.

Kubli et al. (76) described the relationship of human fetal scalp pH with various FHR patterns and demonstrated that the more severe the pattern, the more likely the fetus is to be acidemic. However, the correlation between pH and severity of FHR pattern abnormality had a large standard deviation. The correlation with fetal base deficit was much

tighter. Paul et al. (77) further refined this work. They found that, with both acidosis and depressed Apgar scores, the FHR variability associated with late decelerations had a higher correlation than amplitude of the late decelerations. Many subsequent studies have supported the parallel relationship of ominous FHR patterns and acidosis.

Many studies have linked FHR patterns to Apgar scores, showing generally that the more ominous the tracing, the more likely the outcome of a depressed baby. Because there are really no studies in which fetal monitor patterns are blinded and not acted upon, intervention may have decreased the degree of correlation, because in most patterns a certain time is necessary from the development of intermittent asphyxia to the development of metabolic acidosis. Bisonette (78) has produced one of the most detailed retrospective analyses of FHR patterns and Apgar scores (Table 3.3). Schifrin and Dame (79) attempted to predict Apgar scores from FHR patterns obtained within 30 minutes of delivery without regard to clinical circumstances during labor. When a normal baby was predicted, they were nearly always right; when a depressed baby was predicted, they were more often wrong, but when a baby was born depressed, it was nearly always predicted (Fig. 3.1). Because there are other causes of neonatal depression besides intrapartum hypoxia/asphyxia, one would not expect to find 100% correlation between a predicted healthy baby and a normal Apgar score.

It can be concluded, therefore, that FHR patterns suggesting fetal asphyxia and/or acidosis do correlate with depression at birth. One must be careful to point out that (a) not all abnormal patterns are associated with poor outcome, (b) the extent to which intervention ameliorates or prevents adverse outcome is unknown, (c) electronic fetal monitoring corresponds best and is most valuable when the pattern is reassuring, and (d) fetal heart rate patterns, by themselves, are not predictive of later neurologic outcome (80).

TABLE 3.3. RELATIONSHIP BETWEEN FHR PATTERN AND 1-MINUTE APGAR SCORE

FHR Pattern	Number	Percent	Mean Apgar	Apgar 4–6 (Moderate Depression)		Apgar 0–3 (Marked Depression)	
				Number	Percent	Number	Percent
Normal	322	45.0	8.2	16	5.0	3	0.9
Uncomplicated baseline tachycardia	24	3.4	7.9	1	4.2	1	4.2
Uncomplicated baseline bradycardia	38	5.3	8.1	3	7.9	0	0
Uncomplicated loss of beat-to-beat variation	40	5.6	7.2	7	17.5	2	5.0
Complicated loss of beat-to-beat variation	11	1.5	6.7	2	18.2	2	18.2
Acceleration	52	7.3	8.4	1	1.9	0	0
Early deceleration	122	17.1	8.0	6	4.9	1	0.8
Late deceleration	20	2.8	5.4	7	35.0	5	25.0
Variable deceleration with normal baseline	71	9.9	7.7	9	12.7	2	2.8
Variable deceleration with abnormal baseline	14	2.0	5.9	0	0	7	50.0

FHR, fetal heart rate.
From Bisonette JM: Relationship between continuous fetal heart rate patterns and Apgar score in the newborn. *Br J Obstet Gynaecol* 82:24, 1975, with permission.

Normal Apgar Predicted
1 Min - 93% Correct
5 Min - 99% Correct

Low Apgar Predicted
1 Min - 43% Correct
5 Min - 20% Correct

Low Apgar Baby Delivered
1 Min - 54% Predicted
5 Min - 83% Predicted*

FIGURE 3.1. Reliability of prediction of Apgar score from fetal heart rate tracings. (From Schifrin BS, Dame L: Fetal heart rate patterns. Prediction of Apgar score. *JAMA* 219:1322, 1972.)

CRITERIA NECESSARY TO ASSIGN ACUTE INTRAPARTUM ASPHYXIA AS A CAUSE OF NEONATAL BRAIN DAMAGE

The American College of Obstetricians and Gynecologists (ACOG) issued a technical bulletin in 1992 (34) in which they concluded that for perinatal asphyxia to be linked to a neurologic deficit in the child, all of the following criteria must be present:

1. Profound umbilical artery metabolic or mixed acidemia (pH <7.00)
2. Persistence of an Apgar score of 0 to 3 for longer than 5 minutes
3. Neonatal neurologic sequelae, for example, seizures, coma, hypotonia
4. Multiorgan system dysfunction, for example, cardiovascular, gastrointestinal, hematologic, pulmonary, or renal

In 1995, a policy statement was issued by the Task Force on Cerebral Palsy and Neonatal Asphyxia of the Society of Obstetricians and Gynaecologists of Canada (81) in which they stated that the same criteria as mentioned by ACOG must all be present plus an umbilical artery base defect of ≥16 mmol/L. They stated that if all these criteria are not present, we cannot conclude that hypoxic acidemia existed or had the potential to cause neurologic deficits.

In 1999 Alastair MacLennan published "A template for defining a causal relation between acute intrapartum events and cerebral palsy: international consensus statement," which was a consensus statement of the Perinatal Society of Australia and New Zealand and was endorsed by 21 obstetrical and pediatric societies from around the world and was prepared by 49 people from seven countries (82). The following were the essential criteria to define an acute intrapartum hypoxic event sufficient to cause permanent neurologic impairment contained in this document:

Essential Criteria

1. Evidence of metabolic acidosis in intrapartum fetal, umbilical arterial cord, or very early neonatal blood samples (pH <7.00 and base deficit ≥12 mmol/L)

2. Early onset of severe or moderate neonatal encephalopathy in infants of ≥34 weeks' gestation
3. Cerebral palsy of the spastic quadriparetic or dyskinetic type

Criteria That Together Suggest an Intrapartum Timing but by Themselves Are Nonspecific

1. A sentinel (signal) hypoxic event occurring immediately before or during labor
2. A sudden, rapid, and sustained deterioration of the FHR pattern usually after the hypoxic sentinel event where the pattern was previously normal
3. Apgar scores of 0 to 6 for longer than 5 minutes
4. Early evidence of multisystem involvement
5. Early imaging of evidence of acute cerebral abnormality

While there is almost consistent agreement among the professionals who have looked at these required criteria for hypoxic intrapartum causation of term fetal brain damage, they continue to be debated in the courtroom. In 1997, the NICHD research planning workshop on fetal monitoring (83) concluded that the following patterns are consistent with hypoxia that is predictive of current or impending fetal asphyxia so severe that the fetus is at risk for neurologic and other fetal damage or death:

1. Late decelerations with absent variability
2. Variable decelerations with absent variability
3. Sustained bradycardia with absent variability

They also concluded that patterns with all of the following characteristics confer a high probability of a normally oxygenated fetus.

1. Normal baseline rate
2. Normal (moderate) FHR variability
3. Presence of FHR accelerations
4. Absence of FHR decelerations

There are FHR patterns that meet none of the above ominous or reassuring criteria, and a consensus has not been developed for treatment of patients whose patterns are in between. The use of fetal scalp pH, fetal scalp stimulation, and fetal pulse oximetry discussed later in this book may be helpful in management of such patterns. FHR patterns themselves are not sufficient to indicate damage has occurred but rather are an aid to timing of the hypoxic event if the other criteria are met.

THE IMPACT OF INTRAPARTUM ELECTRONIC FETAL MONITORING

Early studies of electronic fetal monitoring (EFM) indicated a correlation between FHR patterns and fetal pH, Apgar scores, and intrapartum death. Since the clinical introduction of intrapartum electronic FHR monitoring in the late 1960s and early 1970s, there have been a large number of both retrospective and prospective nonrandomized studies (84–96). Initially the nonrandomized, largely retrospective studies indicated a decrease in fetal and neonatal deaths with electronic intrapartum FHR monitoring compared with intermittent auscultation as was done in the early 1970s. Some studies showed better outcome in high-risk EFM fetuses than in low-risk fetuses monitored by intermittent auscultation. At that time, the intrapartum period was regarded as an especially vulnerable time for the fetus, and it was generally believed that most cases of CP were caused by intrapartum asphyxia.

The first randomized prospective trial of intrapartum electronic FHR monitoring was done by Haverkamp (97), and much to the surprise of many, when compared to a one-on-one nurse listening every 15 minutes in the first stage of labor and every 5 minutes in the second stage of labor, outcomes including fetal and neonatal death, Apgar scores, and cord pH values were not different, with excellent results in both groups. The incidence of cesarean birth, however, was significantly increased in the EFM group. A follow-up study by Haverkamp (98), using fetal scalp blood pH before operative intervention, revealed that the excess cesarean birth rate decreased. Since then, there have been a number of prospectively randomized trials that have not shown any advantage to intrapartum EFM over intermittent auscultation with a one-on-one nurse listening every 15 minutes in the first stage of labor and every 5 minutes in the second stage of labor (99–103). One randomized prospective trial by Vintzileos (104) done in Greece, suggested benefit to intrapartum EFM with no hypoxic perinatal deaths and nine per thousand in the intermittent auscultation group. This compared to 0.4 per thousand in the combined auscultation groups from the other prospectively randomized trials, suggesting either a different patient population or different auscultation techniques.

When these randomized prospective trials were completed, long-term neurologic outcome was evaluated in some of the study patients. In the Dublin study by MacDonald and Grant with excellent follow-up, while there were more neonatal seizures in the auscultation group, the incidence of CP was not different between groups (105). A randomized prospective trial was then done by Luthy and Shy (106) in preterm fetuses weighing between 700 and 1,750 g, and again no difference in immediate outcome measures was noted. A 3-year follow-up study on these infants was done by Shy and Luthy (107), and interestingly, the EFM group actually had more cases of CP. This could have been due to the study protocol that required documentation of acidotic fetal scalp pH before intervention in the EFM group, resulting in longer delay to delivery after recognition of the abnormal pattern than in the auscultation group where no pH documentation was required.

The increased cesarean birth rate seen in some of the randomized trials with EFM without apparent benefit continues to be a concern. Because a high percentage of abnor-

mal FHR strips are not associated with bad outcome or fetal acidosis, a technique that will safely reduce the cesarean birth rate among patients with FHR patterns that are concerning would be highly desirable. Fetal pulse oximetry discussed later in this book may provide such a technique.

There have been no trials comparing intrapartum EFM to no monitoring. Another way to look at intrapartum EFM is to point out that it is as good as having a one-on-one nurse listening every 15 minutes in the first stage of labor and every 5 minutes in the second stage of labor. Clearly most busy labor and delivery units cannot provide that type of coverage for all laboring patients. It is the knowledge gained from EFM that is used to do intermittent auscultation, and, in fact, when auscultation is concerning, electronic monitoring is virtually always used before an intervention decision is made.

Thus today we are left with a technique that clearly detects fetal hypoxia even in its earliest stages, but it appears to show no better outcome than intermittent auscultation with a one-on-one nurse listening every 15 minutes in the first stage of labor and every 5 minutes in the second stage. This then leaves us with some questions. Could most fetal asphyxia occur before labor, resulting in an abnormal pattern from the time of admission and a good correlation with outcome but no benefit from intervention? With sudden onset acute intrapartum hypoxia, perhaps fetal damage or death can occur so rapidly that even rapid intervention is not sufficient. Finally, perhaps neurologically abnormal fetuses are more likely to become hypoxic during labor, resulting in FHR patterns that detect the hypoxia but provide no benefit from intervention. Clearly, however, acute intrapartum asphyxia can result in fetal death or later neurologic damage, and in the fetus with a previously normal FHR pattern, acute asphyxia will be detected by FHR change and the potential for intervention with prevention of death or damage exists.

The Effect of Electronic Fetal Monitoring and Dedicated Auscultation on Intrapartum Fetal Mortality

While questions remain regarding the relative value of intrapartum EFM versus auscultation, it is clear that dedicated electronic or auscultatory fetal monitoring during the intrapartum period clearly reduces the intrapartum fetal death rate. Intrapartum fetal death is a clear endpoint that has occurred at a rate between one and four per 1,000 in most obstetric populations. For this reason, a rather large study population would be required to determine the effect of EFM on the intrapartum death rate. The first clinical studies were retrospective and noncontrolled. These studies included over 135,000 patients, approximately one third of whom were electronically monitored (86–96). The intrapartum death rate in these studies was 1.76/1,000 in patients observed during labor with auscultation and 0.54/

TABLE 3.4. INTRAPARTUM FETAL DEATH AND ELECTRONIC FETAL MONITORING: NONRANDOMIZED TRIALS

Primary Author	Year	No EFM	IFD	EFM	IFD	Ratio
Chan et al.[86]	1973	5,427	17	1,162	2	
Kelly and Kulkarni[87]	1973	17,000	15	150	0	
Tutera and Newman[88]	1975	6,179	37	608	1	
Edington et al.[89]	1975	991	4	1,024	0	
Koh et al.[90]	1975	1,161	4	1,080	5	
Shenker et al.[91]	1975	11,599	14	1,950	1	
Lee and Baggish[92]	1976	4,323	15	3,529	1	
Paul et al.[93]	1977	36,724	34	13,344	6	
Amato[94]	1977	2,981	12	4,226	1	
Johnstone et al.[95]	1978	9,099	13	7,313	3	
Hamilton et al.[96]	1978	4,353	11	4,399	1	
Total		99,842	176	38,785	21	
Rate		1.76/1000		0.54/1000		3.26 ($P < .001$)
		Critical no. of subjects for $P < .05$ = 18,046				

EFM, electronic fetal monitoring; IFD, intrapartum fetal death.
From Antenatal Diagnosis. Report of a consensus development conference. NIH Publication no. 79-1973, Bethesda, MD, April 1979.

1,000 in patients followed with EFM ($P < .001$). The intrapartum fetal death ratio calculates to 3.26:1 for auscultated versus electronically monitored patients (Table 3.4). These data were restricted to infants who weighed over 1,500 g at birth and who were corrected for congenital anomalies. These studies can certainly be criticized on several bases, including different time frames in the EFM versus the auscultated groups and no consistent protocols for the use of auscultation. In most of these studies, the electronically monitored patients were higher risk than the auscultated patients, and despite this, the intrapartum stillbirth rate was lower in the high-risk group that was electronically monitored.

Subsequently, eight published randomized controlled trials have compared EFM to auscultation in both high- and low-risk patients and with one exception have shown no difference in intrapartum fetal death (97–104). In Vintzileos' study (104) there was a difference favoring electronically monitored patients and the high hypoxic mortality rate in the auscultated group that may not apply as discussed previously. It is significant that, with the exception of the study by Leveno et al. (103), both groups in each randomized controlled trial had a dedicated one-on-one nurse assigned to the patient and the auscultated groups were followed much more frequently than was commonly practiced in hospitals. This is substantiated by the low combined intrapartum fetal death rate in the auscultated groups: 1.05/1,000 (excluding the Vintzileos [104] study). If the studies by Leveno et al. (103) and Vintzileos (104) are eliminated, thereby including only those with one-to-one nursing providing the auscultation, the intrapartum fetal death rate drops to 0.4/1,000 (Table 3.5). Furthermore, in these studies, abnormal auscultative heart rates were often backed up by electronic FHR monitoring. It is thus evident that

TABLE 3.5. INTRAPARTUM FETAL DEATHS: RANDOMIZED PROSPECTIVE STUDIES[a]

Study Author	Intermittent Auscultation		Continuous EFM	
	Cases	Deaths	Cases	Deaths
Haverkamp et al.[97]	241	0	242	0
Haverkamp et al.[98]	232	0	453	0
Renou et al.[99]	175	1	175	0
Kelso et al.[100]	251	0	252	0
Wood et al.[101]	432	0	445	0
McDonald et al.[102]	4,999	2	4,987	3
Totals	6,155	3	6,554	3

EFM, electronic fetal monitoring.
[a]Does not include study by Leveno et al. (103), which used selective EFM in the control group and Vintzileos (104), where the hypoxic death rate in the auscultated group was an outlier.

either electronic fetal monitoring or dedicated auscultation will reduce the intrapartum fetal death rate compared to less stringent monitoring.

What Are the Risks of Electronic Fetal Monitoring?

There has been much written about the risk of invasive EFM and infection of the fetus and/or mother. Fetal infections have consisted almost exclusively of small scalp infections characterized by erythema and induration requiring no more than local medication and are reported in from 0.3% to 4.5% (108–113) of internally monitored labors.

Maternal infection in patients with internal EFM during labor has been said to be increased in several studies (97,109–111), whereas other studies have indicated no increased risk of maternal infection (86,99). When one examines the reports, it becomes obvious that infection is most pronounced if the patient is monitored and then delivered by cesarean section, as opposed to the patient who is monitored and then delivered vaginally. Scrutiny will reveal that the patient with long labor, many vaginal examinations, prolonged ruptured membranes, and obstructed labor requiring cesarean section is also the most likely patient to be internally monitored for a prolonged time. This association is probably responsible for the presumed cause-effect relationship between EFM and infection following cesarean section. Gibbs et al. (112) looked at all associated factors with postcesarean infection and, using multivariate analysis, found that invasive EFM had little or no effect on infection.

Effect of Electronic Fetal Monitoring on the Cesarean Section Rate

Perhaps the most discussed risk of EFM is the increase in the cesarean section rate that some have attributed to EFM (Table 3.6). Determining the exact contribution, if any,

TABLE 3.6. IMPACT OF EFM ON CESAREAN SECTION RATES: RANDOMIZED PROSPECTIVE STUDIES[a]

Study Author	C-Sections (%)	
	Intermittent Auscultation	Continuous EFM
Haverkamp et al.[97]	7	17
Haverkamp et al.[98]	6	11
Renou et al.[99]	14	22
Kelso et al.[100]	4	10
Wood et al.[101]	2.1	4
McDonald et al.[102]	2.2	2.4

C-sections, cesarean sections; EFM, electronic fetal monitoring.
[a]Does not include study by Leveno et al. (103), which used selective EFM in the control group.

that EFM makes to the overall cesarean section rate is complicated by the fact that many other practices, such as routine cesarean section for breech presentations and abandoning midforceps, have changed during the same period that EFM has been on the increase. Five of the seven randomized controlled trials have shown an increase in the cesarean section rate in the EFM group.

Clearly, there are patients who are allowed to labor because of the fetal monitor, whereas before EFM they would not have even been given a trial of labor. In our practice, this has been best demonstrated in diabetics, patients with clinical abruptions, elderly gravidas, and certain patients with previous intrapartum fetal death where the monitor reassures both the patient and the physician.

Williams and Hawes (114) looked at the impact of EFM on the cesarean section rate in California during 1977. They surveyed 324,085 births and determined that about half the patients in California had electronically monitored labors. They determined the expected perinatal mortality rates for each hospital based on the risk of the population served. They then determined those medical care factors that favorably or unfavorably affected those mortality rates. The most significant factors that favorably affected perinatal mortality were a high cesarean section rate and a high incidence of fetal monitoring. Other factors favorable to an improved perinatal outcome included a neonatal intensive care unit in the hospital, delivery by a trained obstetrician, a perinatal morbidity committee in the hospital, and occurrence of the birth in a nonprofit community hospital with a teaching program. The data, which include a large number of deliveries over a 1-year period from all types of hospitals, suggest that the overall impact of high technology with its probably higher rate of intervention would seem to be justified on the basis of improved perinatal mortality.

THE IMPACT OF ANTEPARTUM FETAL HEART RATE MONITORING

There have been several randomized prospective trials comparing primary antepartum fetal surveillance using the nonstress test to no nonstress test surveillance which have shown no benefit to this form of testing alone (115–118). None of these trials involved long term follow-up. There is only one prospective randomized trial of antepartum surveillance that showed benefit. This was Neldam's study of fetal movement counting that showed a decrease in antepartum fetal deaths in patients instructed in fetal movement counting compared with patients with no fetal movement counting instructions (119). A 1983 study by Beischer et al. did show that when a nonreactive positive spontaneous contraction stress was found, there was a 28% perinatal mortality rate, and 27% of surviving infants were found to have a neurologic handicap (120). Manning looked retrospectively at patients studied with biophysical profile surveillance and found fewer cases of CP when these cases were compared with patients not monitored with biophysical profiles (1.33 vs 4.74 per 1,000) (121,122). Certainly, the potential for benefit of antepartum surveillance would seem high because a majority of stillbirths occur before labor, and even those fetuses with intrapartum hypoxia, more often than not, have evidence of antepartum risk factors. However, because of the high incidence of normal outcome in patients with abnormal antepartum testing, the predictive value of antepartum testing remains poor.

SUMMARY

Intrapartum fetal hypoxia is a clear although infrequent cause of fetal mortality and morbidity that may lead to long-term neurologic damage. Electronic fetal monitoring and dedicated intrapartum auscultation decrease the intrapartum fetal death rate when compared to practices before the introduction of either technique. Most cases of neonatal encephalopathy and cerebral palsy are attributed to causes other than intrapartum hypoxia alone. Electronic FHR monitoring appears to be associated with an increased cesarean section rate in some settings. Current understanding of FHR monitoring patterns seems to be clear with respect to ominous patterns and reassuring patterns, but there are many patterns in between associated with a high degree of disagreement between observers. It is unclear if techniques such as fetal scalp blood pH monitoring, fetal scalp stimulation, or fetal pulse oximetry will result in less unnecessary operative intervention among patients with ambiguous patterns.

REFERENCES

1. Yudkin PL, Johnson A, Clover LM, et al.: Clustering of perinatal markers of birth asphyxia and outcome at age five years. *Br J Obstet Gynecol* 101:774–781, 1994.
2. Behrman RE, Lees MH, Petersen EN, et al: Distribution of circulation in the normal and asphyxiated fetal primate. *Am J Obstet Gynecol* 108:956–969, 1970.
3. Cohn EH, Sacks EJ, Heyman MA, et al.: Cardiovascular responses to hypoxemia and acidemia in fetal lambs. *Am J Obstet Gynecol* 120:817–824, 1974.
4. Peeters L, Sheldon R, Jones M, et al: Blood flow to organs as a function of arterial oxygen content. *Am J Obstet Gynecol* 135:637–644, 1979.
5. Little WJ: On the influence of abnormal parturition, difficult labours, premature birth and asphyxia neonatorum, on the mental and physical condition of the child, especially in relation to deformities. *Trans Obstet Soc London* 3:293, 1862.
6. Windle WF, Becker RF: Asphyxia neonatorum. An experimental study in the guinea pig. *Am J Obstet Gynecol* 45:183, 1943.
7. Windle WF: Neuropathology of certain forms of mental retardation. *Science* 140:1186.
8. Myers RE: Two patterns of perinatal brain damage and their conditions of occurrence. *Am J Obstet Gynecol* 112:246, 1972.
9. Myers RE, Mueller-Huebach E, Adamsons K: Predictability of the state of fetal oxygenation from a quantitative analysis of the components of late decelerations. *Am J Obstet Gynecol* 115:1083, 1973.
10. Freud S: *Die Infantile Cerebrallahmung.* A. Hoelder, Vienna, 1897.
11. Nelson KB, Ellenberg JH: Antecedents of cerebral palsy. Multivariate analysis of risk. *N Engl J Med* 315:81, 1986.
12. Torfs CP, van den BergBJ, Oechsli FW, et al.: Prenatal and perinatal factors in the etiology of cerebral palsy. *J Pediatr* 1990; 116:615-619.
13. Lilienfeld AM, Pasamanick B: The association of maternal and fetal factors with the development of cerebral palsy and epilepsy. *Am J Obstet Gynecol* 70:93, 1.
14. Eastman NJ, DeLeon M: The etiology of cerebral palsy. *Am J Obstet Gynecol* 69:950, 1955.
15. Eastman NJ, Kohl SG, Maisel JE, et al.: The obstetrical background of 753 cases of cerebral palsy. *Obstet Gynecol Surv* 17:459, 1996.
16. Steer CW, Bonney W: Obstetric factors in cerebral palsy. *Am J Obstet Gynecol* 83:526, 1962.
17. Quilligan EJ, Paul RH: Fetal monitoring: is it worth it? *Obstet Gynecol* 45:96, 1975.
18. Badawi N, Kurinczuk, JJ, Keogh JM, et al.: Intrapartum risk factors for newborn encephalopathy: The Western Australia case control study. *BMJ* 1998;317:1554–1558.
19. Paneth N: Birth and the origins of cerebral palsy [Editorial]. *N Engl J Med* 315:124, 1986.
20. Freeman RK: Intrapartum fetal monitoring—a disappointing story. *N Engl J Med* 322:624-626, 1990.
21. Michelis R, Rooschuz B, Dopfer R: Prenatal origin of spastic hemiparesis. *Early Hum Dev* 4:243–255, 1980.
22. Nelson KB, Grether JK: Potentially asphyxiating conditions and spastic cerebral palsy in infants of normal birth weight. *Am J Obstet Gynecol* 179:507–513, 1998.
23. Badawi N, Kurinczuk JJ, Hall D, et al.: Newborn encephalopathy in term infants: three approaches to population based investigation. *Semin Neonatol* 1997;2:181–188.
24. Nelson KB, Ellenberg JH: Epidemiology of cerebral palsy. In: Schoenberg BS, ed. *Advances in neurology,* vol. 19. Raven Press, New York, 1979.
25. Alberman E: Main causes of major mental handicap: prevalence and epidemiology. In: *CIBA Foundation Symposium 59: major mental handicap: methods and costs of prevention.* Elsevier-Excerpta Medica, Amsterdam, 1978.
26. Hagberg G, Hagberg B, Clow I: The changing panorama of cerebral palsy in Sweden, 1954-1970. I. Analysis of the general changes. *Acta Paediatr Scand* 64:187, 1975.
27. Kunban C, Sanocka U, Leviton A, et al.: White matter disorders of prematurity: Association with intraventricular hemorrhage and ventriculomegaly. *J Pediatr* 134:539–546, 1999.
28. Ito T, Kadowaki K, Takahashi H, et al.: Clinical features and cardiotocographic findings for premature infants with antenatal periventricular leukomalacia. *Early Hum Dev* 47:195–201, 1997.
29. Stein Z, Susser M: Mental retardation. In: Last JM, ed. *Public health and preventive medicine.* Appleton-Century-Crofts, New York, 1980.
30. McDonald AD: Severely retarded children in Quebec: prevalence, causes and care. *Am J Ment Defic* 78:205, 1973.
31. Drillien CM: Studies in mental handicap. II. Some obstetric factors of possible aetiological significance. *Arch Dis Child* 43:283, 1968.
32. Warkany J: Mental retardation. In: *Congenital malformations.* Year Book Medical Publishers, Inc, Chicago, 1971:262–267.
33. Drage JS, Kennedy S, Berendes H, et al.: The Apgar score as an

index of infant morbidity. A report from the Collaborative Study of Cerebral Palsy. *Dev Med Child Neurol* 8:141, 1966.

34. American College of Obstetricians and Gynecologists: Fetal and neonatal neurologic injury. ACOG Technical Bulletin 163. Washington DC: ACOG, 1992.

35. Ellenberg J, Nelson K: Birthweight and gestational age in children with cerebral palsy or seizure disorders. *Am J Dis Child* 133:1044, 1979.

36. Nichols PL, Chen TC: *Minimal brain dysfunction: a prospective study.* Erlbaum Associates, Hillsdale, NJ, 1981.

37. Campbell MK, Truls-Ostbye MD, Lorentz M: Post-term birth: risk factors and outcomes in a 10 year cohort of Norwegian births. *Obstet Gynecol* 89:543–548, 1997.

38. Fitzhardinge PM, Steven EM: The small for date infant. II. Neurological and intellectual sequelae. *Pediatrics* 50:50, 1972.

39. Badawi N, Kurinczuk, JJ, Keogh JM, et al.: Antepartum risk factors for neonatal encephalopathy: the Western Australia case-control study. *BMJ* 317:1549–1553, 1998.

40. Hannah ME, Hannah WJ, Hewson SA, et al.: Planned cesarean section versus planned vaginal birth for breech presentation at term: a randomized multicentre trial. Term breech trial collaborative group. *Lancet* 356:1375–1383, 2000.

41. Friedman EA, Niswander KR, Sachtleben MR, et al.: Dysfunctional labor. X. Immediate results to infant. *Obstet Gynecol* 33:776, 1969.

42. Friedman EA, Niswander KR, Sachtleben MR: Dysfunctional labor. XI. Neurologic and developmental effects on surviving infants. *Obstet Gynecol* 33:785, 1969.

43. Friedman EA, Sachtleben MR, Bresky PA: Dysfunctional labor. XII. Long term effects on infant. *Am J Obstet Gynecol* 127:779, 1977.

44. Malamud N: Neuropathology: In: Stevens HA, Heber R, eds. *Mental retardation.* Chicago: The University of Chicago Press, 1964.

45. Leviton A, Nelson KB: Problems with definitions and classifications of newborn encephalopathy. *Pediatr Neurol* 8:85–90, 1992.

46. Dammann O, Leviton A: Role of the fetus in perinatal infection and neonatal brain damage. *Curr Opin Pediatr* 12:99–104, 2000.

47. LiebermanRichardson DK, Lang J, Frigoletto FD, et al.: Intrapartum maternal fever and neonatal outcome. *Pediatrics* 105:8–13, 2000.

48. Impey L, Greenwood C, MacQuillan K, et al.: Fever in labour and neonatal encephalopathy: a prospective cohort study. *Br J Obstet Gynecol* 108:594–597, 2001.

49. Yoon BH, Jun JK, Romero R, et al.: Amniotic fluid inflammatory cytokines (interleukin 6, interleukin 1B, and tumor necrosis factor α), neonatal white matter lesions, and cerebral palsy. *Am J Obstet Gynecol* 177:19–26, 1997.

50. Yoon BH, Romero R, Park JS, et al.: Fetal exposure to an intra-amniotic inflammation and the development of cerebral palsy at the age of three years. *Am J Obstet Gynecol* 182:675–681, 2000.

51. Naccasha N, Hinson R, Montag A, et al.: Association between funisitis and elevated interleukin-6 in cord blood. *Obstet Gynecol* 97:220–224, 2001.

52. Dammann O, Leviton A: Maternal intrauterine infection, cytokines, and brain damage in the preterm newborn. *Pediatr Res* 42:1–8, 1997.

53. Steinborn A, Niederhut A, Solbach C, et al.: Cytokine release from placental endothelial cells, a process associated with preterm labour in the absence of intrauterine infection. *Cytokine* 11:66–73, 1999.

54. Grether JK, Nelson LB: Maternal infection and cerebral palsy in infants of normal birth weight. *JAMA* 278:207–211, 1997.

55. Eschenbach DA: Amniotic fluid infection and cerebral palsy (Editorial). *JAMA* 278:247–248, 1997.

56. Nelson KB, Dambrosia JM, Grether JK, et al.: Neonatal cytokines and coagulation factors in children with cerebral palsy. *Ann Neurol* 44:666–675, 1998.

57. Kraus FT, Acheen VI: Fetal thrombotic vasculopathy in the placenta: cerebral thrombi and infarcts, coagulopathies and cerebral palsy. *Hum Pathol* 30:759–769, 1999.

58. Redline RW, Wilson-Castillo D, Borawski E, et al.: Placental lesions associated with neurologic impairment and cerebral palsy in very low birth weight infants. *Arch Pathol Lab Med* 122:1091–1099, 1998.

59. Kraus FT: Cerebral palsy and thrombi in placental vessels of the fetus. *Hum Pathol* 28:246–248, 1997.

60. Badawi N, Kurinczuk JJ, Mackenzie CL, et al.: Maternal thyroid disease: a risk factor for newborn encephalopathy in term infants. *Br J Obstet Gynecol* 107:798–801, 2000.

61. Perlman JM, Tack EC: Renal injury in the asphyxiated newborn infant: relationship to neurological outcome. *J Pediatr* 113:875–879, 1998.

62. Merritt TA, Farrell PM: Diminished pulmonary lecithin synthesis in acidosis: experimental findings as related to the respiratory distress syndrome. *Pediatrics* 57:32, 1976.

63. Cruz AC, Bohi WC, Birk SA, et al.: Respiratory distress syndrome with mature lecithin/sphingomyelin ratios: diabetes mellitus and low Apgar scores. *Am J Obstet Gynecol* 126:78, 1976.

64. Hobel CJ, Hyvarinen M, Oh W: Abnormal fetal heart rate patterns and fetal acid-base balance in low birth weight infants in relation to respiratory distress syndrome. *Obstet Gynecol* 39:83, 1972.

65. Martin CB, Siassi B, Hon EH: Fetal heart rate patterns and neonatal death in low birthweight infants. *Obstet Gynecol* 44:503, 1974.

66. Ikeda T, Murata Y, Quilligan E, et al.: Histologic and biochemical study of the brain, heart, kidney and liver in asphyxia caused by occlusion of the umbilical cord in near term fetal lambs. *Am J Obstet Gynecol* 182:449–457, 2000.

67. Cohn HJ, Sacks EJ, Heymann MA, et al.: Cardiovascular responses to hypoxemia and acidemia in fetal lambs. *Am J Obstet Gynecol* 120:817, 1974.

68. Perlman JM, Tack EK: Renal injury in the asphyxiated newborn infant: relationship to neurological outcome. *J Pediatr* 113:875–879, 1988.

69. Alward CT, Hook JB, Helmrath TA, et al.: Effects of asphyxia on cardiac output and organ blood flow in the newborn piglet. *Pediatr Res* 12:824, 1978.

70. Towbin A, Turner GL: Obstetric factors in fetal-neonatal visceral injury. *Obstet Gynecol* 52:113, 1978.

71. Braly P, German J, Garite T: Fetal heart rate patterns in infants who develop necrotizing enterocolitis. *Arch Surg* 115:1050, 1980.

72. Modanlou H, Yeh SY, Hon EH, et al.: Fetal and neonatal biochemistry and Apgar scores. *Am J Obstet Gynecol* 117:942, 1973.

73. Low JA, Victory R, Derrick EJ: Predictive value of electronic monitoring for intrapartum fetal asphyxia with metabolic acidosis. *Obstet Gynecol* 93:285–291, 1999.

74. Barcroft J: *Researches on perinatal life.* Blackwell Scientific Publications Ltd, Oxford, 1946:124.

75. Lee ST, Hon EH: Fetal hemodynamic response to umbilical cord compression. *Obstet Gynecol* 22:533, 1963.

76. Kubli FH, Hon EH, Khazin AF, et al.: Observations on fetal heart rate and pH in the human fetus during labor. *Am J Obstet Gynecol* 104:1190, 1969.

77. Paul RH, Suidan AK, Yeh SY, et al.: Clinical fetal monitoring. VII. The evaluation and significance of intrapartum FHR variability. *Am J Obstet Gynecol* 123:206, 1975.

78. Bisonette JM: Relationship between continuous fetal heart rate patterns and Apgar score in the newborn. *Br J Obstet Gynaecol* 82:24, 1975.

79. Schifrin BS, Dame L: Fetal heart rate patterns. Prediction of Apgar score. *JAMA* 219:1322, 1972.

80. Nelson KB, Dambrosia JM, Ting TY, et al.: Uncertain value of electronic fetal monitoring in predicting cerebral palsy. *N Engl J Med* 334:613–618, 1996.

81. Policy Statement-Task Force on Cerebral Palsy and neonatal asphyxia (part I). *SOGC*, December 1996:1267–1279.

82. MacLennan A, for the International Cerebral Palsy Task Force: A template for defining a causal relationship between acute intrapartum events and cerebral palsy-An international consensus statement. *BMJ* 319:1054–1059, 1999.

83. National Institute of Child Health and Human Development Research Planning Workshop. Electronic fetal heart rate monitoring: research guidelines for interpretation. *Am J Obstet Gynecol* 177:1385–1390, 1997.

84. Tejani N, Mann L, Bhakthavathsalan A, et al.: Correlation of fetal heart rate-uterine contraction patterns with fetal scalp blood pH. *Obstet Gynecol* 46:392, 1975.

85. Banta HD, Thacker SB: Costs and benefits of electronic fetal monitoring: a review of the literature. Department of HEW Publication no (PHS) 79-3245, Washington, DC.

86. Chan WH, Paul RH, Toews J: Intrapartum fetal monitoring maternal and fetal morbidity and perinatal mortality. *Obstet Gynecol* 41:7,1973.

87. Kelly VC, Kulkarni D: Experiences with fetal monitoring in a community hospital. *Obstet Gynecol* 41:818, 1973.

88. Tutera G, Newman RL: Fetal monitoring: its effect on the perinatal mortality and caesarean section rates and its complications. *Am J Obstet Gynecol* 122:750, 1975.

89. Edington PT, Sibanda J, Beard RW: Influence on clinical practice of routine intra-partum fetal monitoring. *BMJ* 3:341, 1975.

90. Koh KS, Greves D, Yung S, et al.: Experience with fetal monitoring in a university teaching hospital. *Can Med Assoc J* 112:455, 1975.

91. Shenker L, Post RC, Seiler JS: Routine electronic monitoring of fetal heart rate and uterine activity during labor. *Obstet Gynecol* 46:185, 1975.

92. Lee WK, Baggish MS: The effect of unselected intrapartum fetal monitoring. *Obstet Gynecol* 47:516, 1976.

93. Paul RH, Huey JR, Yaeger CF: Clinical fetal monitoring—its effect on cesarean section rate and perinatal mortality: five-year trends. *Postgrad Med* 61:160, 1977.

94. Amato JC: Fetal monitoring in a community hospital: a statistical analysis. *Obstet Gynecol* 50:269, 1977.

95. Johnstone FD, Campbell DM, Hughes GJ: Antenatal care: has continuous intrapartum monitoring made any impact on fetal outcome? *Lancet* 1(8077):1298, 1978.

96. Hamilton LA, Gottschalk W, Vidyasagar D, et al.: Effects of monitoring high-risk pregnancies and intrapartum FHR monitoring on perinates. *Int J Gynaecol Obstet* 15:483, 1978.

97. Haverkamp AD, Thompson HE, McFee JG, et al.: The evaluation of continuous fetal heart rate monitoring in high risk pregnancy. *Am J Obstet Gynecol* 125:310, 1976.

98. Haverkamp AD, Orleans M, Langendoerfer S, et al.: A controlled trial of the differential effects of intrapartum fetal monitoring. *Am J Obstet Gynecol* 134:399, 1979.

99. Renou P, Chang A, Anderson I, et al.: Controlled trial of fetal intensive care. *Am J Obstet Gynecol* 126:470, 1976.

100. Kelso IM, Parsons RJ, Lawrence GE, et al.: An assessment of continuous fetal heart rate monitoring in labor: a randomized trial. *Am J Obstet Gynecol* 131:526, 1978.

101. Wood C, Renou P, Oates J, et al.: A controlled trial of fetal heart rate monitoring in a low-risk population. *Am J Obstet Gynecol* 141:527, 1981.

102. McDonald D, Grant A, Sheridan-Pereira M, et al.: The Dublin randomized control trial of intrapartum fetal heart rate monitoring. *Am J Obstet Gynecol* 152:524, 1985.

103. Leveno KJ, Cunningham FG, Nelson S, et al.: A prospective comparison of selective and universal electronic fetal monitoring in 34,995 pregnancies. *N Engl J Med* 315:615, 1986.

104. Vintzileos AM, Antsaklis A, Varvarigos O, et al.: A randomized trial of electronic fetal heart rate monitoring versus intermittent auscultation. *Obstet Gynecol* 81:899–907, 1993.

105. Grant A, O'Brien N, Joy MT, et al.: Cerebral palsy among children born during the Dublin randomized trial of intrapartum monitoring. *Lancet* 2:1233–1236, 1989.

106. Luthy DA, Shy KK, van Belle G, et al.: A randomized trial of electronic fetal monitoring in pre-term labor. *Obstet Gynecol* 69:687–695, 1987.

107. Shy KK, Luthy DA,Bennett FC, et al.: Effects of electronic fetal heart rate monitoring a compared with periodic auscultationon the neurologic development of premature infants. *N Engl J Med* 322:588–593, 1990.

108. Cordero L, Hon EH: Scalp abscess: a rare complication of fetal monitoring. *J Pediatr* 78:533, 1971.

109. Gassner CB, Ledger WJ: The relationship of hospital-acquired maternal infection to invasive intrapartum monitoring techniques. *Am J Obstet Gynecol* 126:33, 1976.

110. Hagen D: Maternal febrile morbidity associated with fetal monitoring and cesarean section. *Obstet Gynecol* 46:260, 1975.

111. Wiechetek WJ, Horiguchi T, Dillon TF: Puerperal morbidity and internal fetal monitoring. *Am J Obstet Gynecol* 119:230, 1974.

112. Gibbs RS, Jones PM, Wilder CJY: Internal fetal monitoring and maternal infection following cesarean section: a prospective study. *Obstet Gynecol* 52:193, 1978.

113. Paul RH: Clinical fetal monitoring: experience on a large clinical service. *Am J Obstet Gynecol* 113:573, 1972.

114. Williams RL, Hawes W: Cesarean section, fetal monitoring and perinatal mortality in California. *Am J Public Health* 69:864, 1979.

115. Kidd LC, Patel N, Smith R: Non-stress antenatal cardiotocography—a prospective randomized clinical trial. *Br J Obstet Gynecol* 92:1156, 1985.

116. Flynn A, Kelly J, Mansfield H, et al.: A randomized controlled trial of antepartum non-stress cardiotocography. *Br J Obstet Gynecol* 89:427, 1982.

117. Brown V, Sawyers S, Parsons R, et al.: The value of antenatal cardiotocography in the management of high risk pregnancy: a randomized controlled trial. *Br J Obstet Gynecol* 89:716, 1982.

118. Lumley J, Lester A, Anderson I, et al.: A randomized trial of weekly cardiotocography in high risk obstetrical patients. *Br J Obstet Gynecol* 90:1018, 1983.

119. Neldam S: Fetal movements as an indicator of fetal well-being. *Lancet* 2:1222, 1980.

120. Beischer NA, Drew JH, Ashton PW, et al.: Quality of survival of infants with critical reserve detected by cardiotocography. *Am J Obstet Gynecol* 146:662, 1983.

121. Manning FA, Bondagji N, Harman CR, et al.: Fetal assessment based on the fetal biophysical profile score: relationship of last BPS result to subsequent cerebral palsy. *J Gynecol Obstet Biol Reprod (Paris)* 26:720–729, 1997.

122. Manning FA, Bondaji N, Harman CR, et al.: Fetal assessment based on fetal biophysical profile scoring. VIII. The incidence of cerebral palsy in tested and untested perinates. *Am J Obstet Gynecol* 178:696–706, 1998.

4

INSTRUMENTATION AND ARTIFACT DETECTION

INSTRUMENTATION

For the obstetrician or obstetric nurse to interpret fetal monitor tracings correctly, it is necessary to have some understanding of the processes involved in the acquisition and processing of data relating to fetal heart rate (FHR) and uterine activity. Electronic fetal monitors are designed to interpret accurately in most situations, but there are times when their output can be misleading unless the instruments' limitations are understood. Most errors we see in FHR interpretation are related to the quality of the data acquisition and presentation, and, for this reason, an understanding of this chapter is critical for the clinician using electronic fetal monitoring in the treatment of obstetric patients.

FETAL HEART RATE DERIVED BY DIRECT (INTERNAL) FETAL ELECTROCARDIOGRAPHY

The FHR monitor acquires, processes, and displays an electronic signal. To understand the significance of the FHR display, it is important to understand what the monitor can and cannot count. FHR tracings from a fetal scalp electrode are obtained by measuring the interval between consecutive fetal R waves. Therefore, the fetal electrocardiogram (ECG) signal provides the clinician with a measure of the electrical activity of the fetal heart. It does not necessarily represent mechanical activity. The fetal ECG signal is acquired through a bipolar electrode that penetrates the skin of the fetal scalp (first pole) and that has a second conductor residing in the secretions of the maternal vagina (second pole). It is believed that the circuit is completed through the fetal umbilical cord, placenta, and the maternal circulation and that the potential difference (voltage) being measured is between the two poles. The original electrode was a modified skin clip, but now a spiral electrode is used.

The raw fetal ECG signal is amplified and fed into a beat-to-beat cardiotachometer (Fig. 4.1). The amplifier uses an automatic gain control circuit to boost the fetal ECG signal to a predetermined voltage before electronic counting. All electronic signals are equally strengthened-noise as well as fetal ECG. Once the fetal ECG signal has been amplified, it is filtered, and the interval between R wave peaks is measured. The interval between R waves is processed to a rate in beats per minute (BPM) by computing the reciprocal of the interval. With internal FHR monitors, a new rate is set each time an R wave is detected; as each new wave arrives, the rate is recalculated from the reciprocal of the previous R-R interval. The result of this rate calculation is the plotting of a series of square waves (Fig. 4.2). The minute rate differences between beats are referred to as beat-to-beat or short-term variability and can only be appreciated when the FHR is computed instantaneously by means of a beat-to-beat cardiotachometer. FHR changes with a cyclicity of 3 to 5 per minute are referred to as long-term variability, and those occurring in response to uterine contractions or fetal movement are referred to as periodic. Long-term variability and periodic changes can be detected with Doppler systems, but true short-term variability can be measured only with direct or abdominal fetal ECG systems. The newer fetal monitors have advanced technology allowing for Doppler-derived signal data of significantly improved quality such that, although not exact, the FHR recording is very close to that obtained from direct fetal ECG and visually approximates true short-term variability in many patients.

Most fetal ECG systems will not record R-R intervals less than 250 milliseconds, which corresponds to a rate of 240 beats per minute (BPM). If the FHR exceeds 240 BPM, not even a direct fetal ECG system will count every beat and may halve or not print such rates. This occurs only with fetal supraventricular tachyarrhythmias (paroxysmal atrial tachycardia, atrial fibrillation, or atrial flutter), intermittent premature atrial contractions, or premature ventricular contractions (Fig. 4.3).

An additional instance that may cause confusion is the patient with a cardiac pacemaker. If the transmitted mater-

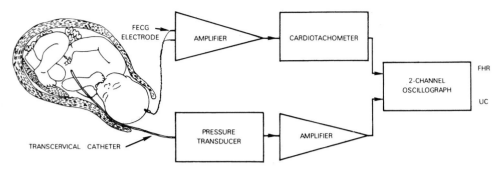

FIGURE 4.1. Schematic diagram of a direct fetal monitoring system. The fetal heart rate is obtained from a fetal scalp electrode and counted in a cardiotachometer. The actual uterine pressure is recorded directly from a transcervical intrauterine catheter. FHR, fetal heart rate; UC, uterine contraction.

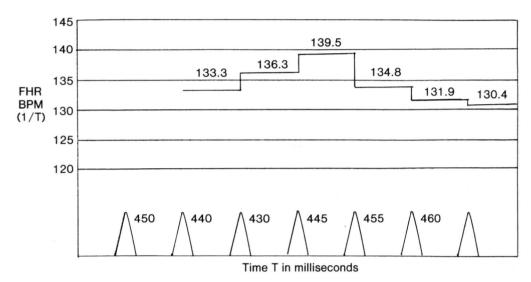

FIGURE 4.2. This schematic represents an enlarged segment of the fetal heart rate tracing. A new rate is set with the arrival of each R wave in the fetal electrocardiogram. This generates a series of square waves that indicate beat-to-beat changes.

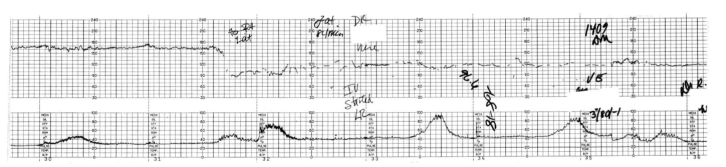

FIGURE 4.3. This is an example of a change in the atrial pacemaker. The fetus is known to have multiple cardiac abnormalities and presented in supraventricular tachycardia with nonimmune hydrops. Cardioversion was achieved successfully with digoxin and quinidine. This tracing is from early labor.

nal pacemaker pulse is at a higher voltage than the fetal R wave, the scalp electrode may record the pacemaker signal (1,2).

In the absence of the fetal ECG signal, such as with a dead fetus, there will usually be no tracing. However, depending on the monitor and the existing maternal R wave, amplification of the incoming signal may continue until, on occasion, counting of the maternal heart rate from the scalp of the dead fetus results (Fig. 4.4) (3,4). This can obviously lead to confusion. When there is any doubt, fetal demise should be confirmed with real-time ultrasound and

in all instances of monitoring, there needs to be documentation of maternal pulse rate as different from the FHR.

DOPPLER ULTRASOUND

In the antepartum period, and often during the intrapartum period, it is neither feasible nor always necessary to use the direct fetal ECG signal to record the FHR. External monitoring using various biophysical modalities has evolved to a point where it currently represents the most

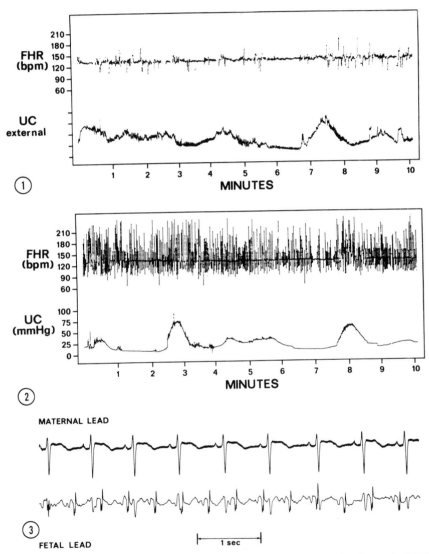

FIGURE 4.4. The **upper panel** shows the heart rate from a fetal scalp electrode (FHR) and maternal leads (MHR) with a dead fetus. Note the two rates are identical in detail. The **lower panel** shows the fetal scalp lead and the maternal lead ECG tracing indicating that the dead fetus is transmitting the maternal ECG to the fetal lead. (from Klapholz H, Schifrin BS, Myrick R et al.: Role of maternal artifact in fetal heart rate pattern interpretation. *Obstet Gynecol* 44:373, 1974, with permission.)

frequent form of FHR monitoring. Doppler ultrasound is the method most commonly used to indirectly record FHR (Fig. 4.5).

The principles underlying the use of Doppler FHR monitoring are described.

Ultrasonic signals can penetrate human tissue. When the transmitted ultrasonic beam encounters an interface of increased density, a portion of the signal is reflected. The angle of reflection varies according to the angle of incidence of the beam. A portion of the signal will be transmitted to the next interface. If the interface is moving, the reflected signal undergoes a frequency change (Doppler shift). The frequency increases if the reflecting interface is moving toward the signal source and decreases if the reflecting interface is moving away from the signal source. An example commonly used to describe the Doppler shift is the audible change in pitch (frequency) noticed by a stationary observer of the whistle from a rapidly moving train. As the train approaches, the whistle gets both louder and higher in frequency. As the train passes and moves away, both loudness and pitch rapidly decline.

The fetal monitor Doppler transducer contains a transmitter, or signal source, and receiver. With all of the first-generation fetal monitors and many second-generation monitors, the signal is transmitted and the reflected signals received continuously by multiple crystals contained in the transducer. A transducer innovation employed by second-generation monitors is pulsed Doppler. The pulsed Doppler transducer alternates the emission of ultrasound waves with the reception of the reflected waves, resulting in a decrease in both the amount and time of exposure of the fetus to ultrasound energy. Ultrasound waves of sufficient intensity will generate heat. Intensities of less than 100 mW/cm^2, regardless of the length of exposure, generate no heat. The amount of energy generated by fetal monitors is only a small fraction of this, with the continuous ultrasound transducers generating intensities of 5 to 12 mW/cm^2 and pulsed ultrasound transducers generating 1.5 to 5 mW/cm^2.

As long as the reflecting interfaces are not in motion, the reflected signal has the same frequency as the transmitted signal. However, if the reflecting interface is the surface of a moving organ such as the fetal heart, there will be a frequency change (Doppler shift) in the reflected signal. The electronic circuitry of the fetal monitor senses this frequency change and converts it to an electronic signal. This signal can then be used as a marker of the fetal heart beat as well as for the creation of fetal heart sounds produced by the monitor. This is the sound that is heard using a Doppler device. A similar shift is created if the Doppler signal is being reflected by any movement such as fetal blood. It is important to understand that with Doppler technology, it is not the actual fetal heart being heard but rather a sound that is created by the device in response to frequency changes generated by a moving interface.

This biphasic signal is immersed in noise created by fetal movements, arterial blood flow, maternal movements, and random muscle contractions. The signal actually received is a composite consisting of bursts with various amplitudes and frequencies. In addition, the actual signal created by the fetal cardiac motion is greatly affected by the position and movement of the transducer with respect to the fetus. With older monitors, the quality of the Doppler-created FHR tracing is directly related to the orientation of the signal to the fetal heart, the amount of fetal movement, and the degree of constant attention by nursing personnel of maintaining an adequate signal while caring for the patient. One potential source of error occurs when the Doppler signal is actually maternal and not fetal heart rate (Fig. 4.6). The maternal pulse should be checked to confirm correct recording of FHR at the initiation of fetal monitoring, with any switching of FHR modes or with any abrupt decrease in FHR, especially in a setting of noncontinuous tracings.

With the evolution of autocorrelation and wide-beam ultrasound transducers in many of the newer monitors,

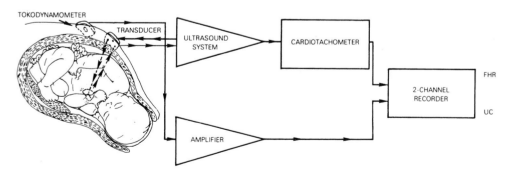

FIGURE 4.5. Schematic diagram of an indirect fetal monitoring system. The fetal ultrasonogram is obtained from an abdominal wall transducer, conditioned, and then counted by a cardiotachometer. The semiquantitative uterine activity is measured by an external tocodynamometer. *UC*, uterine contraction.

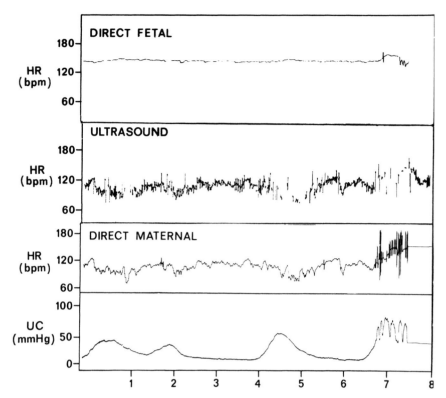

FIGURE 4.6. Simultaneous recording of heart rate *(HR)* from the direct fetal scalp electrode **(upper tracing),** abdominal Doppler **(middle tracing),** and direct maternal **(lower tracing).** Note that the abdominal Doppler signal is recording the maternal heart rate from a maternal vessel in the abdomen. *UC*, uterine contraction. (From Klapholz H, Schifrin BS, Myrick R et al.: Role of maternal artifact in fetal heart rate pattern interpretation. *Obstet Gynecol* 44:373, 1974, with permission.)

great advances have been made in both signal quality and continuity.

FIRST-GENERATION SIGNAL PROCESSING

Fetal monitors obtain the FHR indirectly by use of Doppler ultrasound. To produce an FHR tracing, several modulations of the reflected signal need to be used. As previously discussed, amplification and filtering of the incoming signal within certain frequencies extracts FHR signals from those produced by other moving structures. The filtered signal is converted to an electrical waveform by the transducer, and it is this waveform that is used to generate and display the FHR. Detection of fetal motion with Doppler signal is the same with both the older and newer monitors. It is the process of signal conversion to FHR that differs.

First-generation monitors calculate heart rate by electronic integration and peak detection of the returning Doppler signal. The highest point of the waveform is detected and recorded as a heart beat, even though it may not appear at the same time in each waveform. Despite various electronic logic and filtering processes, this often results in an apparent increase in short-term variability due to a false reproduction of the actual interval from one heart beat or R wave (contraction) to the next (Figs. 4.7–4.9). With signal fading, inconsistent signal shape, and changing signal peaks, the resultant FHR may be, at best, a poor reflection of the true variability of consecutive R-wave intervals. The beat-to-beat variability of the FHR calculated from the fetal ECG usually averages 1 BPM or less (5), but the Doppler signal using the first-generation monitor technology often displays a variability much greater than that and can be very misleading.

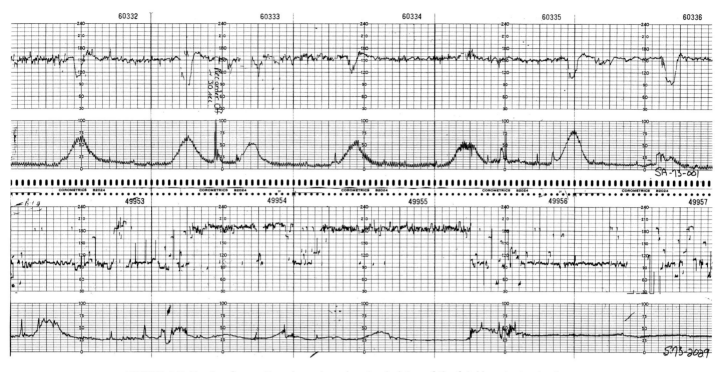

FIGURE 4.7. Tracing from a Doppler system showing halving of the fetal heart rate at rates over 180 beats per minute.

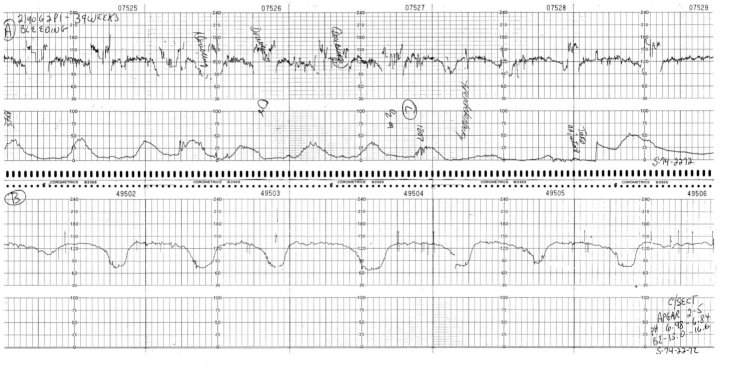

FIGURE 4.8. The **upper tracing** is taken from a Doppler signal source. At first glance, it appears to be a poor-quality erratic tracing, but upon closer examination, the late decelerations can be seen. The fetal heart rate (FHR) doubles whenever it goes below 90 beats per minute, putting the trough of the late decelerations above the baseline. The **lower tracing,** a continuation of the **upper tracing** after the fetal scalp electrode signal source was begun, shows the deep decelerations that were previously unrecognized because of the artifactual doubling of the FHR by the Doppler logic system.

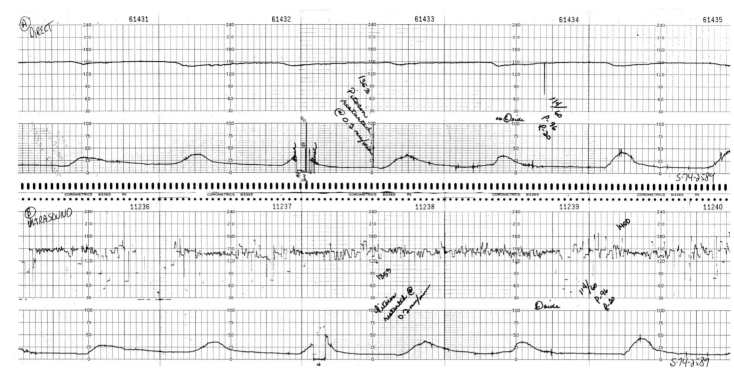

FIGURE 4.9. Simultaneous recordings with Doppler **(lower tracing)** and direct fetal electrocardiogram **(upper tracing)** signal sources. Note the apparent increased variability and obscuring of periodic changes on the Doppler tracing.

AUTOCORRELATION

Although not new in concept, the application of autocorrelation to FHR technology has been made possible by the introduction of high-speed microprocessor integrated circuitry.

The received pattern is broken into very short second envelopes of time made up of 200 to 300 digitalized points (Fig. 4.10). With each consecutive new heart beat waveform, the microprocessor compares the digitalized points to the equivalent points in the preceding envelope. Essentially, auto-

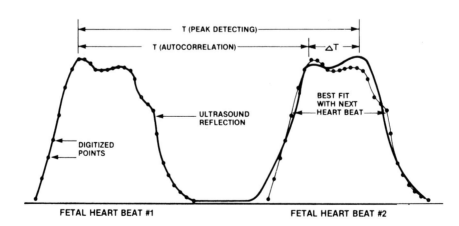

FIGURE 4.10. Schematic representation of consecutive fetal heart beat waveforms demonstrating autocorrelation versus peak detection. (Reproduced with permission of Hewlett Packard Corporation, Bohlinger, Germany.)

correlation is a signal-processing scheme that compares the incoming signal with a time-delayed version of previous signals. Important information has a regular form repeated over time, while random noise has no such regularity. Artifactual waveforms and older points are discarded. The resultant tracing represents a point in each cardiac cycle more accurately than can be done with first-generation monitors. Varying waveform amplitude problems are, therefore, minimized, and markedly less false variability is produced (Fig. 4.11).

As with first-generation monitors, interpretation of the FHR from newer monitors using autocorrelation must be done cautiously. Despite apparent improvement in signal interpretation, autocorrelation is still not a true measure of short-term variability. The possibility for signal loss, doubling, halving, or recording of maternal heart rate or other movements must be kept in mind when reading changes in FHR monitor strips (5,6). Because autocorrelation enhances signal-to-noise levels and periodic phenomena, in the absence of fetal cardiac motion it may produce a false signal and resultant "heart rate" (Fig. 4.12). When doubt is present or diagnosis of fetal distress is suspected, confirmation with auscultation or direct fetal scalp electrode must be done.

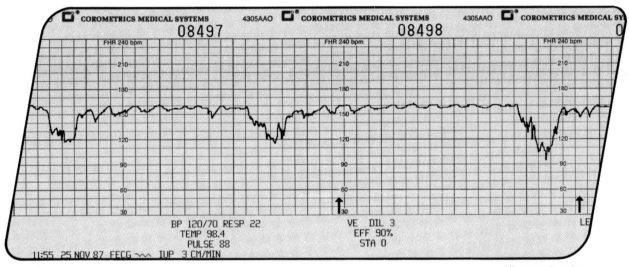

Ultrasound tracing

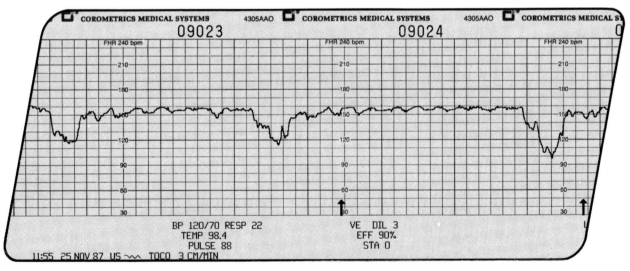

FIGURE 4.11. Example of simultaneous intrapartum fetal heart rate tracings comparing the external monitor with the direct fetal electrocardiogram internal monitor. Autocorrelation has improved the quality of the tracing and eliminated much of the signal loss or error present with many older monitors. (Courtesy of Corometrics Medical Systems, Wallingford, CT.)

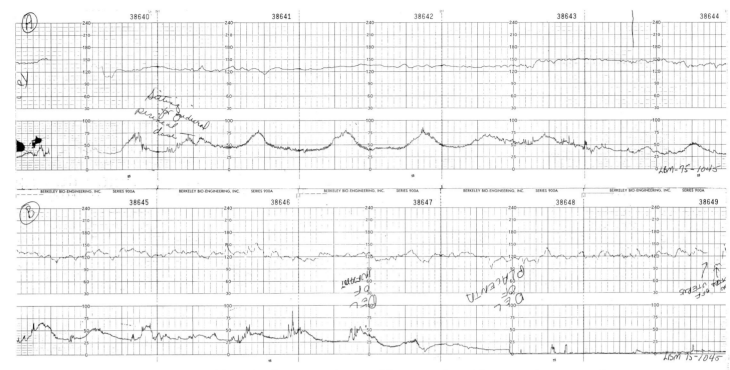

FIGURE 4.12. This tracing shows a Doppler record from a monitor with an excessive amount of electronic logic. Note in the **lower panel** that, even after the delivery of the baby and placenta, an apparent fetal heart rate can still be seen on the tracing.

ABDOMINAL FETAL ELECTROCARDIOGRAPHIC-DERIVED FETAL HEART RATE TRACINGS

Abdominal fetal ECG signals were first recorded by Cremer in 1906 (7). The original application of this method was to diagnose fetal life. Later, Larks and Dasgupta (8) and Hon and Hess (9) showed that the presentation of the fetus could be predicted by the polarity of the fetal QRS complex in relation to the maternal abdomen. With a breech presentation, the fetal ECG complex would be similar in polarity to that of the mother; with a cephalic presentation, the R-wave would be opposite that of the maternal polarity. In addition, abdominal fetal ECG tracings could be used to diagnose twins by comparing the fetal complexes and determining two separate rate patterns among the fetal complexes. From the maternal abdomen, the fetal ECG complex is much smaller than the maternal ECG (Fig. 4.13). Often, if the electrical noise level is high, one may not be able to see a fetal ECG signal.

Due to the weakness of the fetal ECG signal before 30 weeks' gestation, the interference created by the electromyographic muscle noise of the maternal abdominal wall, and the frequency of coincidence of maternal and fetal ECG signals, abdominal ECG plays little role in modern

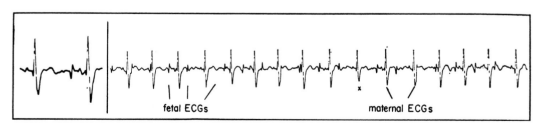

FIGURE 4.13. An abdominal tracing showing the large maternal electrocardiogram complexes and the clear but much smaller fetal complexes. (From Hon EH, Lee: *Am J Obstet Gynecol* 87:804, 1963, with permission.)

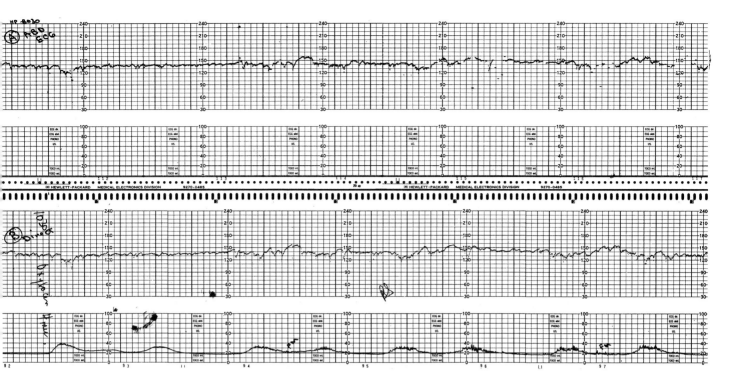

FIGURE 4.14. Simultaneous fetal heart rate tracings derived from abdominal electrocardiogram (ECG) (**upper panel**) and scalp ECG (**lower panel**).

FHR monitoring other than in arrhythmia detection. However, before the introduction of autocorrelation and improved Doppler technology with the newer monitors, abdominal fetal ECG-derived tracings were the most accurate recordings of FHR signal in many patients (Fig. 4.14). Several attempts have been made, with varying degrees of success, to reliably obtain FHR variability indirectly using the abdominal fetal ECG modality (10,11).

PHONOCARDIOGRAPHICALLY DERIVED FETAL HEART RATE

Phonocardiography was the first method used to record FHR electronically. As the fetal heart beats, closure of the valves may be detected by listening with a suitable stethoscope through the mother's abdominal wall. With ventricular systole, the closure of the atrioventricular valves produces the first heart sound. This mechanical energy may be sensed by a microphone and amplified, producing an electrical signal that may then be reconverted to sound or used to produce a phonocardiogram, an oscillographic tracing of the heart sounds. The amplified electrical signal can also be used as a counting source for an FHR monitor. The phonocardiographic signal is clearer than the Doppler signal,

resulting in less artifactual "jitter." For this reason, phonocardiography historically was widely used for antepartum FHR monitoring.

The main drawback to phonocardiographically derived FHR systems is that they are extremely sensitive to ambient noise such as maternal bowel sounds, voices in the room, certain air-conditioning systems, and, especially, noise produced by any motion of the microphone or of the bed clothing against the microphone. In addition, any fetal kicking or motion produces a very loud noise that will saturate the automatic gain system on the monitor's amplifier, resulting in complete loss of recording for several seconds while waiting for the amplifier to reopen. For this reason, a manual gain control offers a great advantage when using abdominal fetal phonocardiography for recording heart rate. Also, because of the high sensitivity to ambient noise, the technique is unsatisfactory for monitoring during the active phase of labor (Fig. 4.15). The current role of phonocardiographic FHR recording is quite limited but should be considered if abdominal fetal ECG and Doppler do not produce satisfactory recordings. Today, it would have to be considered below Doppler in a ranking of preferred methods of antepartum FHR recording. Both abdominal fetal ECG and phonocardiographic FHR are rarely employed means of fetal monitoring, but are of historic significance.

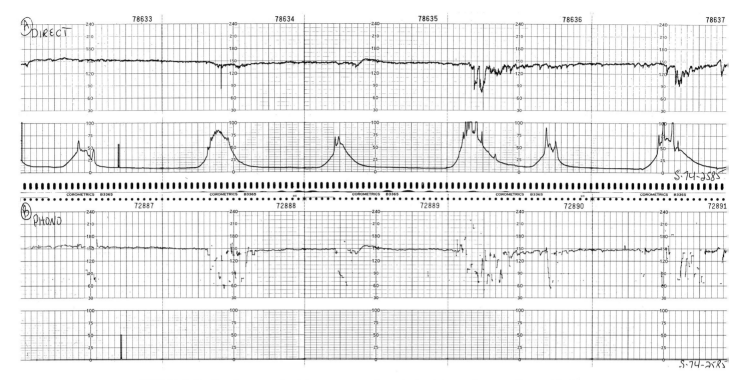

FIGURE 4.15. Simultaneous fetal heart rate tracings derived from phonocardiographic (**upper tracing**) and scalp electrocardiogram (**lower panel**). Note the signal loss during contractions with the phono recording.

SCALING FACTORS

The choice of vertical and horizontal scaling directly affects the appearance of the FHR and uterine contraction tracings. In the United States, the standard factors are 30 BPM/cm on the vertical scale and 3 cm/minute on the horizontal scale. In Europe, standard factors are 20 BPM/cm (vertical) and 1 or 2 cm/minute (horizontal). The European scaling factors accentuate apparent FHR variability and tend to make periodic changes appear more abrupt than American scaling factors. Although we think that 1 cm/minute tracings are harder to read than the same tracings at 3 cm/minute, the slower rate of tracing is commonly used in Europe, South America, and certain centers in this country. Figure 4.16 shows how paper speed can significantly alter the appearance of a tracing.

APPLICATION OF MONITORING DEVICES

Uterine Contraction Monitors

Clinically, uterine contractions can be monitored by two techniques: external tocodynamometry or intrauterine pressure measurement. Both methods have advantages and disadvantages, and one or the other are more applicable in certain clinical situations. This section will deal with the methodology involved in the clinical application of these techniques.

Intrauterine Pressure Monitoring

The pregnant uterus is a closed, fluid-filled space. Hydrostatic pressure within the uterus should be equal at all points. Intrauterine pressure has historically been determined with the use of an open-ended, fluid-filled catheter placed through the cervix and externally attached to a strain gauge transducer. Pascal's law dictates that assuming such a monitoring system is a closed system, the baseline tone as well as the intrauterine pressure during a contraction will be transmitted directly to the external strain gauge pressure transducer. With such a system, both technical and logistic problems exist, such as catheter occlusion by solid matter, kinking or entrapment of catheter between the uterus and the fetus, as well as introduction of artifact secondary to maternal movement and catheter manipulation (12). An alternative type of intrauterine pressure device was introduced in 1987. This device has a micro-pressure transducer located at the tip of the catheter, which is inserted through the cervix into the uterine cavity. Such a device eliminates most of the problems associated with the fluid-filled devices used for uterine pressure monitoring. Most devices currently employed to monitor intrauterine pressure come

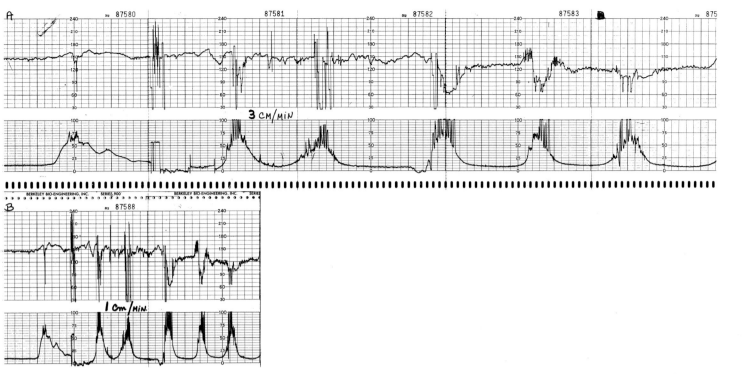

FIGURE 4.16. Tape-recorded fetal heart rate and uterine contraction patterns were played back simultaneously to monitors running at 3 cm/minute (**upper tracing**) and 1 cm/minute (**lower tracing**).

from one of the manufacturers of these transducer-tipped catheters (see Figs. 5.3, 5.4).

The pressure within the uterine cavity is directly proportional to the uterine wall tension and inversely proportional to the diameter of the uterus. Thus, the larger the uterus, the lower the intrauterine pressure for a given uterine wall tension. Clinical support of this concept is reflected in the fact that pressure in the nonpregnant uterus may exceed 200 mm Hg during menstrual contractions, whereas intrauterine pressure with twins may never exceed 35 or 40 mm Hg, even in active labor. The usual pressures observed in the pregnant uterus during active labor at term are in the range of 50 to 100 mm Hg at the peak of contractions, with a baseline tone of 5 to 12 mm Hg.

Insertion of the uterine pressure catheter is accomplished by introducing it, while within the sterile introducer tube, just inside the uterine cervix and next to the presenting part (Fig. 4.17). The flexible intrauterine catheter is usually advanced into the uterus quite easily, but, on occasion, resistance will be met. In this situation, one should move the introducer 90 degrees in its orientation to the cervix and try again. Usually, one begins posterior to the presenting part, but the catheter can be inserted anywhere in the 360-degree circumference of the cervix. When the catheter advances easily, it should be inserted to the mark on the catheter that should be just visible at the introitus. All sys-

tems for measuring intrauterine pressure must be zeroed, which is the referencing of the pressure to 0 mm Hg while the system is open to air. Any reconnection of the patient to the monitor requires re-zeroing. It is expected that there will be a baseline uterine tone, so if the monitor is registering zero or a negative number, the calibration is incorrect.

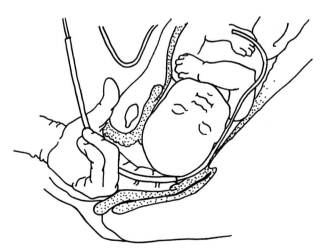

FIGURE 4.17. Technique of transcervical insertion of uterine catheter. Note that the introducer is only inserted about 1 cm inside the cervix.

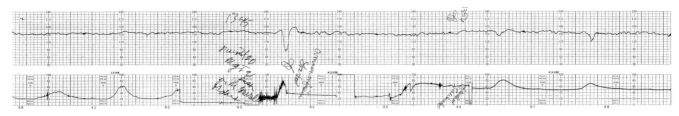

FIGURE 4.18. Amnioinfusion effect on uterine tone. Note the significant change in the baseline uterine tone associated with initiation of amnioinfusion. This results from the hydrostatic pressure of the infusate and must be considered in assessing the actual intrauterine pressure.

Replacement of the catheter is necessary if a good recording does not result from simple manipulation.

Another modification of the intrauterine pressure catheter allows for amnioinfusion while simultaneously recording contraction strength directly (see Fig. 5.5). The accuracy of pressure monitoring is not lessened with this catheter and allows for continuous amnioinfusion without artifactual elevation of baseline uterine pressure or a need for the placement of a second catheter for infusion. If one is using a single lumen catheter for pressure readings and simultaneous amnioinfusion, there is an elevation of the apparent baseline uterine tone (Fig 4.18). However, this is actually the result of the hydrostatic pressure from the infusate and is readily confirmed by interrupting the infusion and confirming true baseline and peak contraction strength.

The Spiral Fetal Scalp Electrode

The most commonly used fetal electrode consists of a spiral or corkscrew-shaped device placed inside two concentric tubes, with the wires trailing through the center tube (Fig. 4.19). After clearly identifying the presenting part, the whole assembly is inserted through the vagina and cervix against the fetus. The inner tube is then rotated clockwise one full turn so that the electrode tip penetrates the fetal presenting part (Fig. 4.20). The wires are then attached to the leg plate, which is usually placed on the mother's thigh (Fig. 4.21). The leg plate is then attached to the fetal monitor.

If the signal is not adequate, efforts should be made to be certain that the electrode is attached to the fetal presenting part and that the leg plate is appropriately grounded.

Precautions that should be taken when inserting an internal electrode include the following:

1. Use sterile technique.
2. Do not attempt placement if unsure of the exact site of placement.
3. Do not place over facial structures.
4. Avoid the genitalia in breech position.
5. Never try to reinsert an electrode by twisting manually. Sometimes the spiral is stretched out, and the depth of insertion may exceed the safe depth set on nonstretched electrodes.

FIGURE 4.19. Example of the fetal spiral electrode. (Tyco Healthcare-Kendall LTP, Chicopee, MA.)

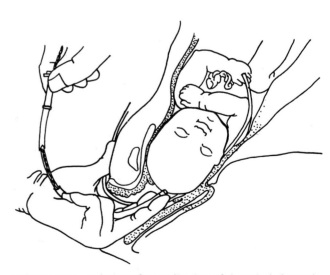

FIGURE 4.20. Technique for application of the spiral electrode.

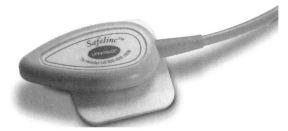

FIGURE 4.21. Example of leg plate that is attached to the patient's upper thigh. The scalp electrode wires connect directly to this plate. (Tyco Healthcare-Kendall LTP, Chicopee, MA.)

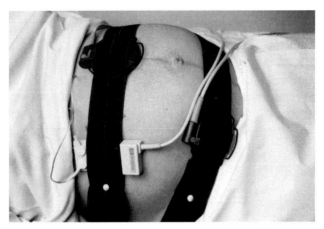

FIGURE 4.22. Maternal electrocardiogram, external tocodynamometer, and ultrasound fetal heart rate transducer on patient.

6. Do not rotate the spiral more than 360 degrees, as tissue injury may result.
7. Do not use in a patient who has active herpes, hepatitis, or human immunodeficiency virus infection.

When removing the electrode, twist the wires counterclockwise simultaneously. This can be done just before or after delivery of the neonate. At cesarean section, the electrode should be removed through the vagina before delivery if possible.

Following delivery, the area of electrode placement in the baby's scalp should be cleaned in the nursery.

The External Tocodynamometer

If the membranes are not yet ruptured, the external tocodynamometer allows the patient's uterine activity to be monitored in a nonquantitative way. This is quite satisfactory for patients who are progressing well. Occasionally, FHR decelerations may be observed in a patient when contractions are not recorded with an external tocotransducer. Intrauterine pressure monitoring may clarify the timing of the decelerations with respect to uterine activity.

External tocotransducers come in many different sizes and shapes and are attached by means of an elastic belt around the patient's abdomen. When the uterus contracts, the change in shape and rigidity slightly depresses a plunger, causing a change in the voltage of a small electrical current. These voltage changes are proportional to the uterine activity and are represented qualitatively by the fetal monitor as contractions. Because this method does not reflect the true intrauterine pressure, avoid detecting only the peaks by adjusting the pen position to set the uterine activity channel at about 25 relative units between contractions. Positioning of the external tocotransducer is important because if not placed over the proper part of the uterus, uterine activity may not be detected at all. Palpate to find where contractions are the most easily felt and place the transducer with careful attention to adjustment of the elastic belt to an appropriate tension (Fig. 4.22). In the presence of maternal obesity or a small uterus, the external tocotransducer is very poor at picking up uterine activity (Fig. 4.23). Palpate and pay attention to both the patient's complaints of contractions and any evidence of FHR decelerations sugges-

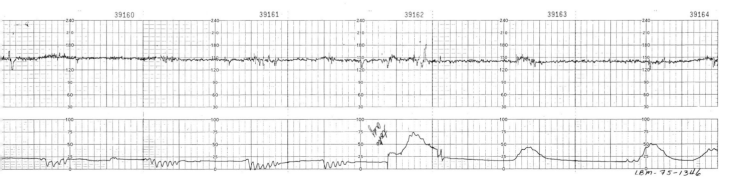

FIGURE 4.23. This tracing shows that contractions were evident only as irregular areas on the pressure tracing until the tocodynamometer was adjusted and repositioned. Subsequent contraction recording is satisfactory.

tive of undetected uterine activity. While the external tocotransducer estimates the frequency and duration of contractions fairly well, the baseline tone and actual contraction amplitude cannot be measured with the external tocotransducer. Monitoring with a tocotransducer provides real-time pressure measurements of uterine activity compared to a baseline. Newer monitors have simplified the technology of establishing baseline, and this can be accomplished either manually or automatically. One should follow the specific instructions with the type of monitor used in order to obtain as accurate information as possible with external tocotransducers.

The Doppler Transducer

The Doppler transducer is usually secured to the patient with an adjustable elastic strap that encircles the maternal abdomen. Selection of the optimum location for the transducer should proceed in the following manner:

1. Place the retaining strap under the patient in the supine position.
2. Place an adequate amount of ultrasonic coupling gel over the transducer face and apply to the maternal abdomen.
3. Begin searching for the strongest signal by listening with the monitor audio turned on. In cephalic presentation, this is usually found to be below the umbilicus; with a breech it may be higher on the maternal abdomen. It is often best to locate the fetal back with Leopold's maneuvers and place the transducer over this area. Use of real-time ultrasound can also assist in confirming fetal position and heart location.
4. When the optimal area is located, secure the transducer to the retaining strap and adjust for final placement at the location where the signal is clearest and the monitor is able to record well.

Because the Doppler transducer both transmits ultrasonic beams and receives the reflected signals, the angle of the transducer is important. By the laws of physics, the beam is reflected from a moving interface with the angle of incidence equaling the angle of reflection. Therefore, the beam will only return to the transducer when it is arranged perpendicular to the moving interface. Because of this, the transducer should be tilted (Fig. 4.24) to get the optimal signal, then moved to a point where the tangential placement allows reception of the reflected beam without transducer tilt. Once the transducer placement is optimal, it is necessary to constantly recheck the signal. If the fetus moves or the mother changes position, the signal may be lost and the transducer may have to be repositioned. With newer monitors using wide-beam ultrasound and autocor-

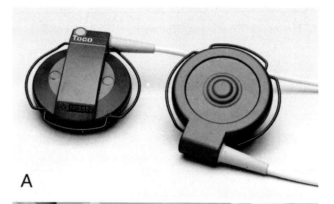

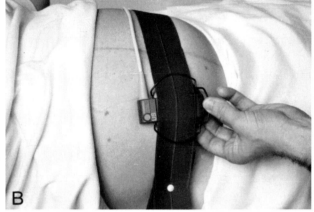

FIGURE 4.24. Newer monitors have dramatically improved the quality of the external mode. **A:** Both sides of the external toco-dynamometer transducer. **B:** Demonstration of the placement of the ultrasound fetal heart rate (FHR) transducer over the area of the maternal abdomen that gives the best FHR signal.

relation, obtaining a continuous, reliable fetal cardiac tracing is less problematic.

NETWORKING OF FETAL HEART RATE MONITORING

Until recently, the majority of both antepartum and intrapartum FHR monitoring was performed in the confines of the hospital. With the high cost of monitors and expertise required for the accurate generation and interpretation of data, antepartum FHR monitoring has typically been centralized to the hospital's labor and delivery unit or fetal diagnostic center. Smaller, less expensive, and very reliable monitors are now being marketed for physician use in the office. The small size and light weight of the units make it possible to provide antepartum FHR monitoring services to patients in their homes. This is of benefit to patients who need frequent monitoring yet should remain at bedrest (e.g., preterm premature rupture of membranes, multiple gestations). Data can now be collected through networking of FHR monitoring via transmission over telephone lines to the receiver of a medical center. While the patient remains on the monitor, data can be interpreted and proper instructions given regarding further testing or immediate patient evaluation.

ADVANCES IN FETAL MONITORING EQUIPMENT

In addition to the previously described autocorrelation improvements in Doppler signal processing, the newer fetal monitors provide features that represent further improvement over the first-generation monitors. Depending upon the particular model, these features may include the processing of returning signal from specific depths (ranged-

directional Doppler), fetal arrhythmia detection, maternal ECG monitoring, blood pressure, pulse and pulse oximetry, and monitoring for twins. Certain equipment allows for patient-related information (vital signs, cervical dilatation, medications). Remote internal or external FHR monitoring via radiowave telemetry allows for maternal ambulation without loss of continuous monitoring data. Central monitoring of multiple FHR tracings has also evolved. This feature allows for the immediate assessment of several laboring patients in a centralized area, ideally without the loss of close intrapartum patient contact by both nurse and physician (Fig. 4.25). Further monitoring advances include the widespread use of modern computer data storage and retrieval technology for FHR monitor strips. The ability to reliably record, store, retrieve, and reproduce the hard-copy tracing represents a tremendously important advance in this field.

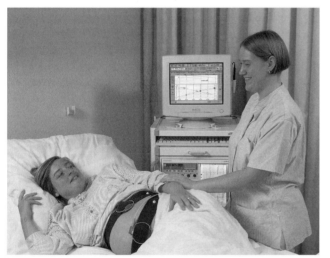

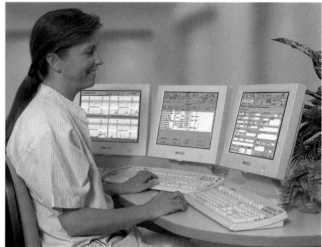

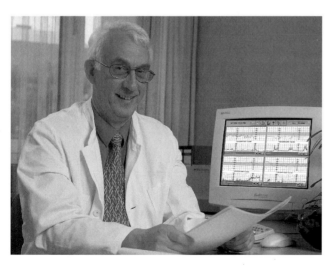

FIGURE 4.25. Example of centralized monitoring in a labor and delivery suite. This allows the physician or nurse to observe simultaneously the fetal heart rate (FHR) tracing of several patients. In addition, a terminal can be placed in the physician's office to allow for instant access to the FHR data. (Koninklijke Philips Electronics, the Netherlands).

FUTURE APPROACHES TO FETAL MONITORING

Fetal Systolic Time Interval Monitoring

The electromechanical interval of the cardiac cycle is that time which elapses between initiation of the electrical impulse and the beginning of mechanical activity. This period is also known as the isometric phase of the cardiac cycle because there is no motion during this interval. This pre-ejection period, from the onset of ventricular depolarization (indicated by the Q wave on the electrocardiogram) to the opening of the aortic valve, is the most extensively studied fetal systolic time (ST) interval. A second ST interval, which has been studied primarily in animals, is the ventricular ejection time. This is the time required for the ventricle to eject blood into the great vessels and is measured from the opening to the closing of the aortic valve. The ST interval is influenced by a number of factors, including fetal condition. Studies suggest that the fetus with either a prolonged or shortened antepartum pre-ejection period has a significantly greater chance of poor outcome (13–15). Murata et al. (16,17) have shown very good correlation between the pre-ejection period and the pH in animal fetuses. Thus far, however, there is no reported experience in which ST intervals have been used in the management of the human fetus.

Analysis of the Fetal Systolic Time Waveform

It is well established that analysis of the ST waveform of the electrocardiogram provides accurate and valuable information regarding myocardial response to workload usually induced with exercise. Experimental data derived from hypoxic fetal lambs reveal changes in both the ST segment and amplitude of the T-wave. This has been quantified by the T-wave to QRS amplitude ratio (T/QRS) and is associated with metabolic changes such as catecholamine release, myocardial glycogenolysis, and metabolic acidosis (18). ST-segment depression was the most common change reported in growth-restricted fetal guinea pigs exposed to hypoxia, perhaps resulting from anaerobic metabolism and endocardial cell hypoxia (19). Such observations have resulted in the development of an electronic FHR monitor (i.e., cardiotocograph) plus ST-waveform analyzer (STAN) (20,21). Westgate et al. (22) have reported on a randomized controlled trial comparing intrapartum monitoring with electronic fetal monitors in combination with ST-waveform analysis. These authors reported a 46% reduction in operative interventions for fetal indications in those laboring patients receiving the added ST-waveform analysis. Further modification of the STAN technology uses digital signal processing and automatic assessment of ST-segment changes. Amer-Wahlin et al. (23) reported a Swedish ran-

domized controlled trial similar in design to that of Westgate et al., but using the modified STAN technology. They report a significant reduction in umbilical artery metabolic acidosis and of operative delivery for fetal indications in term laboring patients when using this modified STAN technology compared with those patients receiving electronic fetal monitoring alone. Whether the wider application of STAN technology is warranted or not can only be determined with further clinical study, but this may represent a valuable addition to the science of FHR monitoring.

REFERENCES

1. Goodlin RC, Cheatham JP: Electronic fetal monitor paced by maternal implanted pacemaker. *Am J Obstet Gynecol* 153:570, 1985.
2. Westgren M, Ingemarsson I: Maternal pacemaker activity mimicking fetal heart during labor. *Z Geburtshilfe Perinatal* 184:443, 1980.
3. Schneiderman CI, Waxman B, Goodman CJ Jr: Maternal-fetal electrocardiogram conduction with intrapartum death. *Am J Obstet Gynecol* 113:1130, 1972.
4. Lackritz R, Schiff I, Gibson M, et al.: Decelerations on fetal electrocardiography with fetal demise. *Obstet Gynecol* 51:367, 1978.
5. Fukushima T, Flores CA, Hon EH, et al.: Limitations of autocorrelation in fetal heart rate monitoring. *Am J Obstet Gynecol* 153:685, 1985.
6. Amato J: Fetal heart rate monitoring. *Am J Obstet Gynecol* 147:967, 1983.
7. Cremer M: *Munch Med Wochenschr* 53:811, 1906.
8. Larks SD, Dasgupta K: Fetal electrocardiography with special reference to early pregnancy. *Am Heart J* 56:701, 1958.
9. Hon EH, Hess OW: The clinical value of fetal electrocardiography. *Am J Obstet Gynecol* 79:1012, 1960.
10. Nageotte MP, Freeman RK, Freeman AG, et al.: Short-term variability assessment from abdominal electrocardiogram during the antenatal period. *Am J Obstet Gynecol* 145:566, 1983.
11. Oldenburg JT, Macklin M: Changes in the conduction of the fetal electrocardiogram to the maternal abdominal surface during gestation. *Am J Obstet Gynecol* 129:425, 1977.
12. Devoe LD, Gardner P, Dear C, et al.: Monitoring intrauterine pressure during active labor: A prospective comparison of two methods. *J Reprod Med* 34: 811–814, 1989.
13. Murata Y, Martin C: Systolic time intervals of the fetal cardiac cycle. *Obstet Gynecol* 44:224, 1974.
14. Wolfson R, Zador I, Pillay S, et al.: Antenatal investigation of human fetal systolic time intervals. *Am J Obstet Gynecol* 129:203, 1977.
15. Murata Y, Martin C, Ikenoue T, et al.: Antepartum evaluation of the pre-ejection period of the fetal cardiac cycle. *Am J Obstet Gynecol* 132:278, 1978.
16. Murata Y, Martin C, Ikenoue T, et al.: Cardiac systolic intervals in fetal monkeys: pre-ejection period. *Am J Obstet Gynecol* 132:285, 1978.
17. Murata Y, Miyake K, Quilligan E: Pre-ejection of cardiac cycles in fetal lamb. *Am J Obstet Gynecol* 133:509, 1979.
18. Greene KR, Dawes GS, Lilja H, et al.: Changes in the ST waveform of the lamb electrocardiogram with hypoxia. *Am J Obstet Gynecol* 144:950–957, 1982.
19. Widmark C, Jansson T, Lindecrantz K, et al.: ECG waveform, short term heart rate variability and plasma catecholamine con-

centrations in response to hypoxia in intrauterine growth retarded guinea pig fetuses. *J Dev Physiol* 15:161–168, 1991.

20. Lilja H, Karlsson K, Lindecrantz K, et al.: Microprocessor based waveform analysis of the fetal electrocardiogram during labor. *Int J Gynecol Obstet* 1989; 30: 109-116

21. Arulkumaran S, Lilja H, Lindecrantz K, et al.: Fetal ECG waveform analysis should improve fetal surveillance in labor. *J Perinat Med* 18:13–22, 1990.

22. Westgate J, Harris M, Curnow JSH, et al.: Plymouth randomized trial of cardiotocogram only versus ST waveform plus cardiotocogram for intrapartum monitoring: 2400 cases. *Am J Obstet Gynecol* 169:1151–1160, 1993.

23. Amer-Wahlin I, Hellsten C, Noren H, et al.: Cardiotocogram only versus cardiotocography plus ST analysis of fetal electrocardiogram for intrapartum fetal monitoring: a Swedish randomized controlled trial. *Lancet* 358:534–538, 2001.

UTERINE CONTRACTION MONITORING

In discussions on the benefits of fetal monitoring, uterine contraction monitoring is most often ignored. The initial development of fetal heart rate (FHR) monitoring was concerned with detecting fetal distress. Contraction patterns were included so that the various decelerative patterns could be timed in relation to contractions. With the use of monitors in labor, however, it became apparent that one principle benefit of such routine monitoring was the data it provided relative to uterine activity.

Uterine activity may be assumed to be adequate if progress in labor, as defined by progressive cervical dilatation and descent, is occurring. Failure to progress in labor may be due to inadequate uterine contractions. On the other hand, excessive uterine activity, as in abruptio placenta, may cause inadequate placental perfusion, and thus give rise to fetal hypoxia. When it is necessary to induce or augment labor, the clinician must be especially aware of uterine activity, because it could lead to fetal distress or even uterine rupture. Any of these conditions require close monitoring of uterine contractions.

Manual palpation has been the traditional method of monitoring contractions. This method can be used to measure contraction frequency and duration, but it can measure intensity only relatively. It is time-consuming, requires constant attendance, and provides no permanent record. The process becomes tedious and, at best, what occurs in most cases is intermittent manual palpation for short intervals. The fetal monitor provides us with a tool that can significantly improve our ability to accurately monitor uterine contractions.

PHYSIOLOGY OF UTERINE CONTRACTIONS

Uterine contractions have as a primary function the expulsion of the intrauterine contents. Uterine activity before the onset of active labor may prepare the uterus and cervix for labor. The uterus is a smooth muscle organ that, during pregnancy, is progressively stretched. Contractions may be a physiologic response to this stretch, perhaps dampened by mechanisms that normally inhibit the premature onset of labor. Two types of preparatory contractions have been described by Caldeyro-Barcia and Poseiro (1). The first are small, weak contractions of short duration, localized to isolated small areas of the uterus, and occurring about once a minute. These high-frequency, low-intensity contractions begin in early pregnancy and seem to disappear near term. They may be related to or may be the same as the localized periodic thickening of the uterine wall frequently seen on routine ultrasound during early gestation (2,3). The second are the better-known Braxton-Hicks contractions. These have a higher magnitude of strength (10 to 20 mm Hg), are more generalized, and have a frequency that increases from one contraction per hour at 30 weeks to as often as every 5 to 10 minutes at term. This background frequency is greater with multiple gestations and the vast majority of the time are not perceived by the patient (4). The transition into the regular rhythmical contractions of labor may be insidious or abrupt, and the exact control remains unknown.

Contractions must be defined by their characteristics of frequency, duration, strength (amplitude), uniformity, and shape. During normal labor, the strength of contractions varies from an average of 30 mm Hg in early labor to 50 mm Hg in later first stage and 50 to 80 mm Hg during the second stages. The uterus is not a flaccid sac but has baseline tone. At and near term, this baseline tone is generally 8 to 12 mm Hg, with values in excess of 20 mm Hg defined as hypertonus (or, redundantly, baseline hypertonus). The smaller nonpregnant uterus will generate very large uterine pressures because, according to the law of Laplace, at a given amount of uterine wall tension, the amount of intracavitary pressure is inversely proportional to the radius of the cavity. This is true for the uterus only to a point, however. With excessively large volumes, as in polyhydramnios, tonus may begin to rise because of excessive stretching of the muscle fibers (5).

Once actual labor begins, contractions become more frequent, more coordinated, and stronger. The propagation of uterine contractions is the result of pacemaker-like activity originating usually from the area of the uterotubal junction. For the contraction to fulfill its purpose most efficiently (i.e., expulsion of the fetus via cervical dilation and fetal descent), the contraction must start in the fundus and progressively propagate toward the cervix. Reynolds et al. (6) described this as "fundal dominance," which, simply stated, means that, because of the lesser curvature at the fundus and the greater muscle mass, the strength of contractions is greatest at the fundus and least at the cervix. Caldeyro-Barcia and Poseiro (1) further refined this description. They described a triple descending gradient of wave propagation, intensity, and duration, such that the origin of the contraction is in the fundus and the direction of the contractile wave is toward the cervix. Not only is the contraction more intense in the fundus, but the duration of the contraction is progressively shorter from the fundus to midcorpus to cervix.

MONITORING OF UTERINE ACTIVITY

External Monitoring

Contractions are most conveniently monitored externally with a tocodynamometer. Mechanical devices for monitoring contractions externally were introduced as early as 1861. Murphy (7) described a ring tocodynamometer and, subsequently, Reynolds et al. (8) used three such instruments on various portions of the uterus to describe normal contraction physiology. The tocodynamometer or "toco" is essentially a weight with a centrally placed pressure sensitive button secured to the abdominal wall with a strap (Fig. 5.1). The toco is positioned near the fundus and adjusted to a position that results in the best contraction recording. A sensitivity calibration device, present either on the toco or, more commonly, on the monitor itself, is adjusted to place the resting pressure at 15 to 20 mm Hg to obtain the best tracing. It must always be remembered that the contraction strength is only relatively accurate and varies greatly with maternal position, relative obesity, and the tightness of the belt. These factors also affect the sensitivity of the recording. The duration of the contraction will appear to vary:

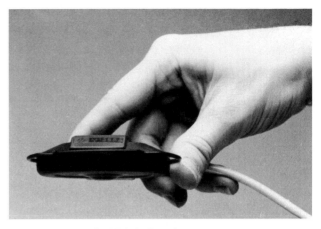

FIGURE 5.1. Tocodynamometer.

The more sensitive the toco, the longer the apparent duration (Fig. 5.2). With external contraction monitoring, frequency is most accurately, duration less accurately, and intensity least accurately recorded.

The external technique has the advantage of being non-invasive, thus being applicable for patients with intact membranes, that is, the antepartum patient, the patient in premature labor, or the patient during the early intrapartum period. There are, however, disadvantages. Patient mobility is limited. Often, the best tracings are obtained with the patient supine. This leads nurses and physicians to encourage laboring in this less desirable position. More recently, fetal monitors have been introduced that allow for ambulation while recording contractions with a tocodynamometer. Generally, external monitors are more uncomfortable for the patient. Some obese patients give poor to nonexistent tracings. The limitations with regard to intensity and duration have been discussed. At times, when FHR patterns

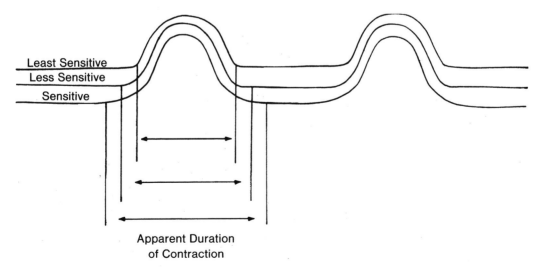

FIGURE 5.2. This drawing illustrates the correlation between the sensitivity of the contraction-monitoring device and the apparent duration of the contraction. The less sensitive the monitoring technique, the shorter the apparent duration of the contraction.

consistent with fetal distress occur and position is changed, loss of a previously good contraction tracing results, thus making decelerations difficult to time or record at all.

Internal Monitoring

According to the law of Pascal, pressure within a fluid-filled closed spheroid is equal at all points. This describes the uterus quite well; therefore, the pregnant uterus is ideal for contraction pressure monitoring. As early as 1872, Schatz (9) used a hydrostatic bag in the lower uterine segment for pressure recording after the membranes had ruptured. In 1927, Bourne and Burn (10) used the hydrostatic bag extraovularly (between the membranes and the lower uterine segment). Alvarez and Caldeyro-Barcia (11) described a transabdominal technique for inserting open fluid-filled catheters in the amniotic cavity to record contractions. Other techniques, including electrohysterography and intramyometrial pressure recording, have been reported. In 1952, Williams and Stallworthy (9) suggested the use of a Drew-Smythe metal cannula (originally designed for high amniotomy) as a guide to introduce a polyethylene tubing transcervically into the amniotic cavity. This was the forerunner for the technique now commonly used for internal contraction monitoring. Currently, sterile disposable kits are available with flexible plastic catheters and guides for internal contraction monitoring. A newer modification, with the pressure-sensing device located in the catheter tip, has possible advantages over the original (Figs. 5.3 and 5.4). In addition, newer double-lumen catheters are being studied to allow for simultaneous amnioinfusion and contraction monitoring (Fig. 5.5). The details of insertion, instrumentation, and calibration are described in Chapter 4. This

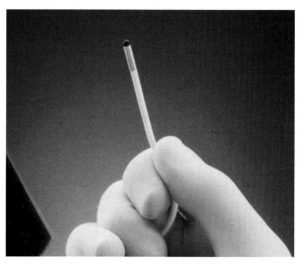

FIGURE 5.4. Close-up of catheter tip showing pressure sensor. (Viggo-Spectramed, Oxnard, CA.)

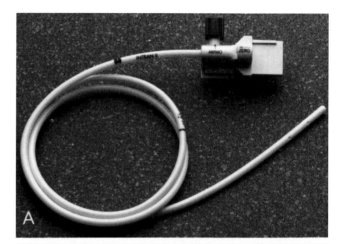

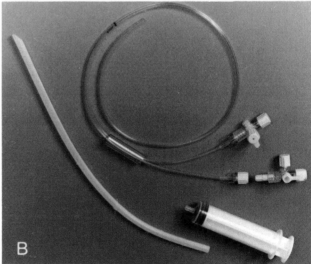

FIGURE 5.5. Two examples of double lumen catheters allowing simultaneous amnioinfusion and uterine contraction monitoring. **A:** Catheter with pressure sensor tip. (Utah Medical Products, Inc.) **B:** Double lumen with fluid column for measuring uterine contractions. (Gish Biomedical, Inc., Santa Ana, CA.)

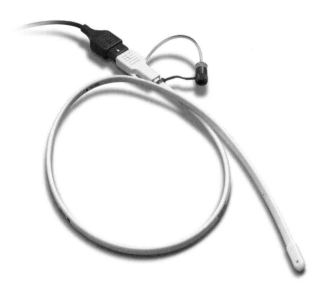

FIGURE 5.3. Internal pressure catheter with pressure-sensing device in tip. There is no need to fill catheter with fluid when using this technology. (Tyco Healthcare-Kendall LTP, Chicopee, MA.)

method can be used to define and record accurately the frequency, duration, strength, and tonus of the uterus and its contraction. It is less confining and more comfortable for the patient and is unaffected by position, except as contraction pressures actually change with position change.

Regarding the value of internal pressure monitoring, the literature is somewhat controversial. The clinician must wait for membrane rupture or perform amniotomy to use commonly available internal techniques. There is some evidence that internal monitoring is associated with an increased risk of infection, although these data are often confounded by the fact that many patients with internal pressure monitoring have protracted labors, prolonged rupture of membranes and frequent pelvic examinations. Uterine perforation has been described but is usually caused by insertion of the less flexible catheter guide. To avoid this complication, the guide should never be inserted much beyond the edge of the cervix. For the patient, there can be some discomfort associated with introduction of the catheter. The alternative to electronic contraction monitoring is manual palpation or reliance on the patient's sensation. Caldeyro-Barcia and Poseiro (1) have said that intrapartum contractions are palpable to the examiner at a minimum pressure of 10 mm Hg, and that the patient senses the pain of contractions at a minimum of 15 mm Hg. As with external monitoring, palpation and patient sensation will be reliable with regard to frequency but will be less so for duration and intensity (Fig. 5.6).

QUANTITATION OF UTERINE ACTIVITY

For many reasons, it may be important to quantitate the amount of uterine activity per unit of time. The most practical reason would be to determine, in evaluating poor progress in labor, whether uterine contractions are sufficient. Because failure to progress with a clinically adequate pelvis and inadequate contractions is an indication for

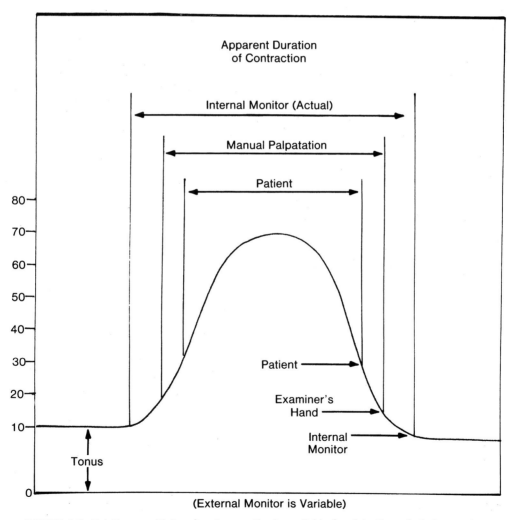

FIGURE 5.6. Relative sensitivity of various methods available for detection of uterine contractions.

oxytocin, adequate uterine activity must be defined. In 1957, Caldeyro-Barcia et al. (5) defined the Montevideo unit as the product of the average contraction peak in millimeters mercury multiplied by the number of contractions in 10 minutes. Schifrin (12) defined adequate uterine activity in labor to be greater than 200 Montevideo units. This has been the quantitation measure most extensively used by investigators, although it does have the limitation of not including contraction duration in its calculation. To overcome this problem, El-Sahwi et al. (13) defined the Alexandria unit as the average contraction peak amplitude (in millimeters mercury), multiplied by the average duration (in minutes), multiplied by the average number of contractions in 10 minutes. Both methods are very time-consuming. Miller et al. (14) described a computerized method of quantitating uterine activity by integrating the entire area under the curve (Fig. 5.7). Besides inadequate uterine activity, abnormal rhythmicity or excessive uterine activity may cause problems. These can occur spontaneously or in pregnancies complicated by premature labor, polyhydramnios, or placental abruption. During antepartum testing, uterine hyperstimulation can result from excessive breast stimulation or oxytocin administration. The terminology, which is not universally agreed upon, is described in Figure 5.8.

There are two characteristics of these nonsynchronous abnormal contraction patterns. The first is their effect on the progress in labor, and this will depend on cause. Some abnormal patterns may be noted with protracted active phases of labor or secondary arrest of labor (15). In these

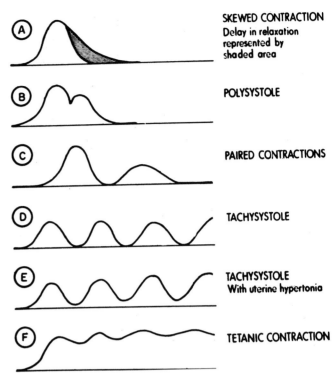

FIGURE 5.8. Abnormal contraction patterns. (From Stookey RA, Sokol RJ, Rosen MJ: Abnormal contraction patterns in patients monitored during labor. *Obstet Gynecol* 42:359, 1973.)

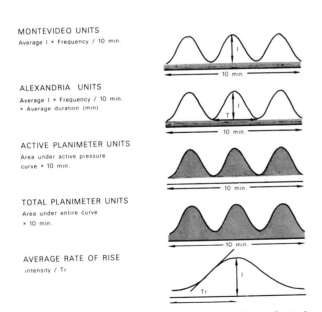

FIGURE 5.7. Available methods for quantitation of uterine activity. (From Miller FC, Yeh SY, Schifrin BS, et al.: Quantitation of uterine activity in 100 primiparous patients. *Am J Obstet Gynecol* 124:398, 1976.)

cases, the patterns may be the result, rather than the cause, of abnormal labor. Other causes may include injudicious oxytocin administration, polyhydramnios, and placental abruption, in which case the effect of these contraction patterns on labor is to shorten it. The other consideration is the effect that these contraction patterns may have on intervillous blood flow, fetal oxygenation, and FHR. Intramyometrial pressure is usually approximately two to three times that of intraamniotic pressure. Mean arterial blood pressure is about 85 to 90 mm Hg in labor. Therefore, the duration that intraamniotic pressure exceeds 30 to 40 mm Hg (corresponding to myometrial pressures in excess of mean arterial pressure) determines how long the maternal spiral arteries are compressed and, therefore, how long. Another important aspect is how much relaxation time is available for recovery. The effects that these contraction patterns may have on the fetus are most immediately reflected in heart rate and may be manifested by increased variability, delayed (late) decelerations, or prolonged decelerations (Fig. 5.9). Shenker (16) suggested that the most frequent cause of late decelerations is excessive uterine activity. If these excessive contractions and their resultant fetal hypoxia are prolonged, fetal acidemia may result, manifesting FHR changes in the form of decreased variability and persistent late decelerations.

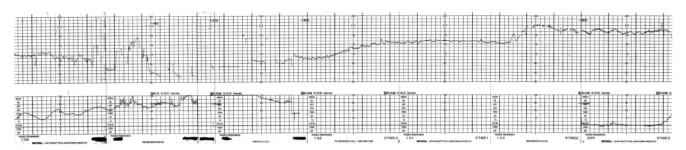

FIGURE 5.9. Note the changes of the fetal heart rate following a tetanic uterine contraction. In this example, there a temporary rise in the baseline heart rate with subsequent return to a normal baseline and evidence of late decelerations.

OTHER FACTORS AFFECTING UTERINE CONTRACTION

To understand and correct abnormal contraction patterns and heart rate reactions to them, it is important to be aware of the intrinsic and extrinsic factors that affect uterine contractility. These factors may manifest themselves by decreasing or increasing contraction strength, frequency, or both. Intrinsic factors include pathologic state and maternal position. The most common diseases which alter uterine contractions include polyhydramnios, preeclampsia, abruption, and, perhaps, amnionitis. Abruption usually causes the greatest degree of hyperactivity (Fig. 5.10). Polysystole, tachysystole, hypertonus, or any form of hyperactivity may be seen. With abruptio placenta, it may be the uterine hyperactivity, loss of placental surface area, or both, that results in the fetal distress that is often seen. Even in patients without complaints of severe pain or evidence of vaginal bleeding, the finding of frequent spontaneous contractions, often without return to baseline, in the presence of abnormal FHR patterns makes the diagnosis of abruption a strong consideration. With pregnancies complicated by preeclampsia or eclampsia, Alvarez et al. (17) have pointed out that uterine tonus is unaffected but that frequency and intensity of contractions are often increased. Polyhydramnios has a variable effect on tonus until the uterus is severely stretched and baseline tone is often low to low normal. However, if the hydramnios worsens, a hypertonus may develop. Uterine contractions may be quite prolonged with hydramnios (Fig. 5.11).

Position has a relatively consistent effect on uterine activity. It is clear that uteroplacental perfusion is poorer in the supine position than in either lateral position. Caldeyro-Barcia et al. (18) have shown that, generally, when the patient is turned from her back to her side, contractions become stronger and less frequent (Fig. 5.12). Finally, maternal pushing efforts during labor are commonly seen on contraction tracings and can add 20 mm Hg or more to the recorded intensity of contractions. They are usually seen as rapid, brief elevations of intra-

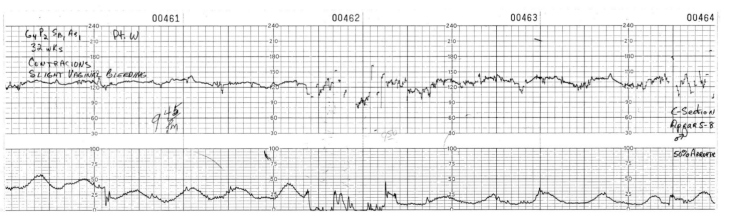

FIGURE 5.10. This example of uterine hyperactivity in the form of tachysystole was seen in a patient in premature labor with vaginal bleeding. In this case, it is very difficult to interpret the occurrence of late decelerations. Both fetal heart rate and contractions are being monitored externally. The cause of uterine hyperactivity and late decelerations was a 50% abruptio placenta.

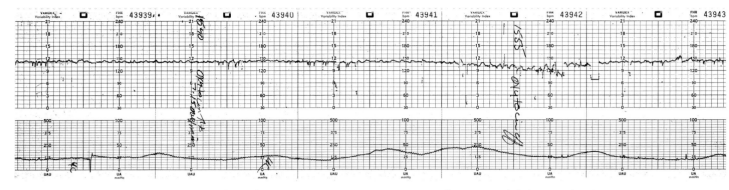

FIGURE 5.11. Prolonged uterine contraction seen in an externally monitored diabetic with polyhydramnios. Labor is being augmented with oxytocin. Such prolonged contractions in response to oxytocin are commonly seen with polyhydramnios.

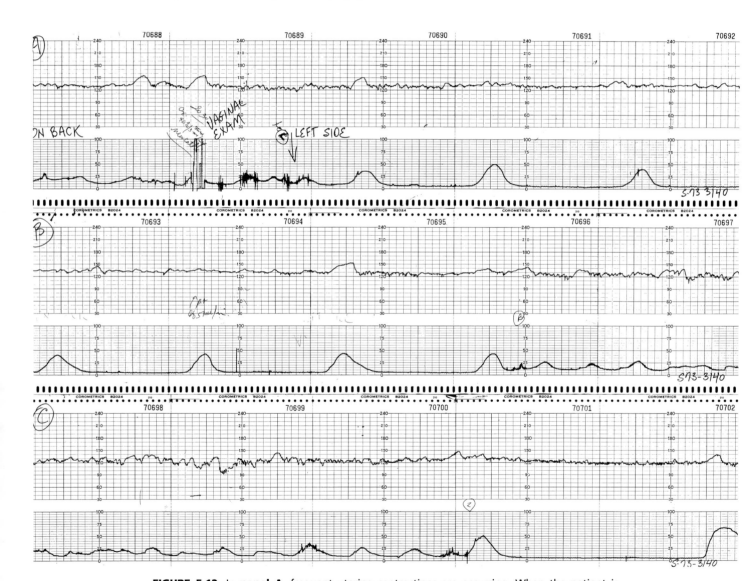

FIGURE 5.12. In **panel A**, frequent uterine contractions are occurring. When the patient is turned to her left side, the contractions become less frequent and increase in strength. In **panel B**, the patient has turned and is lying on her back. The contractions have become more frequent and smaller. Finally, again with the patient on her left side in **panel C**, the contractions are spaced out as before in **panel A**.

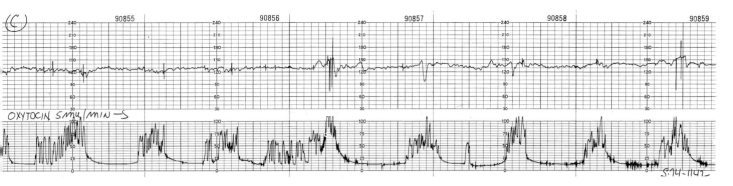

FIGURE 5.13. Small spikes (intermittent short elevations of pressure) seen on top of uterine contractions represent maternal pushing.

uterine pressure superimposed on the uterine contraction (Fig. 5.13).

There has always been conjecture and debate as to whether oxytocin reproduces a physiologic contraction pattern. Much of this debate stems from the fact that many clinicians use dose rates far in excess of physiologic values. Caldeyro-Barcia et al. (19), Caldeyro-Barcia and Poseiro (20), and Poseiro and Noriega-Guerra (21) have shown that oxytocin both accelerates and coordinates uterine contractions, and that at physiologic doses of 1 to 8 mU/minute, this occurs without elevation of tonus. These studies have shown no difference between contractions, with or without oxytocin, with data from intraamniotic pressure, intramyometrial pressure, and electrohysterography. Alvarez and Cibils (22) have shown that both types of contractions have equivalent efficiency in producing cervical dilatation. When doses of oxytocin exceed physiologic requirements, how-

ever, all forms of hyperactivity as well as hypertonus can be seen. Seitchik and Castillo (23) report that the majority of uterine hypercontractility episodes can be avoided by a slow increase (intervals not less than 30 minutes) in oxytocin of 1.0 mU/minute from an initial rate of 1.0 mU/minute. Steady progress in labor, as defined by progressive cervical dilatation, occurs in 95% of patients with an infusion rate less than or equal to 6 mU/minute. Other protocols using a more aggressive use of oxytocin have been proposed for labor augmentation (24–26). Termed "active management of labor," these approaches use oxytocin in a more rapidly increasing dosage and achieve much higher total amounts of drug being administered than with the protocol suggested by Seitchik and Castillo. The success in labor augmentation with oxytocin may be more related to the timing of initiation and achieving of an adequate labor pattern than the actual amount used. Many other drugs affect uterine activity. The more common ones are listed in Table 5.1.

TABLE 5.1. DRUGS AFFECTING UTERINE CONTRACTIONS

Stimulating drugs
  Acetylcholine
  Ergonovine
  Estrogen
  Norepinephrine
  Oxytocin
  Propranolol
  Prostaglandins
  Quinine
  Sparteine sulfate
  Vasopressin
Inhibiting drugs
  β-Sympathomimetics
    Ritodrine, calcium-channel blockers, Orciprenaline,
      Isoxsuprine, Salbutamol, Fenoterol, Epinephrine, etc.
  Diazoxide
  Ethanol
  Halothane
  Magnesium sulfate
  Progesterone
  Prostaglandin inhibitors

SUMMARY

The study of fetal monitoring is incomplete without detailed knowledge of uterine activity and its effects on fetal oxygenation and heart rate. Most significant periodic changes in the FHR occur at or after the time of the uterine contraction. The intent of this chapter has been to describe the details of contraction monitoring and the physiologic mechanisms of labor so that the reader might better be able to integrate this knowledge and understand the physiologic and pathophysiologic basis of fetal monitoring.

REFERENCES

1. Caldeyro-Barcia R, Poseiro JJ: Physiology of the uterine contraction. *Clin Obstet Gynecol* 3:386, 1960.
2. Sample WF: The unsoftened portion of the uterus: a pitfall in grayscale ultrasound studies during mid-trimester pregnancy. *Radiology* 126:227, 1978.

3. Buttery B, Davison G: The dynamic uterus revealed by time lapse echography. *J Clin Ultrasound* 6:19, 1978.

4. Newman RB, Gill PJ, Katz M: Uterine activity during pregnancy in ambulatory patients: comparison of singleton and twin gestations. *Am J Obstet Gynecol* 154:530, 1986.

5. Caldeyro-Barcia R, Pose SV, Alvarez H: Uterine contractility in polyhydramnios and the effects of the withdrawal of the excess of amniotic fluid. *Am J Obstet Gynecol* 73:1238, 1957.

6. Reynolds SRM, Hellman LM, Bruns P: Patterns of uterine contractility in women during pregnancy. *Obstet Gynecol Surv* 3:629, 1948.

7. Murphy D: *Uterine contractility.* Lippincott, New York, 1947.

8. Reynolds SRM, Heard OO, Bruns P: Recording uterine contraction patterns in pregnant women; applications of strain gauge in multi-channel tocodynamometer. *Science* 106:427, 1947.

9. Williams EA, Stallworthy JA: A simple method of internal tocography. *Lancet* 330, 1952.

10. Bourne AW, Burn JH: Dosage and action of pituitary extract in labour with note on action of adrenalin. *J Obstet Gynecol Br Emp* 34:249, 1927.

11. Alvarez H, Caldeyro-Barcia R: Contractility of the human uterus recorded by new methods. *Surg Gynecol Obstet* 91:1, 1950.

12. Schifrin BS: The case against pelvimetry. *Contemp Obstet Gynecol* 4:77, 1974.

13. El-Sahwi S, Gaafar A, Toppozada HK: A new unit for evaluation of uterine activity. *Am J Obstet Gynecol* 98:900, 1967.

14. Miller FC, Yeh SY, Schifrin BS, et al.: Quantitation of uterine activity in 100 primiparous patients. *Am J Obstet Gynecol* 124:398, 1976.

15. Stookey RA, Sokol RJ, Rosen MJ: Abnormal contraction patterns in patients monitored during labor. *Obstet Gynecol* 42:359, 1973.

16. Shenker L: Clinical experience with fetal heart rate monitoring of 1000 patients in labor. *Am J Obstet Gynecol* 115:1111, 1973.

17. Alvarez H, Pose SV, Caldeyro-Barcia R: La contractilidad uterina en la toxemia gravidica. *Proc First Peruv Cong Obstet Gynecol* 2:281, 1959.

18. Caldeyro-Barcia R, Noriega-Guerra L, Cibils LA, et al.: Effects of position change on the intensity and frequency of uterine contractions during labor. *Am J Obstet Gynecol* 80:284, 1960.

19. Caldeyro-Barcia R, Sica-Blanco Y, Poseiro JJ, et al.: A quantitative study of the action of synthetic oxytocin on the pregnant human uterus. *J Pharmacol Exp Ther* 121:18, 1957.

20. Caldeyro-Barcia R, Poseiro JJ: Oxytocin and contractility of the human pregnant uterus. *Ann NY Acad Sci* 75:813, 1959.

21. Poseiro JJ, Noriega-Guerra L: Dose response relationships in uterine effect of oxytocin infusion. In: *Oxytocin.* Pergamon Press, London, 1960.

22. Alvarez H, Cibils LA: Cervical dilation and uterine work in labor induced with oxytocin. In: *Oxytocin.* Pergamon Press, London, 1960.

23. Seitchik J, Castillo M: Oxytocin augmentation of dysfunctional labor. I. Clinical data. *Am J Obstet Gynecol* 144:899, 1982.

24. O'Driscoll K, Stronge JM, Minogue M: Active management of labor. *BMJ* 3:135, 1983.

25. Thorp JA, Boylan PC, Parisi VM, et al.: Effects of high-dose oxytocin augmentation on umbilical cord blood gas values in primigravid women. *Am J Obstet Gynecol* 159:670, 1988.

26. Neuhoff D, Burke MS, Porreco RP: Cesarean birth for failed progress in labor. *Obstet Gynecol* 73:915, 1989.

BASIC PATTERN RECOGNITION

The evaluation of the fetus during labor by electronic fetal heart rate (FHR) monitoring is a complex process. Patterns that are known to be reassuring have a highly reliable correlation with normal oxygenation and a vigorous baby at birth; these must be distinguished from nonreassuring patterns so that action may be taken to reverse the problem, find alternatives to provide reassurance, or intervene operatively before damage or death can occur. Many factors must be weighed to determine if the pattern is reassuring or nonreassuring. The FHR is evaluated for baseline rate, variability, and presence of accelerations or decelerations, and the progression of each. Contraction frequency and strength must be considered. The patient's parity, her rate of progress in labor, the estimated time of delivery, and maternal and obstetric complications are all factored into this rather complex equation.

Quantifying various parameters of fetal well-being by means of mathematical and statistical computations of the FHR is difficult. This is because the interpretation of FHR tracings is both a study of pattern recognition and a process of evaluating multiple clinical and heart rate variables in determining the status of fetal oxygenation. Previous chapters have dealt with the basic understanding of the physiology and technology of electronic FHR monitoring. This chapter will be devoted to pattern recognition.

Efforts to arrive at universal nomenclature and criteria for various FHR patterns have not been uniformly successful. In 1997, a workshop convened by the NICHD published a document in an attempt to create more consistent and uniform terminology and guidelines for interpreting FHR patterns. For most patterns, they are consistent with the terminology used in this textbook, but where they differ, this will be pointed out and the reasons explained (1).

PATIENT IDENTIFICATION

Many modern monitoring systems have electronic storage of patient information and electronic fetal monitoring (EFM) tracings. These systems require patient data entry before starting the monitor on a new patient. However, hospitals continue to store paper records for back-up medical records, for teaching purposes, or because some information (e.g., continuous fetal pulse oximetry data) may not be stored on the digital record. Therefore, it is important to appropriately label the paper record as well. Monitors should be identified numerically and tracings labeled accordingly. Should a technical problem occur, it can be traced to the correct monitor. Also, different monitors may have different logic and other technical characteristics, and when a facility has various brands, the clinician can better interpret the tracing by taking the make and model into consideration.

BASELINE FETAL HEART RATE

The normal baseline FHR ranges from 120 to 160 beats per minute (BPM). The NICHD defined baseline FHR changes as those that last more than 10 minutes. Changes of shorter duration are called "periodic changes." While it is appropriate to attempt to create a defined duration of a periodic change, for which a more sustained rate becomes a baseline change, this is often inconsistent with what is the obvious physiologic explanation for a prolonged periodic change. For example, a profound hypotensive episode that results in a prolonged deceleration will ultimately return to the original baseline when the insult is reversed. Thus the deceleration may have lasted longer than 10 minutes and, according to the previous NICHD definition, would now be called a bradycardia, but it was truly not a baseline change. Similarly, a fetus that is unusually active may have an acceleration that lasts considerably longer than 10 minutes but returns to the original baseline when the fetus returns to a more quiet state.

Fetal Tachycardia

Fetal tachycardia is defined as a baseline heart rate in excess of 160 BPM. Factors associated with or causing tachycardia are listed in Table 6.1. Because tachycardias represent increased sympathetic and/or decreased parasympathetic autonomic tone, they are generally associated with a loss of variability (Fig. 6.1). Most fetal tachycardias do not reflect

TABLE 6.1. CAUSES OF FETAL TACHYCARDIA

Fetal hypoxia
Maternal fever
Parasympatholytic drugs
   Atropine
   Hydroxyzine hydrochloride (Atarax or Vistaril)
   Phenothiazines
Maternal hyperthyroidism
Fetal anemia
Fetal sepsis
Fetal heart failure
Chorioamnionitis
Fetal cardiac tachyarrhythmia
β-Sympathomimetic drugs

a hypoxic fetus, particularly when present in a term gestation. In a preterm fetus or when seen in a term pregnancy without an obvious explanation (e.g., maternal fever), close evaluation is critical.

Fetal Bradycardia

Bradycardia is a baseline FHR of less than 120 BPM (the NICHD used <110 BPM). Bradycardia, within the range of 80 to 120 BPM with good variability is generally reassuring (Fig. 6.2). Slowing of the baseline heart rate is most likely in response to an increased vagal tone (2). Fetal bradycardia that is first noted at the initiation of monitoring may be difficult to distinguish from a prolonged deceleration. Generally, prolonged decelerations are associated with loss of variability and their rate fluctuates up and down rather than remaining consistent, unless rates below 70 BPM are seen.

Actual baseline FHRs of less than 70 BPM are generally seen without variability and may represent congenital heart block (Fig. 6.3). Persistent bradycardia from complete atrioventricular dissociation should alert the clinician to the possible diagnosis of maternal connective tissue disease,

most often systemic lupus erythematosus, which results in fetal heart block and bradycardia consequent to transplacental passage of maternal antibodies that have an affinity for fetal cardiac conduction fibers (3). Structural cardiac defects and cytomegalovirus infections are also potential etiologies of congenital heart block. To reliably establish that fetal cardiac activity is present and that the persistent bradycardia is due to fetal heart block, confirmation with real-time ultrasound is necessary. Ultrasound allows for a further advantage in that cardiac structure can be carefully evaluated as well (see Chapter 7). However, ultrasound is really only an option in the antepartum period because it may not be possible to take the time required to make this evaluation in labor where an ominous prolonged deceleration may require urgent operative intervention. When the diagnosis of complete fetal heart block is made antenatally, the problem then becomes how to monitor the fetus in labor because the normal alterations in FHR in response to hypoxia and other central nervous system (CNS) input cannot be transmitted to the ventricles. Thus, in this situation, the FHR cannot be used as a way to monitor for fetal hypoxia and acidosis. Three options are reasonable in this situation. Intermittent scalp pH is theoretically an option, but the need for repeating the test every 30 minutes makes this option unrealistic except in very rapid labors. In the past, an elective cesarean section was often undertaken, simply because there had been no other way to monitor the fetus. More recently, fetal pulse oximetry has provided a logical option, and limited data suggest that this is a safe and effective way of monitoring patients whose fetal arrhythmia prevents adequate FHR monitoring (4).

Mild degrees of baseline bradycardia are often seen in the second stage of labor. When fetal bradycardia occurs in the second stage, it is reassuring if variability is maintained and the heart rate does not decrease below 80 to 90 BPM. Rare causes of fetal bradycardia are maternal hypothermia, prolonged hypoglycemia, beta-blocker therapy, and fetal panhypopituitarism with brain-stem injury (5). Maternal heart

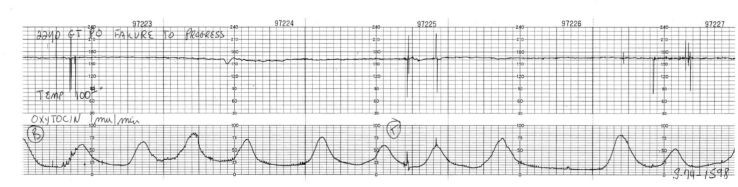

FIGURE 6.1. Fetal tachycardia, fetal heart rate 165 beats per minute. This tachycardia is associated with maternal fever (note temperature [100.4°F]). Also note the associated loss of variability. The absence of associated decelerations and presence of an explanation (fever) makes hypoxia an unlikely cause.

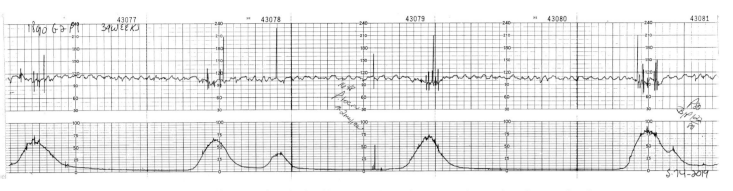

FIGURE 6.2. Fetal bradycardia. The fetal heart rate is 110 beats per minute. There is normal variability present by direct internal scalp electrode monitoring. Four hours later, the patient delivered a 3,025 g baby with Apgar scores of 9 at 1 minute and 10 at 5 minutes. Mother and baby did well.

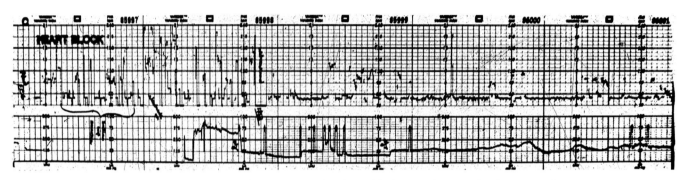

FIGURE 6.3. Fetal bradycardia due to complete heart block. Note the rate of 50 beats per minute with lack of variability.

rate will, on occasion, be transmitted and recorded as FHR when using direct (electrode) or Doppler monitoring. Persistent bradycardia requires careful evaluation to ensure that it is not the maternal heart rate being recorded in the presence of a fetal demise. Real-time ultrasound can establish the correct diagnosis and thus avoid unnecessary and potentially dangerous therapy in the presence of an already dead fetus.

Variability

In determining the immediate fetal status, the most important single FHR characteristic is variability. Normal variability is a reflection of intact neurologic modulation of the FHR and of intact or normal cardiac responsiveness. The two components are short-term and long-term variability (Fig. 6.4). Short-term variability is the beat-to-beat irregu-

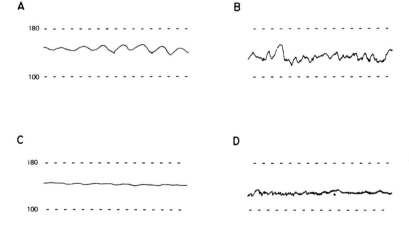

FIGURE 6.4. Long-term variability (LTV) is demonstrated in **A** and **B** and is absent in **C** and **D**. Short-term variability (STV) alone is shown in **D** and its concurrent presence with LTV is shown in **B**. Absence of both LTV and STV is seen in **C**. (From Zanini B, Paul RA, Huey JR: *Am J Obstet Gynecol* 136:43, 1980, with permission.)

larity caused by the normal variance in intervals between consecutive cardiac cycles. It is a consequence of the constant "push-pull" effect of sympathetic and parasympathetic nervous system input. Long-term variability is the waviness of the FHR tracing, generally at a frequency of 3 to 5 cycles/minute. With older EFM systems, using external Doppler, FHR variability could not be accurately determined because Doppler monitoring can artifactually increase FHR variability due to the imprecision of the signal. With newer Doppler signal processing systems, however, variability can be accurately assessed. Although there is utility in distinguishing between long- and short-term variability in research settings because mathematical quantification of these two types are different, there is no current evidence that the distinction between the two has any clinical relevance. Perhaps the single exception to this is the sinusoidal tracing that is absent short term but uniformly increased long-term variability. Increased variability has been shown in animals to be a sign of mild hypoxia (6). However, when FHR variability is normal or increased, fetal pH is usually normal.

As gestation advances and the fetal autonomic nervous system matures, the baseline FHR decreases and both short- and long-term variability increase. This is thought to reflect an increase in vagal control of cardiovascular reflexes. Decreased variability is generally seen with prematurity or anything that causes fetal CNS depression. Fetal hypoxia is the most worrisome cause; however, any condition that depresses the CNS can also decrease variability (Table 6.2). In labor it is critical to carefully review the strip for the presence or absence of nonreassuring decelerations (persistent late, nonreassuring variable, or prolonged) when decreased variability is seen. It is highly unlikely that decreased or absent variability reflects CNS depression due to hypoxia and acidosis unless the decelerations verify that ongoing hypoxia is present. This is analogous to backing up the nonreactive nonstress test (NST) with a contraction stress test (see Chapter 12). The exception to this rule may occur in the fetus who presents in labor with a flat baseline without decelerations, as one cannot rule out an hypoxic insult immediately prior to the initiation of electronic monitor-

TABLE 6.2. CAUSES OF DECREASED FHR VARIABILITY

Hypoxia/acidosis
Drugs
  CNS depressants
  Parasympatholytics
Fetal sleep cycles
Congenital anomalies
Extreme prematurity
Fetal tachycardia
Preexisting neurologic abnormality

CNS, central nervous system; FHR, fetal heart rate.

TABLE 6.3. EXAMPLES OF DRUGS CAUSING DECREASED FETAL HEART RATE VARIABILITY

Analgesics/narcotics
  Demerol
  Heroin
  Nisentil
  Morphine
Barbiturates
  Phenobarbital
  Secobarbital
Tranquilizers
  Diazepam
Phenothiazines
  Largon
  Phenergan
Parasympatholytics
  Atropine
General anesthetics

ing. Especially in the absence of nonreassuring decelerations, other causes of CNS depression should be considered. Certain drugs may be responsible (Table 6.3), particularly drugs that depress the CNS (Fig. 6.5) and drugs with autonomic blocking effects. Parasympathetic blocking drugs decrease variability while increasing baseline heart rate. Sympatholytic drugs (e.g., beta-adrenergic blockers) also decrease variability but decrease baseline heart rate.

Baseline heart rate variability is also associated with fetal wakefulness. When the fetus is sleeping, there is decreased variability (Fig. 6.6). When FHR variability spontaneously decreases in labor without associated nonreassuring decelerations, it is a benign finding. Usually the variability will spontaneously return to its previous level after a reasonable time, although the duration of fetal sleep states in labor is not as consistent as in the antepartum period. Stimulation of the fetus by manipulation of the uterus or noise may arouse the fetus and cause the variability to return. The new onset of loss of variability in the absence of periodic FHR decelerations with contractions is not a sign of fetal hypoxia.

From an intrapartum monitoring perspective, the most ominous cause of decreased variability is fetal hypoxia or asphyxia. FHR decelerations precede the loss of variability. In the presence of nonreassuring heart rate patterns, such as persistent late decelerations, loss of variability is associated with a high incidence of fetal acidosis and low Apgar scores (7) (Fig. 6.7), particularly in the case of preterm infants (8). A most difficult heart rate pattern to interpret is the persistently flat baseline (absent variability) seen in the fetus with a normal baseline heart rate and no decelerations. This may represent a previous insult to the fetus that has since been corrected but has resulted in persistent neurologic damage. Also, this pattern may be seen in fetuses with significant congenital anomalies, especially of the central nervous and cardiac systems. Extreme prematurity is associated with

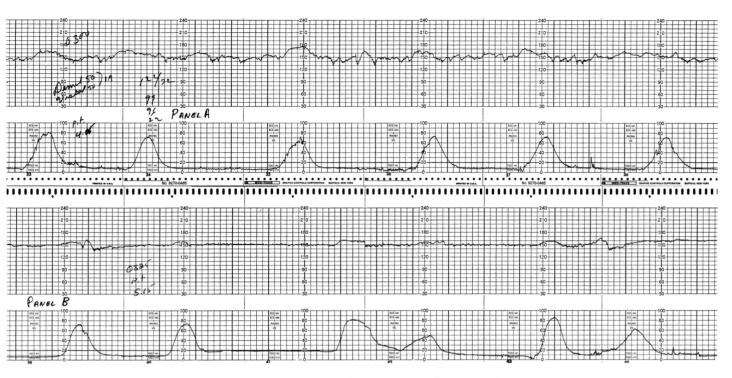

FIGURE 6.5. Narcotics are among the most frequent causes of decreased fetal heart rate variability in labor. In **A**, Demerol and Vistaril are given intramuscularly. At the beginning of **B**, about 20 minutes later, there is a noticeable decrease in variability without a change in baseline heart rate.

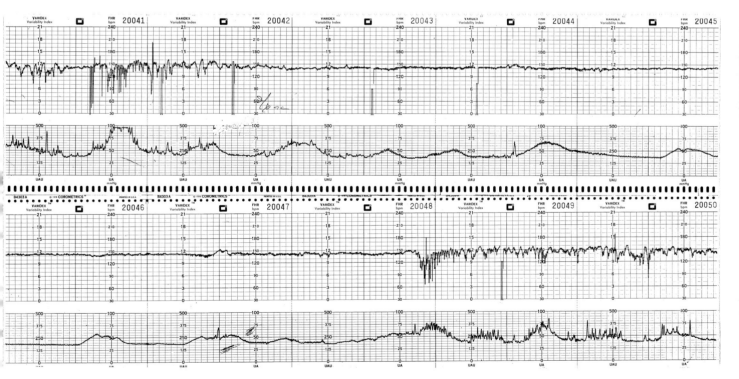

FIGURE 6.6. Spontaneous changes in variability occur normally in labor. Note the abrupt decrease in variability at **panel 20042**, which again abruptly returns to normal at **panel 20048**. This decreased variability lasted 20 to 30 minutes. There were no medications used. A vigorous normal baby was subsequently delivered.

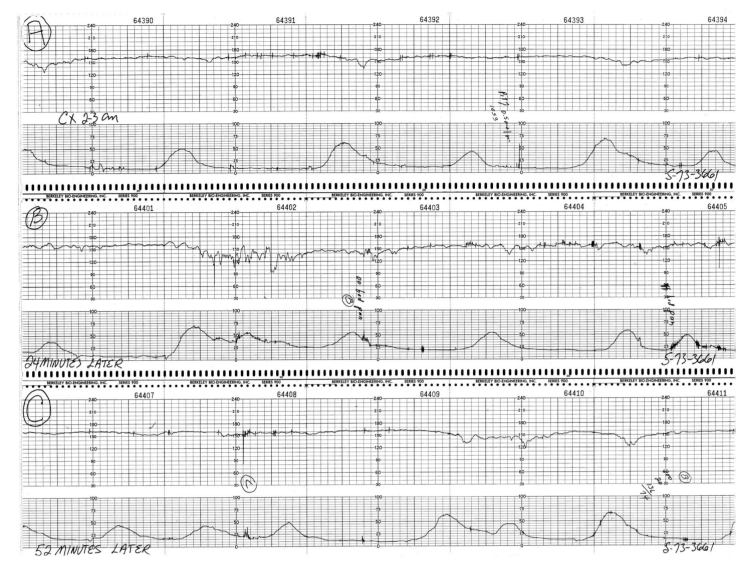

FIGURE 6.7. Persistent late decelerations are seen after most contractions. At **panel 64407** and after, variability is notably decreased. There is an associated fetal tachycardia.

decreased variability and nonreactive FHR patterns. Also, these patterns can be idiopathic and occur in a subsequently vigorous and healthy neonate (9). Table 6.3 lists the causes of decreased variability.

PERIODIC CHANGES

Tachycardia, bradycardia, and alterations in variability involve baseline FHR changes. Periodic changes are transient heart rate accelerations or decelerations that ultimately return to the original or a newly established baseline heart rate. Generally, these periodic changes occur in response to contractions and may also be seen with fetal movement.

Decelerations

There are four principal types of decelerations named according to shape and temporal relationship to contractions. These are early, late, and variable and prolonged decelerations.

Early Decelerations

Early decelerations are uniformly shaped decelerations of gradual onset and gradual return to baseline (Fig. 6.8). They begin early in the uterine contraction cycle, have their nadir at the peak of the contraction, and return to baseline before completion of the contraction. Acceleration of the heart rate generally does not precede or follow early deceleration. An important characteristic of early

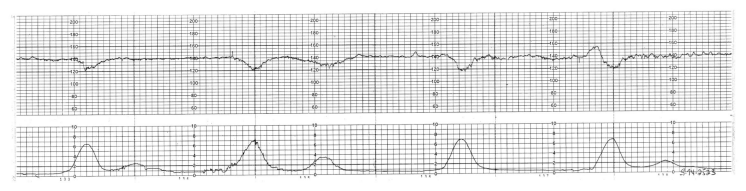

FIGURE 6.8. Early decelerations are seen with each contraction on this panel. They are uniform, mirror the contractions, and decelerate only 10 to 20 beats per minute.

deceleration is the minimal amplitude. The degree of FHR slowing is generally proportional to the strength of the contraction but rarely falls below 100 to 110, or 20 to 30 BPM below baseline. Early decelerations are thought to be caused by fetal head compression, with altered cerebral blood flow precipitating cardiac slowing through a vagal reflex. Early deceleration is generally seen in the active phase of labor, between 4 and 7 cm of cervical dilation. It is not associated with tachycardia, loss of variability, or other heart rate changes. Early deceleration is a reassuring FHR pattern and is not associated with fetal hypoxia, acidosis, or low Apgar scores.

Late Decelerations

In shape and uniformity, late decelerations are similar to early decelerations, but the timing is delayed relative to the uterine contraction (Fig. 6.9). The onset of the deceleration is often seen 30 seconds or more after the onset of the contraction. The nadir of the deceleration occurs after the contraction peak, and usually the return to baseline occurs after the contraction is over. In recognizing late decelerations, several important characteristics in addition to the timing are important. The descent and return are gradual and smooth.

There are usually no accelerations seen preceding or following the deceleration. The FHR rarely falls more than 30 to 40 BPM below baseline and usually not by more than 10 to 20 BPM. Late decelerations are significant and nonreassuring when they are persistent and not correctable. Variability is often increased during the deceleration. Most late decelerations are vagally mediated and result from relative or absolute fetal hypoxia, usually from inadequate oxygen exchange within the placenta provoked by uterine contractions. Although late decelerations may be associated with hypoxia, acidemia, and hypotension, only a decrease in fetal oxygen tension is essential for late decelerations to occur. The degree of this hypoxia and the appearance of late decelerations are related to many factors, including, on occasion, the strength and duration of the uterine contraction (Fig. 6.10). There may be a correlation between the magnitude of late decelerations (amount of slowing) and the degree of hypoxia, but this is not always the case, as the most depressed fetuses may have only shallow late decelerations. Persistent late decelerations are significant and potentially ominous. The association of late decelerations with loss of variability and/or elevation of baseline FHR is of more significance than the decelerations alone and reflects fetal intolerance to the hypoxic stress of uterine contractions.

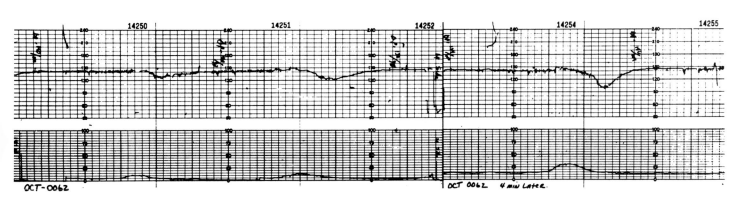

FIGURE 6.9. Late decelerations are seen after each of the three contractions. They are uniform, smooth, and drop only 20 to 30 beats per minute below baseline. There are no associated accelerations.

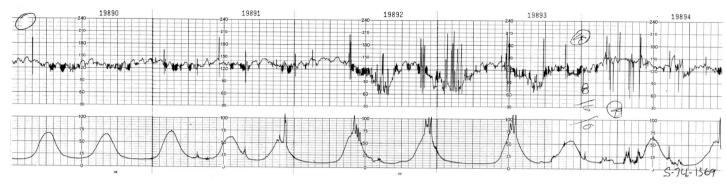

FIGURE 6.10. Late decelerations are seen occasionally only with the stronger contractions. In this panel, late decelerations are seen only with those contractions that exceed 70 mm Hg (internal pressure catheter and electrode).

The cause of late decelerations is uteroplacental insufficiency (UPI) elicited by intervillous stasis occurring during uterine contractions, and the factors which lead to this hypoxia may be intrinsic or extrinsic to the placenta. Decreased uterine blood flow is a much more common cause of late deceleration than poor exchange from other causes. Causes of decreased flow include supine hypotension and decreased uterine artery perfusion secondary to epidural or spinal anesthesia. The most common cause of late deceleration is uterine hyperactivity or hypertonus, often as a result of excessive oxytocin stimulation. Late decelerations seen in association with vaginal bleeding and/or spontaneous uterine hyperactivity may be the result of premature placental separation (abruptio placentae) (Fig. 6.11). Several disease states, including chronic hypertension, postmaturity, intrauterine growth restriction (IUGR), diabetes mellitus, pregnancy-induced hypertension/preeclampsia, and collagen vascular disease, may compromise placental exchange. The decreased intervillous blood flow associated with contractions (labor) may further aggravate this exchange and produce late decelerations. Because each contraction can produce hypoxic stress, the persistence

of late deceleration may precipitate metabolic acidosis. The most important two variables to watch for at this point are loss of accelerations and the loss of variability (Fig. 6.12). Tachycardia may also occur with the development of fetal acidosis, although for unknown reasons, this is not as consistently seen as it is with progressively severe variable decelerations. Decreased variability and fetal tachycardia are important signs of developing acidosis, and their presence with persistent late decelerations correlates highly with neonatal depression.

Variable Decelerations

The most frequently seen FHR deceleration pattern in labor is variable decelerations. This aptly named pattern is variable in nearly all respects: shape, duration, intensity, and timing relative to uterine contractions. It is commonly the result of umbilical cord compression but can result from any interruption of umbilical blood flow that is acute and intermittent. Other causes of interruption of cord flow include cord stretch and cold (e.g., rapid infusion of room-temperature amnioinfusion). In addition, head compres-

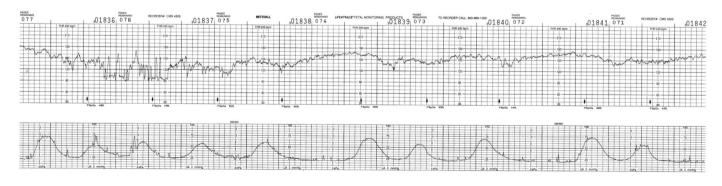

FIGURE 6.11. Late decelerations are seen after each contraction in this externally monitored patient, a term gestation admitted with vaginal bleeding. Note also the frequent/tachysystolic contraction pattern seen with the first five contractions. At cesarean section, a large abruption was found subsequent to delivering a 3,500 g female with Apgar scores of 7 at 1 minute and 8 at 5 minutes.

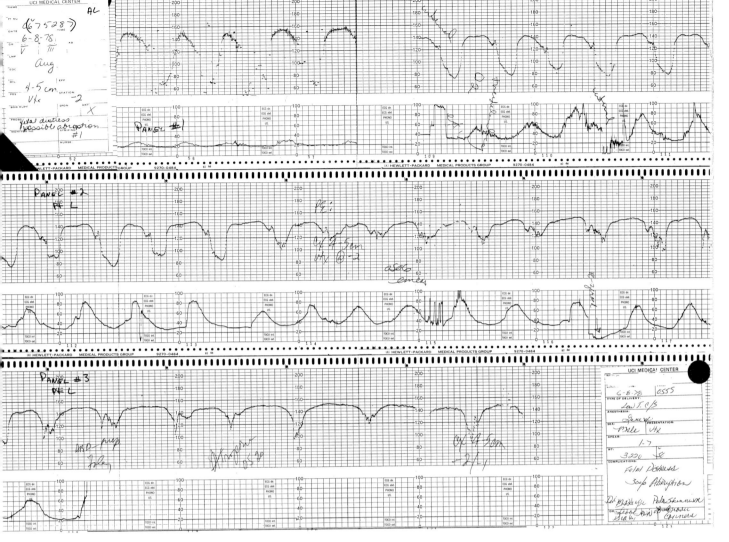

FIGURE 6.12. This is a gravida 5, para 3 admitted at term with contractions and minimal vaginal bleeding. On internal monitor (second half of **panel 1**), persistent late decelerations are noted that fail to respond to oxygen and position change. Variability is poor throughout and the baseline heart rate gradually increased from 140 to 155 beats per minute. In the presence of late decelerations, poor variability and rising baseline rate are signs of fetal intolerance to hypoxia and developing acidosis. In this case, a female with Apgar scores of 1 at 1 minute and 7 at 5 minutes was delivered. The 30% abruption is the cause of the late decelerations.

sion may also produce or alter the shape, depth, and duration of variable decelerations. Because cord compression during labor occurs most often during uterine contractions, variable decelerations usually coincide with uterine contractions (Fig. 6.13). This is, however, an inconsistent occurrence, and such decelerations may be seen with one but not the subsequent contraction. Characteristically, these decelerations are very abrupt in both onset and return to baseline. Small abrupt accelerations of the FHR usually precede and/or follow these decelerations. Variable decelerations are also occasionally observed during antepartum monitoring with fetal movement. There appears to be an association between the presence of variable decelerations on antepar-

tum monitoring and both oligohydramnios and fetal distress in labor. The degree of oligohydramnios correlates with the frequency of severe variable decelerations in labor (10). Assessment of amniotic fluid volume should be considered in antepartum patients with frequent variable decelerations during FHR testing and in patients with variable decelerations occurring relatively early in labor.

It is useful to think of four potential groups of causes of variable decelerations, because these groups aid in understanding the pathophysiology, determining the best method(s) for correction, and predicting the most likely progression (Table 6.4). Variable decelerations that begin early in the active phase of labor are often associated with

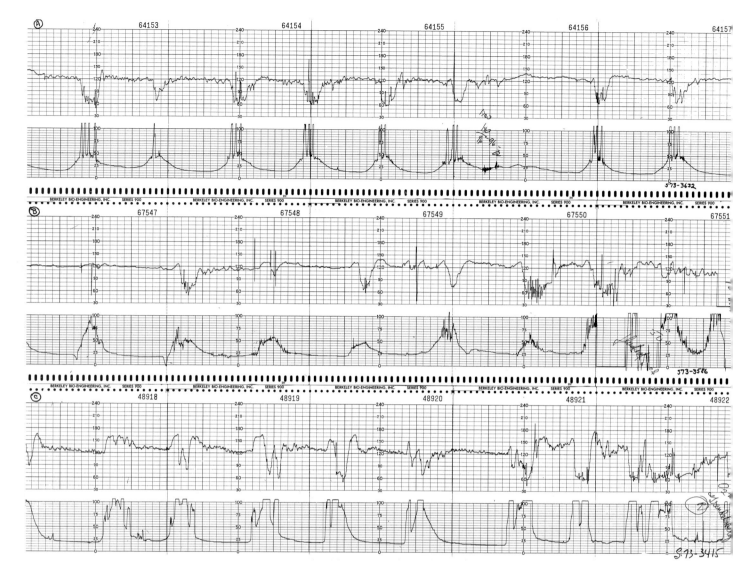

FIGURE 6.13. Typical variable decelerations are seen in this patient in the second stage of labor. Although all are occurring with contractions, they are variable in depth, duration, and shape. They are abrupt in onset and return to baseline. There are accelerations seen preceding and following most of these decelerations.

TABLE 6.4. CAUSES OF VARIABLE DECELERATIONS AND THEIR RELATIONSHIPS TO LABOR

Oligohydramnios
  Onset usually in the early active phase of labor or after membrane rupture
Descent
  Onset usually at 8–10 cm of dilation
  Often associated with nuchal cords
  Aggravated by pushing efforts
Cord prolapse
  Sometime after rupture of membranes
  Associated with unengaged station or abnormal presentation
Unusual causes
  True knots, short cords, limb entanglement, occult prolapse, etc.
  Onset and progression variably related to labor

and caused by oligohydramnios (Fig. 6.14). These will not likely respond to position change but may well be reversed or ameliorated by amnioinfusion if they progress to require intervention. Those developing during or just before the onset of the second stage of labor are most likely due to umbilical cord stretch or compression. This time in labor coincides with an acceleration of descent of the fetal presenting part, and these decelerations are most commonly seen in association with cord encirclement about the fetal neck (nuchal cords). It is presumed that in such circumstances the variable decelerations are due to cord stretch as the fetus descends. Such events are so common that experienced labor and delivery nurses know it is time to examine the patient because the new appearance of variable deceleration often heralds the onset of the second stage (Fig. 6.15)

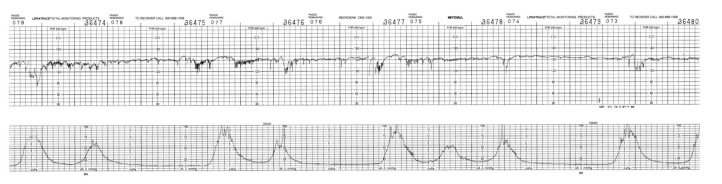

FIGURE 6.14. This nulliparous patient is at 41½ weeks in early labor. Note the occasional mild variable decelerations. The amniotic fluid volume on ultrasound was noted to be markedly reduced. Subsequently, at the time of amniotomy, thick meconium was noted and amnioinfusion was started. Variable decelerations appearing in early labor are unusual, and oligohydramnios should always be considered as an etiology of the cord compression.

Rarely the appearance of variable decelerations can announce the presence of umbilical cord prolapse, and this is another important reason to examine the patient. The final category of causes of cord compression can be thought of as "unusual cords" including such things as short cords, true knots, cord entanglement about fetal small parts, occult cord prolapse, etc. The course of cord compression is most unpredictable in such circumstances.

The vast majority of variable decelerations are not associated with significant hypoxia or, acidosis. Thus the challenge of evaluating and managing these patterns depends on the ability to distinguish between patterns that do and do not require further evaluation and management. In terms of fetal compromise, any insult should vary directly with the duration and degree of cord compression. With persistent mild degrees of cord compression, a mild respiratory acido-

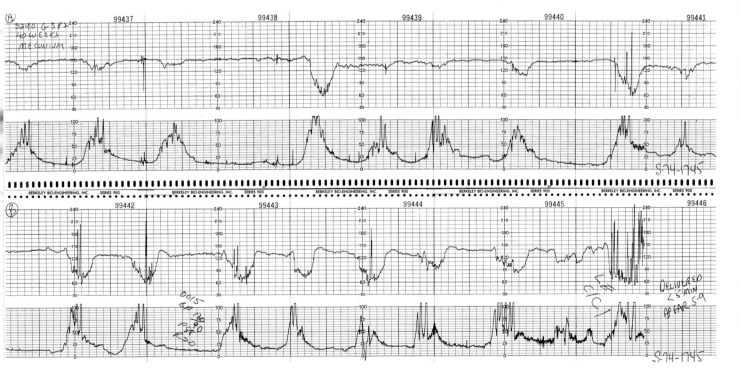

FIGURE 6.15. Variable decelerations here, as they often do, herald the onset of the second stage of labor in **panel A**. Maternal pushing can be detected by the short spikes on top of the contractions. The reason for this is probably a nuchal cord that is stretched during descent of the fetal vertex. Although the decelerations become larger and more regular, baseline heart rate and variability remain unchanged and reassuring. A term-size infant with Apgar scores of 5 at 1 minute and 9 at 5 minutes was delivered less than 5 minutes after the monitor was removed and there was indeed a tight nuchal cord.

sis may develop from carbon dioxide (CO_2) retention. However, if placental function is adequate and contractions are not too frequent, this CO_2 retention should clear rapidly with reversal of the respiratory acidosis. Should cord compression be prolonged and/or repetitive, progressive fetal hypoxia and resultant metabolic acidosis may also develop. For these reasons, variable decelerations have been graded as mild, moderate, or severe. The more severe the variable deceleration pattern, and the more prolonged and sustained it becomes, the more likely the result will be the delivery of a depressed newborn. Kubli et al. (11) graded variable decelerations on the basis of the level and duration of decelerations, without considering other parameters. Mild variable decelerations have a duration of less than 30 seconds, regardless of level, or a deceleration not below 70

to 80 BPM, regardless of duration (Fig. 6.16). Moderate variables have a level less than 80 BPM regardless of duration (Fig. 6.17). Severe variables are less than 70 BPM for greater than 60 seconds (Fig. 6.18). With variable decelerations, unlike late decelerations where hypoxia is the actual cause, the depth and duration of the decelerations correlate to the degree of hypoxia, but are not always indicative of hypoxia, because they are initially caused by a baroreceptor reflex (Fig. 6.19). To evaluate how a given fetus is responding to or tolerating these variable decelerations, other parameters of the FHR tracing require evaluation. Loss of variability and baseline tachycardia suggest possible progressive neurologic depression from hypoxia and acidosis (Fig. 6.20). In the presence of variable decelerations that are persistent, deeper, and of greater duration, the development of

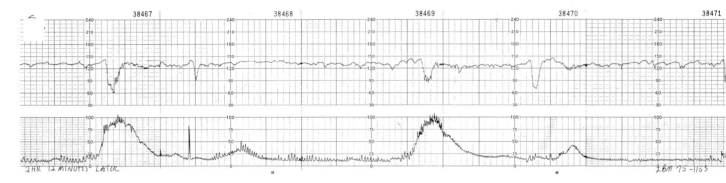

FIGURE 6.16. Mild variable decelerations are seen in this patient in early labor. They are occurring with contractions and probably with fetal movement. Baseline heart rate and variability are normal.

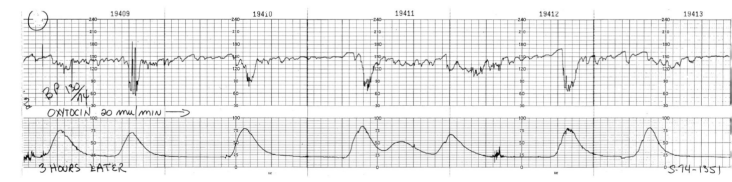

FIGURE 6.17. Moderate variable decelerations are seen in this panel. Baseline heart rate and variability are normal.

FIGURE 6.18. Severe variable decelerations are seen in a 14-year-old primigravida admitted at 43 weeks with meconium-stained amniotic fluid. Variable decelerations are seen throughout, becoming progressively deeper and more prolonged. Baseline heart rate is somewhat erratic from 140 to 180 beats per minute. Increased heart rate variability seen in **G** and **H** probably represents early hypoxia between contractions. A 2760-g infant with Apgar scores of 6 at 1 minute and 5 at 5 minutes was delivered. The low 5-minute Apgar score may have been caused by meconium in the airway and difficult ventilation.

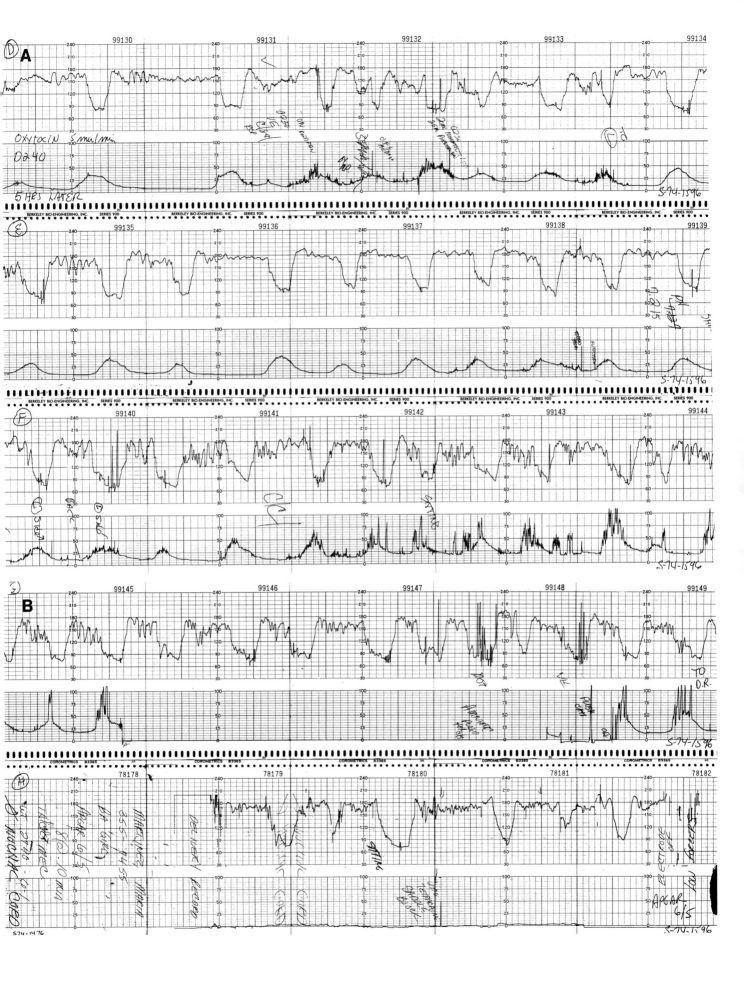

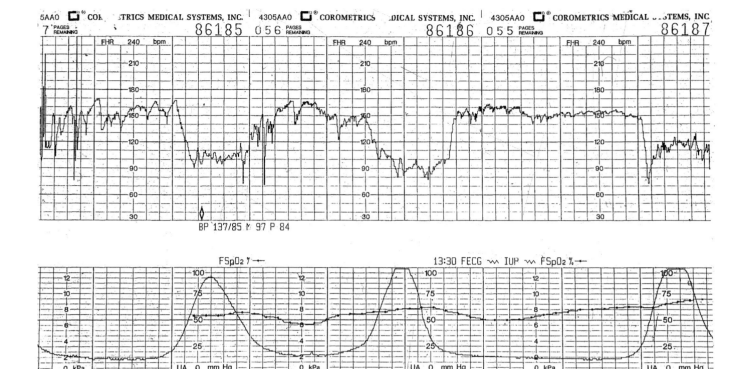

FIGURE 6.19. These deep variable decelerations dropping to 80 beats per minute and lasting up to 1 minute are seen in conjunction with a fetal pulse oximeter that is showing normal fetal oxygen saturation values between 50% and 60%. Because the inciting stimulus of a variable deceleration is the increase in peripheral vascular resistance in the fetal circulation, and a slowing of the fetal heart rate that is the result of a baroreceptor reflex, even marked decelerations are often not associated with hypoxia.

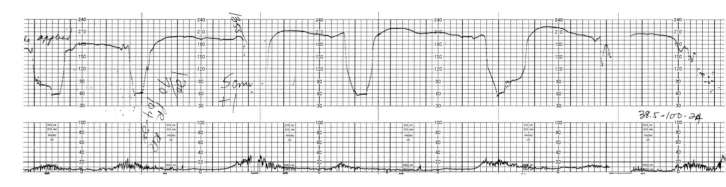

FIGURE 6.20. Severe ominous deceleration is seen with increasing heart rate to 210 beats per minute and virtually absent variability. A premature baby was delivered by cesarean section with Apgar scores of 1 at 1 minute and 2 at 5 minutes.

these additional warning signs, in the absence of other causes such as drugs, is an important sign that the fetus is not tolerating the intermittent cord compression. The other sign of fetal intolerance to cord compression is a slow return of the variable deceleration pattern to baseline heart rate (Fig. 6.21). Usually, variable decelerations are very abrupt in both their descent and return to baseline. Should the return to baseline persistently become more gradual, the indication is that progressive hypoxia is developing. It is

probable that this slow return represents a component of late deceleration that would be consistent with a developing fetal hypoxia. Sometimes, distinct variable decelerations are followed by distinct late decelerations when simultaneous cord compression and primary UPI are occurring (Fig. 6.22). With mild variable decelerations, especially without tachycardia or loss of variability, it is unlikely that the cord compression has caused the hypoxia and late decelerations. Therefore, a placental perfusion or exchange problem prob-

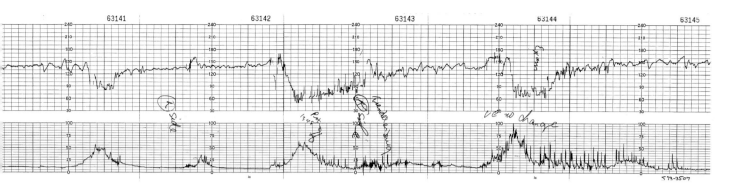

FIGURE 6.21. Severe decelerations are seen with slow return to baseline. Baseline heart rate and variability are normal.

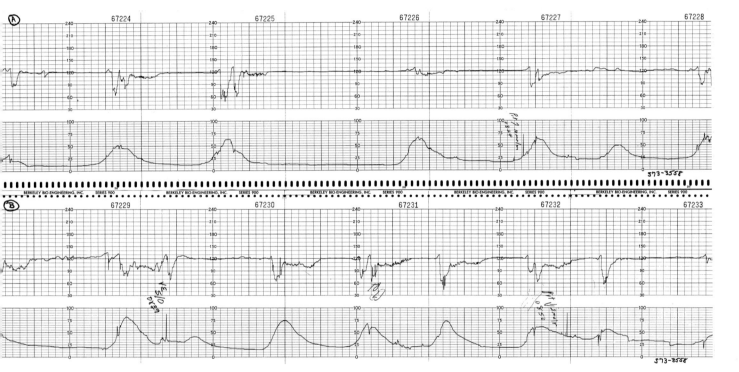

FIGURE 6.22. Mixed mild variable and late decelerations are seen with most contractions. With such mild variable decelerations, it is unlikely that progressive cord compression has caused the hypoxia, but a coexistent uteroplacental insufficiency probably exists. Poor variability suggests acidosis may also be present.

ably coexists with cord compression. Variable decelerations with slow return to baseline is one of the most confusing and difficult patterns to interpret and manage. These patterns may or may not be associated with fetal hypoxia. Recent human data, using fetal pulse oximetry, have shown that when this pattern is preceded in its development by late or severe variable decelerations, then it is a sign of progressive hypoxia; but when slow return to baseline is associated with neither, then it is no more often associated with hypoxia than if the variable decelerations with which it occurs did not have a slow return to baseline (12).

As variable decelerations become more severe and hypoxia is present or more severe, and especially as acidosis develops, additional FHR changes are common. The variable deceleration pattern will begin to appear smoother and rounded or blunted (Fig. 6.23). This change can be partially reproduced with atropine or may be seen in a very premature fetus. In extreme situations, with severe and progressive variable deceleration, the contraction may be followed by a blunt acceleration described by Goodlin and Lowe (13) as "overshoot." This is a transient smooth acceleration lasting more than a minute and occurring after severe variable

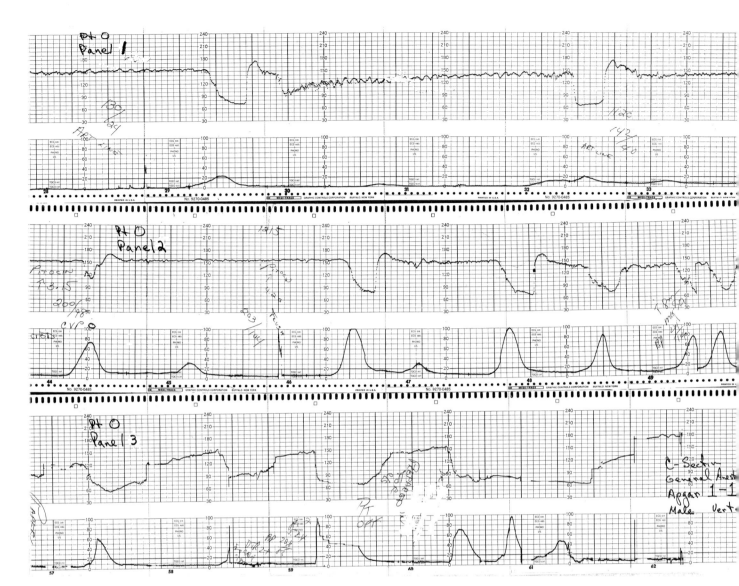

FIGURE 6.23. Severe variable decelerations are seen throughout these three panels. The blunted (rounded and not abrupt) accelerations seen following the decelerations are not the usual abrupt acceleration and may represent overshoot. Variability is progressively lost and decelerations become ominously prolonged. Delivery in this 30-week severe preeclamptic was by cesarean section and a severely depressed neonate with Apgar scores of 1 at 1 minute and 1 at 5 minutes was delivered.

decelerations. There is no acceleration preceding the deceleration. The overshoot lacks abruptness, is without short-term variability within the acceleration, and returns to baseline very gradually. This pattern is only seen with variable decelerations, usually with a flat baseline and with blunted changes as previously described.

Another finding that may occur when variable decelerations approach 50 to 60 BPM is transient cardiac asystole. Junctional rhythms are common if the FHR decreases below 70 BPM, with ventricular escape beats seen on occasion. Prolonged asystole is quite unusual and sudden death exceedingly rare. These do not seem to alter the likelihood that the decelerations correlate with hypoxia and acidosis over and above the appearance of the remainder of the pattern.

Rather than attempting to quantify variable decelerations and using this as some means to determine intrapartum management, we view variable decelerations as reassuring or nonreassuring. Reassuring variable decelerations have the following components:

1. The deceleration lasts no more than 30 to 45 seconds.
2. There is a rapid return to baseline from the nadir of the deceleration.

3. Average short-term variability of the baseline FHR is present (not absent or increased), and normal baseline FHR continues.
4. The baseline rate is not increasing.

Nonreassuring variable decelerations are those that become deep and long lasting and have delayed return to baseline with or without overshoot. Absence of short-term variability or an increasing baseline FHR are nonreassuring signs. In contrast to late decelerations, what makes variable decelerations so difficult to manage is their unpredictability. Because the second stage precedes delivery by only a relatively short time, and intervention is usually immediately possible should truly ominous patterns develop, more prolonged and deeper variable decelerations can be tolerated. This is true as long as the baseline heart rate is not rising and variability is maintained (Fig. 6.15). Because cord compression is more frequent in the second stage and is likely to be more severe, having to deal with this issue in practice is a very common problem. To what extent head compression is involved in the production of these decelerations is not totally clear; however, the depth and progression of many of these decelerations do make it clear that cord compression is the main component, and referring to these second-stage decelerations as early deceleration is inappropriate. If loss of variability and/or an increasing baseline develop with the more severe second-stage variable decelerations, expeditious delivery definitely becomes warranted (Fig. 6.24).

Prolonged Decelerations

Prolonged decelerations are isolated decelerations lasting more than 2 minutes. They are difficult to classify in terms of pathophysiology because they may be seen in a multitude of situations. As might be expected, cord compression can cause prolonged decelerations. This is generally seen either with progression of severe variable deceleration or with sudden occult cord prolapse (Fig. 6.25), but may also occur solely as recurrent prolonged decelerations. Profound placental insufficiency may cause prolonged decelerations. This is most characteristically seen with hypotension from the supine position or following epidural or spinal anesthesia (Fig. 6.26).

Hypertonic or tetanic uterine contractions may precipitate UPI-induced prolonged decelerations (Fig. 6.27). Tetanic uterine contractions can be seen with oxytocin, breast hyperstimulation, abruptio placenta, or with uterine artery vasospasm. Cocaine ingestion has been implicated in

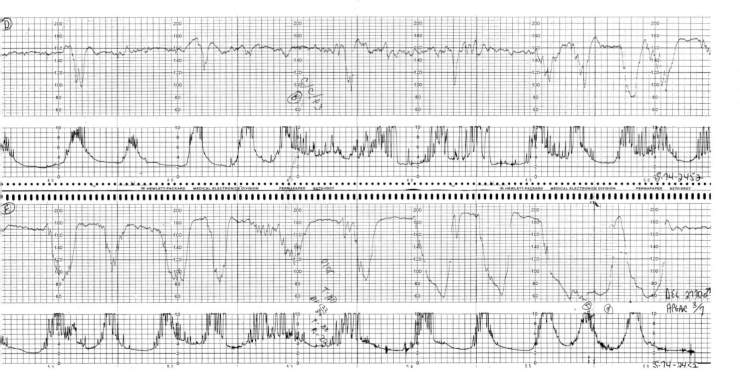

FIGURE 6.24. The patient is being monitored with an internal electrode and intrauterine catheter. There is a rapid progression of variable decelerations from mild to severe. The baseline heart rate rises from 150 beats per minute (BPM) at the beginning to 190 BPM. The heart rate variability is normal at the beginning of the tracing but is markedly decreased just before delivery. The patient was delivered by low forceps of a 2,770-g male with Apgar scores of 3 at 1 minute and 7 at 5 minutes and a single loop of tight nuchal cord.

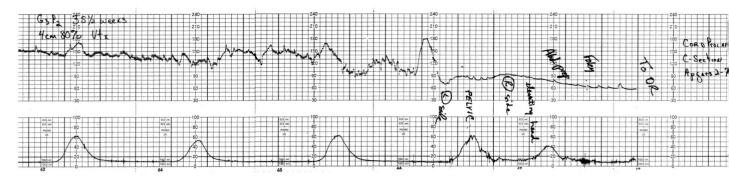

FIGURE 6.25. A sudden prolonged deceleration is seen in this patient in the early active phase of labor. An immediate pelvic examination revealed cord prolapse, and cesarean section was performed.

the development of vasospasm and abruptio placenta. Maternal hypoxia causing such decelerations might be seen with seizures, respiratory depression secondary to a high-spinal anesthetic, or following an overdose of narcotics or magnesium sulfate. Frequently, prolonged decelerations of the FHR, especially when the duration is more than 4 to 5 minutes, are associated with a rebound tachycardia and loss of variability (Fig. 6.28). This may be due to release of fetal epinephrine or may reflect some degree of fetal CNS depression or injury. If the original insult does not recur

immediately, and the fetus was well-oxygenated before the insult, the placenta is very effective in resuscitating the fetus. Generally allowing placental resuscitation is a better choice than operative intervention in these situations. The loss of variability and tachycardia are not necessarily prognostically ominous because the insult may no longer be present and the placenta can effectively restore the fetus to its normal well-oxygenated state. Occasionally, in addition to the loss of variability and tachycardia seen after such prolonged decelerations, there may be a period of late

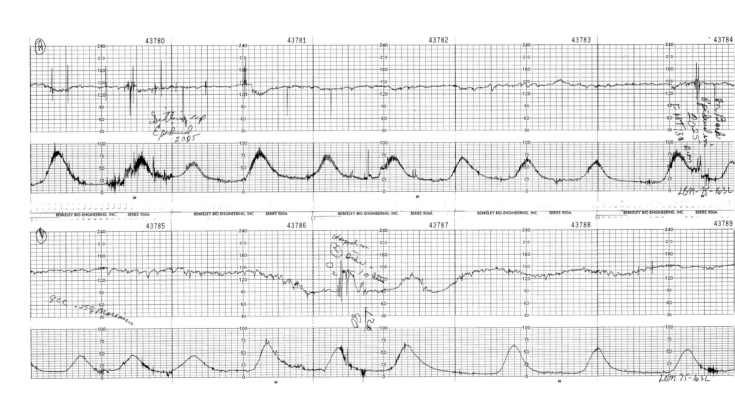

FIGURE 6.26. A prolonged deceleration is seen after injection of epidural anesthesia with Marcaine. This is followed by several late decelerations, often seen following such epidural-induced decelerations. The pattern subsequently returned to normal and a vigorous newborn was delivered vaginally.

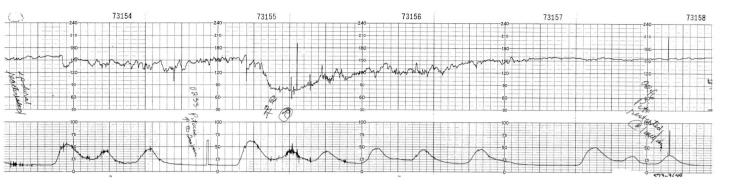

FIGURE 6.27. Here a prolonged deceleration is seen associated with excessive uterine activity secondary to oxytocin hyperstimulation. Again, a rebound tachycardia with decreased variability follows the prolonged deceleration. Pitocin was stopped and restarted at a lower rate and the heart rate subsequently returned to normal.

decelerations. These usually clear spontaneously with in utero recovery of the fetus.

Prolonged decelerations may not always return to baseline. When seen following a protracted course of severe variable decelerations or a prolonged period of recurrent late decelerations, such a prolonged deceleration may occur just before fetal death (Fig. 6.29). Recurrent prolonged decelerations without apparent etiology probably represent cord compression and are the most difficult of all patterns to manage. This is because one cannot prognosticate fetal tolerance based on previous performance of the FHR in labor or on such parameters of the FHR as variability. Such prolonged decelerations may just continue to recur, and prolonged cord compression may cause fetal death.

There are a few other, more benign, causes of prolonged declarations that merely represent an active fetal vagus nerve

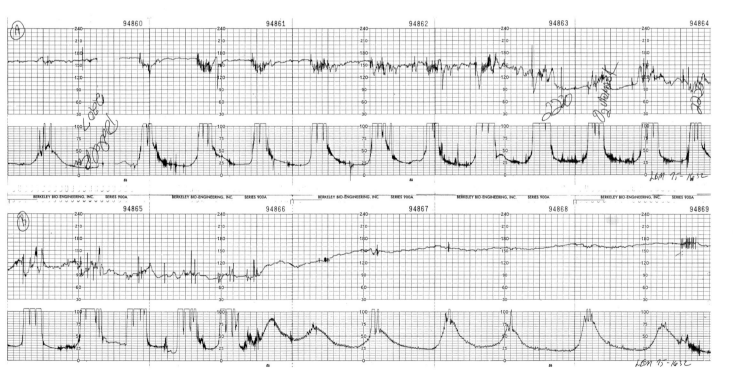

FIGURE 6.28. A prolonged deceleration from a baseline heart rate of 160 to 90 beats per minute (BPM) is seen lasting 12 minutes in the second stage of labor. An apparent cause is not present. Tachycardia to 170 BPM and decreased variability are seen after this deceleration. Also, some subtle late decelerations are probably present during this time. Again, the heart rate pattern returned to normal. No further significant decelerations recurred and a vaginal delivery of an Apgar 7 infant occurred approximately 15 minutes later.

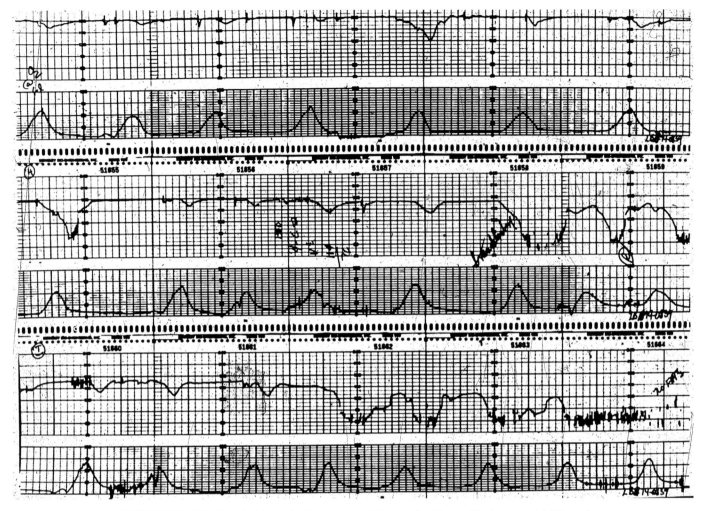

FIGURE 6.29. This fetus in labor is having recurrent late decelerations with absent variability and tachycardia. At the end of the strip a terminal bradycardia is seen immediately preceding the demise of the fetus.

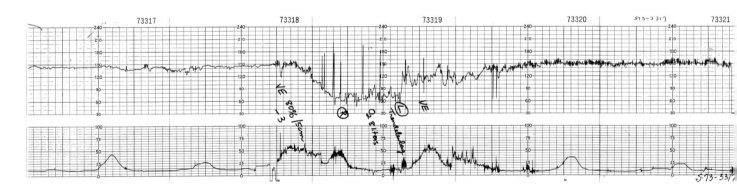

FIGURE 6.30. A prolonged deceleration is seen after a pelvic examination. Also, note the uterine hyperactivity commonly seen following a pelvic examination (Ferguson reflex?). This probably represents a fetus with an active vagal reflex.

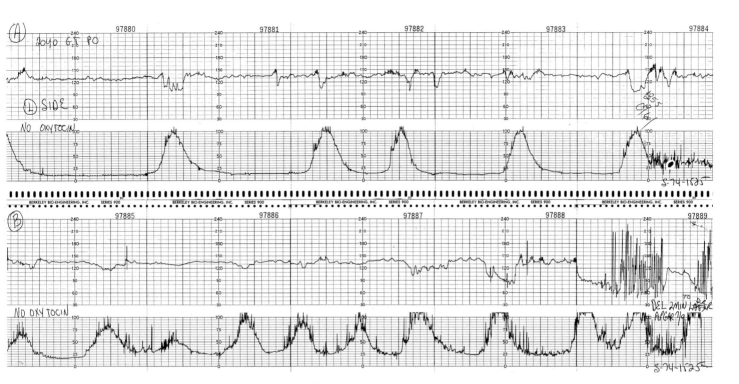

FIGURE 6.31. In this case, a prolonged deceleration is seen at the end of **panel B**. This patient progressed rapidly from 6 cm at the end of **panel A** to delivery 2 minutes after the end of panel B. Such prolonged decelerations should incite performance of a pelvic examination, not only to rule out cord prolapse, but as is often the case, to check for rapid descent as occurred here.

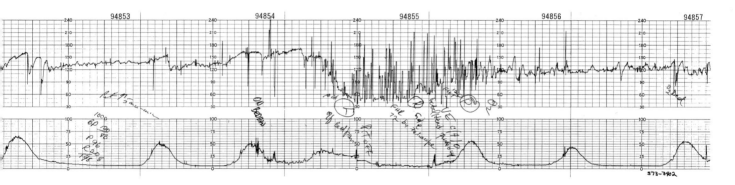

FIGURE 6.32. Here, a prolonged deceleration occurs while the patient is on a bedpan. Again, a fetal vagal reflex may cause decelerations with maternal Valsalva.

and not fetal hypoxia. Occasionally, such decelerations are associated with pelvic examination (Fig. 6.30), application of scalp electrode, rapid descent of the fetus through the birth canal (Fig. 6.31), or with sustained maternal Valsalva maneuver (Fig. 6.32). Such decelerations generally do not last more than a few minutes and are not usually followed by tachycardia or loss of variability. Because these prolonged decelerations are thought to be vagally mediated, therapy with atropine has been suggested. However, this treatment is not recommended, because there is not an associated increase in fetal cardiac output or oxygenation (14).

Accelerations

Because periodic changes are defined as transient changes above and below the baseline, accelerations are the counterpart of decelerations. Accelerations of the FHR occur most commonly in the antepartum period, in early labor, and in association with variable decelerations. There are at least two physiologic mechanisms responsible for accelerations. Accelerations associated with fetal movement or uterine contractions (Fig. 6.33) seem to have the same significance as FHR variability in that their presence represents fetal alertness or arousal states. The other cause of accelerations seems to be partial umbilical cord occlusion. If the low-pressure umbilical vein is compressed and the higher pressure umbilical artery remains patent, a period of decreased placental return and fetal hypotension results in baroreceptor response. The normal baroreceptor response to hypotension or decreased cardiac return is an increase in heart rate, with a resultant acceleration.

The presence of FHR accelerations in the intrapartum period is reassuring. These accelerations may occur with contractions, fetal movement, or without apparent stimulus. In addition, as with decelerations, accelerations may be seen in response to pelvic examination and stimulation of the fetal head (Fig. 6.34). Virtually all of these accelerations are associated with fetal movement. Indeed, as described in Chapter 8, accelerations with intrapartum pelvic examination reflect normal fetal pH. This is the rationale for using spontaneous or stimulus-produced accelerations in the presence of otherwise nonreassuring FHR patterns to reassure the clinician that the baby is neither depressed nor acidotic. It cannot be emphasized

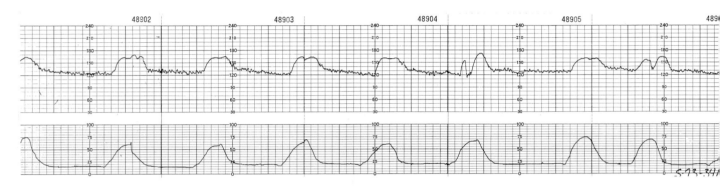

FIGURE 6.33. Accelerations of the fetal heart rate are seen with each contraction. Baseline heart rate and variability are normal. Such a pattern is reassuring.

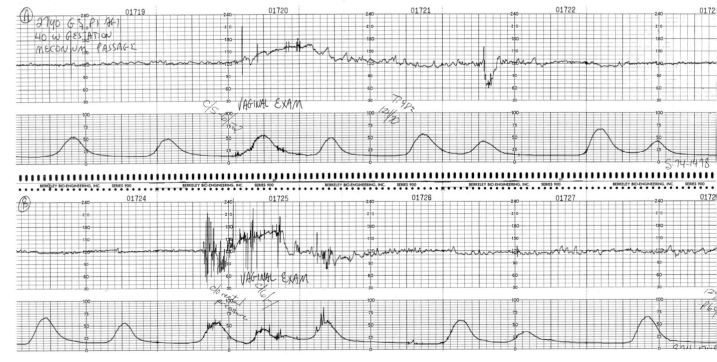

FIGURE 6.34. Just as a vaginal examination may precipitate prolonged deceleration (Fig. 6.30A), a vaginal examination may stimulate the fetal heart rate to accelerate as occurs in both panels.

enough, however, that the absence of FHR accelerations in the intrapartum period is not in and of itself alarming as long as variability is normal and there are no deceleration patterns indicative of possible fetal hypoxia. Thus in labor, fetuses are often inactive, and long periods with the absence of accelerations occur that do not, in and of themselves, constitute a nonreassuring scenario. One other problem created by accelerations of the FHR is that, at times, it is difficult to be sure whether one is dealing with decelerations or with accelerations with return to baseline (Fig. 6.35). This is especially true in the beginning of the monitoring period when the baseline has not been established. This is an important practical problem because there may be cases of misinterpretation with intervention for fetal distress when, in reality, there were no decelerations but rather accelerations mistaken for baseline heart rate and return to baseline mistaken for decelerations. There are three clues to help avoid this difficulty. First, accelerations and decelerations are rounded at their peak, whereas the baseline tends to be flat. Second, with accelerations especially, there is usually a period preceding or following without periodic changes when the baseline may be more clearly determined. Third, accelerations are almost always associated with fetal movement that can be documented by patient symptoms, palpation, or ultrasound.

Unusual Patterns

Sinusoidal Pattern

Originally described in separate reports from Shenker (15) in 1973 and Kubli et al. in 1972 (16), the sinusoidal FHR is a rare but distinct baseline pattern. Observed in antepartum, intrapartum, and neonatal FHR monitoring, this pattern is strongly associated with fetal hypoxia, often resulting from severe fetal anemia (Fig. 6.36). This fetal anemia may result from Rh sensitization, fetal-maternal hemorrhage, or in utero fetal hemorrhage and has an associated increased perinatal morbidity and mortality. The sinusoidal FHR pattern has been reported following the intrapartum administration of the analgesics alphaprodine (Nisentil) (17), butorphanol (Stadol) (18), or meperidine (Demerol) (19), and in association with amnionitis (20). In the absence of acidosis or anemia, sinusoidal heart rate following analgesic administration does not appear to have an ominous significance for the fetus, and the mechanism of this heart rate change is unclear. Many times, benign FHR patterns with increased long-term variability may be easily confused with sinusoidal patterns (Fig. 6.37).

The ability to correctly recognize and manage a sinusoidal pattern unrelated to previous analgesia use is of critical importance. Despite numerous publications on the def-

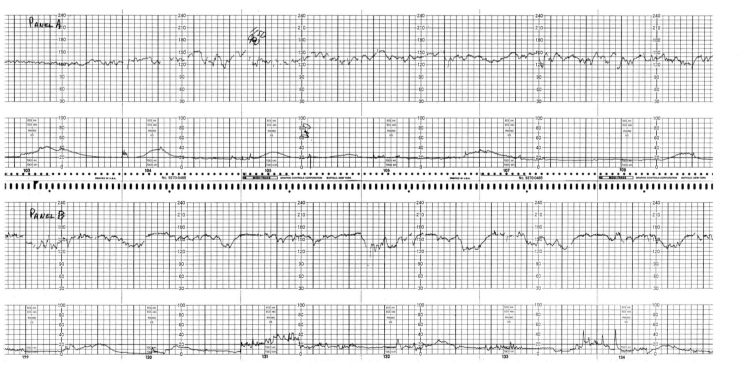

FIGURE 6.35. In **panel B**, accelerations with a return to baseline could easily be confused for late decelerations. Looking back at **panel A**, it can be seen that the real baseline heart rate is 120 to 130 beats per minute. Also, note that the return to baseline tends to be flat rather than rounded at the nadir as late decelerations would be.

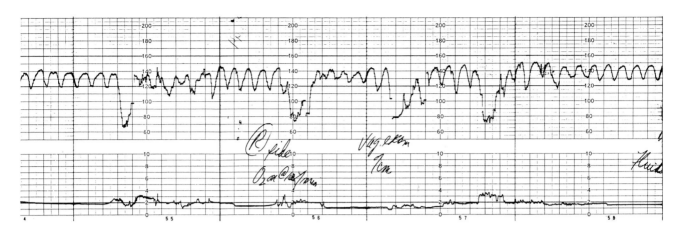

FIGURE 6.36. Intrapartum sinusoidal fetal heart rate (FHR) pattern. There are also moderate variable decelerations present. (From Klavin M, et al.: Clinical concepts of FHR monitoring. Hewlett-Packard Co., Boston, 1977:106, with permission.)

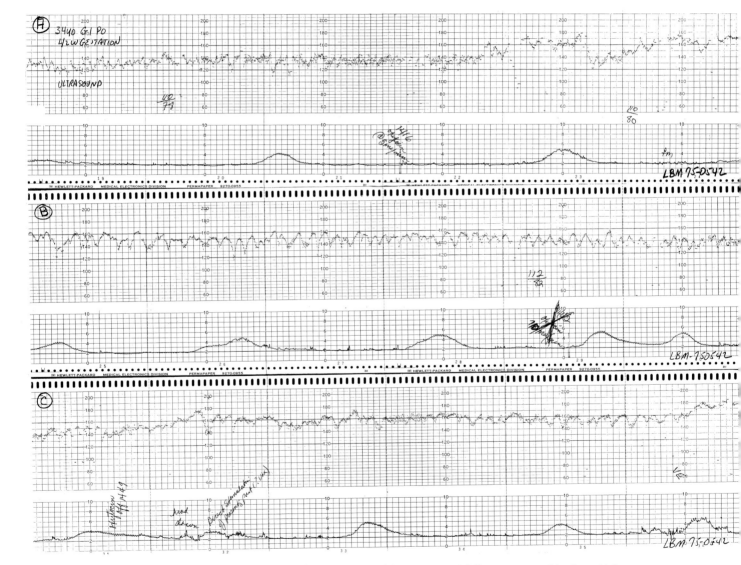

FIGURE 6.37. As seen in **panel B**, exaggerated long-term variability may resemble sinusoidal heart rate patterns. The presence of short-term variability within the pattern, and the normal patterns before and after **B**, distinguish this pseudosinusoidal pattern from a true sinusoidal one.

inition, pathogenesis, and clinical significance of the sinusoidal heart rate pattern, confusion continues regarding the features of sinusoidal heart rate associated with poor perinatal outcome. We consider that the following heart rate features must be present: (a) stable baseline heart rate of 120 to 160 BPM with regular oscillations, (b) amplitude of 5 to 15 BPM (rarely greater), (c) frequency of 2 to 5 cycles/minute (as long-term variability), (d) fixed or flat short-term variability, (e) oscillation of the sinusoidal wave from above and below a baseline, and (f) absence of FHR accelerations (21).

The exact pathophysiology of sinusoidal heart rate remains unknown. The association of fetal anemia with the sinusoidal heart rate is well documented for the human fetus. Young et al. (22) clinically demonstrated an inverse correlation between sinusoidal heart rate amplitude and fetal pH. A derangement of nervous control of the heart secondary to central or peripheral ischemia is hypothesized to result in sinusoidal heart rate (23–25). Murata et al. (26) have reported in an animal model an association between sinusoidal heart rate and plasma arginine vasopressin concentration. Chemical or surgical vagotomy with subsequent infusion of arginine vasopressin produces a sinusoidal pattern. Arginine vasopressin is elevated following hemorrhage or acidosis, and perhaps secondary to direct or indirect effects of this hormone on calcium transfer in the sinus node, sinusoidal heart rate results.

Wandering Baseline

A very rare FHR abnormality is seen when it is impossible to establish the baseline. Although falling within the defined normal limits of 120 to 160 BPM, this baseline wanders and does not remain steady. This rare abnormality is seen in the absence of short-term variability and is highly suggestive of a neurologically abnormal fetus. This wandering baseline will occasionally be seen as a preterminal event (Fig. 6.38).

Lambda Pattern

First described by Aladjem et al. (27), the "lambda pattern" is an FHR pattern involving an acceleration followed immediately by a deceleration (Fig. 6.39). Although neither rare nor ominous, the problem with this pattern is the potential for confusing it with late deceleration or other abnormal patterns (28). This pattern most typically appears early in labor and does not persist. The appearance of this pattern does not predict an increased likelihood of subsequent development of nonreassuring variable or other con-

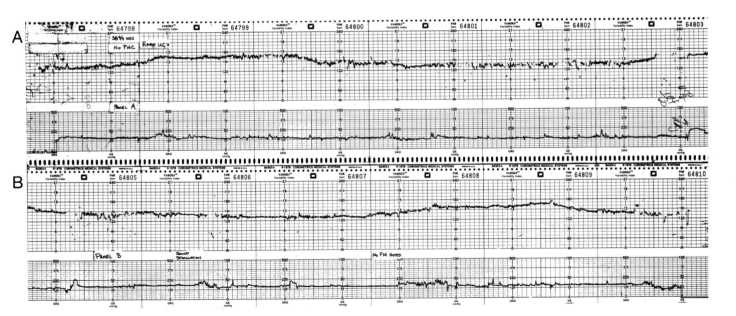

FIGURE 6.38. As seen in **panel A**, when evaluated in early labor, this patient was thought to have a reassuring tracing on the basis of a prolonged acceleration. However, as the monitoring was continued, there was no evidence of true reactivity **(panel B)**. The patient stated that fetal movement had been decreased for 2 weeks. A biophysical profile found no evidence of fetal breathing, tone, or movement. Artificial rupture of membranes revealed thick yellow meconium. Subsequently, persistent late decelerations were noted and emergency cesarean section was performed. The infant was depressed (Apgar scores 2 and 3 at 1 and 5 minutes) but not acidotic (umbilical pH 7.30). Seizure activity was noted in the delivery room. A head computed tomography scan and ultrasound revealed a large cystic area in the left brain consistent with a porencephalic cyst. This example of a wandering baseline resulted from significant preexisting central nervous system insult.

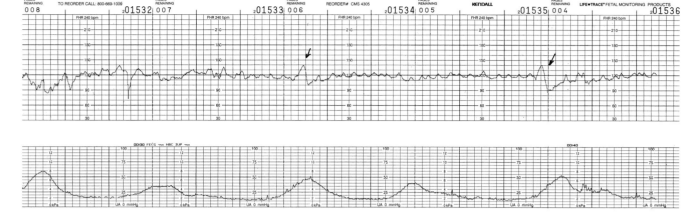

FIGURE 6.39. The complex of an acceleration immediately followed by a variable deceleration has been termed the "Lambda" pattern. Generally, this is similar to a variable deceleration. Such patterns are, benign, often confused with late decelerations, but in general are not persistent and do not portend the appearance of a subsequently nonreassuring tracing.

cerning patterns. The mechanism responsible for causing this pattern is unknown but may result from intermittent mild cord compression or stretch.

CONCLUSION

A knowledge of the physiology and pathophysiology of the FHR, coupled with experience in pattern recognition, is essential for the appropriate use of electronic FHR monitoring. Pattern recognition is a process of recognizing FHR changes, such as decelerations, that suggest the type of pathophysiologic process occurring, determining how the fetus is tolerating that process at any given moment by such parameters as variability and baseline heart rate, and of prognosticating how long such a process might be allowed to continue without significant fetal depression or damage by the severity, repetitiveness, and duration of the pattern. Unfortunately, such a process is difficult to analyze quantitatively, making the task of pattern recognition and integration all the more important.

REFERENCES

1. National Institutes of Child Health and Human Development Research Planning Workshop: Electronic fetal heart rate monitoring: Research guidelines for interpretation. *Am J Obstet Gynecol* 177:1385, 1997.
2. Young B, Katz M, Klein S, et al.: Fetal blood and tissue pH with moderate bradycardia. *Am J Obstet Gynecol* 135:45, 1979.
3. Shenker L: Fetal cardiac arrhythmias. *Obstet Gynecol Surv* 34:561, 1979.
4. Dildy GA: Intrapartum fetal pulse oximetry in the presence of fetal cardiac arrhythimia. *Am J Obstet Gynecol* 169:1609, 1993.
5. Marsh TD, Lagrew DC, Cook LN, et al.: Unexplained fetal baseline bradycardia in congenital panhypopituitarism. *Am J Obstet Gynecol* 156:977, 1987.
6. Druzin ML, Ikenoue T, Murata Y, et al.: A possible mechanism for the increase in fetal heart rate variability following hypoxemia. Presented at the Society for Gynecologic Investigation, San Diego, California, 1979.
7. Paul RH, Suidan AK, Yeh SY, et al.: Clinical fetal monitoring. VII. The evaluation and significance of intrapartum baseline FHR variability. *Am J Obstet Gynecol* 123:206, 1975.
8. Bowes W, Gabbe S, Bowes C: Fetal heart rate monitoring in premature infants weighing 1500 grams or less. *Am J Obstet Gynecol* 137:791, 1980.
9. Garite TJ, Linzey EM, Freeman RK, et al.: Fetal heart rate patterns and fetal distress in fetuses with congenital anomalies. *Obstet Gynecol* 53:716, 1979.
10. Vintizileos AM, Campbell WA, Nochimson DJ, et al: Degree of oligohydramnios and pregnancy outcome in patients with premature rupture of membranes. *Obstet Gynecol* 66:165, 1985.
11. Kubli FW, Hon EH, Khazin AE, et al.: Observations on heart rate and pH in the human fetus during labor. *Am J Obstet Gynecol* 104:1190, 1969.
12. Henigsman S, Garite T, Patillo C, et al: Fetal pulse oximetry defines which variable decelerations with slow return to baseline are associated with hypoxia. *Am J Obstet Gynecol* 185:S131, 2001.
13. Goodlin RC, Lowe EW: A functional umbilical cord occlusion heart rate pattern: the significance of overshoot. *Obstet Gynecol* 42:22, 1974.
14. Parer JT: Effects of atropine on heart rate and oxygen consumption of the hypoxic fetus. *Gynecol Invest* 8:50, 1977.
15. Shenker L: Clinical experience with fetal heart rate monitoring of 1000 patients in labor. *Am J Obstet Gynecol* 115:1111, 1973.
16. Kubli F, Ruttgers H, Haller U, et al.: Die antepartale fetale Herzfrequenz. II. Verhalten von Grundfrequenz, Fluktuation and Dezerationo bei antepartalem Fruchttod, Z. *Gerburtshilfe Perinatol* 176:309, 1972.
17. Gray J, Cudmore D, Lether E, et al.: Sinusoidal fetal heart rate pattern associated with alphaprodine administration. *Obstet Gynecol* 52:678, 1978.
18. Angel J, Knuppel R, Lake M: Sinusoidal fetal heart rate patterns associated with intravenous butorphanol administration. *Am J Obstet Gynecol* 149:465, 1984.
19. Epstein H, Waxman A, Gleicher N, et al.: Meperidine induced sinusoidal fetal heart rate pattern and reversal with naloxone. *Obstet Gynecol* 59:225, 1982.

20. Gleicher N, Runowicz C, Brown B: Sinusoidal fetal heart rate patterns in association with amnionitis. *Obstet Gynecol* 56:109, 1980.

21. Modanlou H, Freeman RK: Sinusoidal fetal heart rate pattern: its definition and clinical significance. *Am J Obstet Gynecol* 142:1033, 1982.

22. Young B, Katz M, Wilson S: Sinusoidal fetal heart rate. I. Clinical significance. *Am J Obstet Gynecol* 136:587, 1980.

23. Baskett T, Koh K: Sinusoidal fetal heart rate pattern: a sign of fetal hypoxia. *Obstet Gynecol* 44:379, 1974.

24. Cetrulo C, Schifrin B: Fetal heart rate patterns preceding death in utero. *Obstet Gynecol* 48:521, 1976.

25. Richter R, Hohl M, Hammacher K, et al.: Significance of oscillation frequency in intrapartum fetal monitoring. *Obstet Gynecol* 50:694, 1977.

26. Murata Y, Miyake Y, Yamamoto T, et al.: Experimentally produced sinusoidal fetal heart rate pattern in the chronically instrumented fetal lamb. *Am J Obstet Gynecol* 153:693, 1985.

27. Aladjem S, Feria A, Rest J, et al.: Fetal heart rate responses to fetal movements. *Br J Obstet Gynaecol* 84:487, 1977.

28. Brubaker K, Garite TJ: The lambda fetal heart rate pattern: An assessment of its significance in the intrapartum period. *Obstet Gynecol* 72:881, 1988.

7

FETAL CARDIAC ARRHYTHMIAS

Fetal cardiac arrhythmias occur in one form or another in a significant number of pregnancies. The documentation of various fetal arrhythmias has increased subsequent to the more extensive application of antepartum and intrapartum electronic fetal heart rate (FHR) monitoring. The importance of recognition of an abnormal cardiac rhythm, correct diagnosis of arrhythmia type, associated incidence of underlying heart disease, and the need for appropriate medical intervention depends on the specific type of arrhythmia present. Diagnosis can be established through the use of both M-mode and real-time ultrasound (1,2). In the absence of signs of failure (i.e., cardiac enlargement or hydrops) or evidence of FHR abnormalities suggestive of hypoxia, most fetal cardiac arrhythmias are benign, do not require immediate delivery, and are not associated with structural fetal cardiac abnormalities. Many arrhythmias, particularly those diagnosed during the intrapartum period, such as premature atrial contractions (PAC) and premature ventricular contractions (PVC), do not persist in the neonatal period and rarely require medical therapy. PACs and PVCs are, for the most part, entirely benign and do not require any special attention. However, certain types of arrhythmias are of clinical significance for both mother and fetus. Supraventricular tachycardias and fetal heart block may be associated with previously undiagnosed fetal compromise, maternal disease, or both, and frequently require active management.

FETAL TACHYCARDIA

The three general types of fetal tachycardia are sinus tachycardia, atrial flutter/fibrillation, and supraventricular tachycardia.

Sinus Tachycardia

Sinus tachycardia is defined as FHR above 160 beats per minute (BPM) and is usually secondary to maternal fever, drugs (i.e., atropine, β-sympathomimetics), amnionitis, congenital infection, or hyperthyroidism (Fig. 7.1). Although benign, on occasion sinus tachycardia accompanied by late or severe variable decelerations may be a sign of early fetal hypoxia (3). Recognition of the cause of tachycardia and differentiation from supraventricular tachycardia is of obvious importance. Tachycardia is not a sign of fetal hypoxia unless it is associated with ominous decelerations.

Atrial Flutter/Fibrillation

The antepartum diagnosis of atrial flutter or fibrillation is rare. A monotonous atrial rate that varies between 400 and 500 BPM is seen with this form of supraventricular tachyarrhythmia in the fetus. The ventricular rate is much lower, due to an accompanying atrioventricular (AV) block. If the AV block is fixed, a regular ventricular rate of 60 to 200 BPM is seen. If the block is intermittent, the ventricular rate will vary widely. Atrial flutter and fibrillation are serious arrhythmias; nonimmune hydrops can occur and a concomitant severe congenital heart defect is found in as many as 20% of cases (4). These arrhythmias are most resistant to in utero therapy and are associated with a very high fetal and neonatal mortality rate. Atrial fibrillation is rarer in the fetus than atrial flutter. Treatment with digoxin and/or verapamil may increase the degree of atrioventricular block but rarely corrects the atrial arrhythmia. However, control of ventricular rate does not necessarily improve fetal hydrops. This may require restoration of a 1:1 atrioventricular conduction. The use of type I antiarrhythmic agents (e.g., flecainide, quinidine, procainamide) should be considered as well in such patients.

Supraventricular Tachycardia

Thought to be the most frequent form of fetal tachyarrhythmia, supraventricular tachycardia can occur for short periods and be of no clinical significance, or can persist for long periods and lead to high output failure, nonimmune hydrops fetalis, and fetal death (5,6). Defined as an FHR greater than 220 BPM with no variability or conduction abnormality, supraventricular tachycardia can be suspected on cardiac auscultation and confirmed with M-mode echocardiography and pulsed-Doppler flow-velocity waveforms (7). Real-time ultrasound often will demonstrate

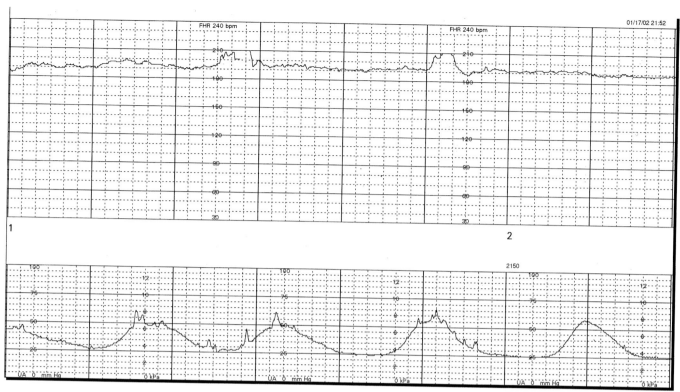

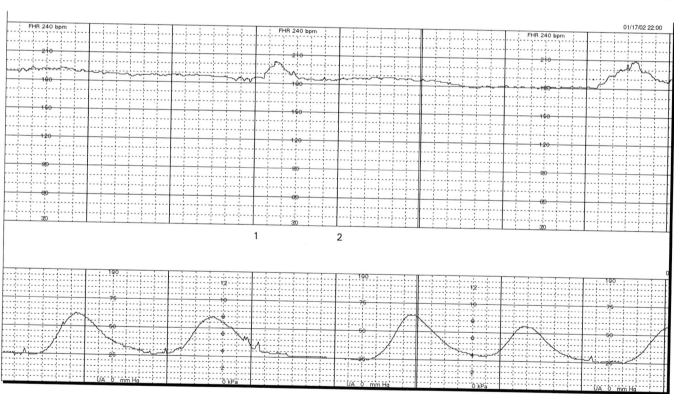

FIGURE 7.1. Sinus tachycardia. This example of fetal tachycardia is present in a patient with a fever and presumptive diagnosis of chorioamnionitis. Note the absence of decelerations, which is a reassuring finding regarding fetal oxygenation. *(Continued on next page)*

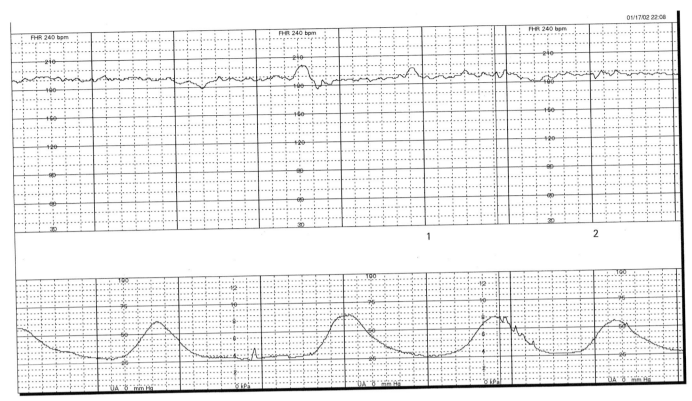

FIGURE 7.1. *(continued)*

varying degrees of cardiac failure. Although there may be no evidence of effusions or hydropic changes coexistent with supraventricular tachycardia, rapid progression can be seen in as little as 36 hours of continued tachyarrhythmia. More commonly, this is not a continuous but rather intermittent arrhythmia for which the term (paroxysmal) atrial tachycardia was used in the past.

Supraventricular tachycardia (SVT) may be a manifestation of atrial flutter or fibrillation and, in theory, results from one of two mechanisms. The first is increased automaticity of an ectopic pacemaker (other than the normal sinus nodal pacemaker) above the bundle of His. The second, and more likely, mechanism in fetal and childhood SVT is reentrant tachycardia resulting from a circular "circus movement" of electrical activity, most commonly within the AV node. Less commonly, but seen in the Wolff-Parkinson-White (WPW) syndrome, this movement is due to an accessory conduction pathway (bundle of Kent). Both types of reentrant tachycardia are thought to result from an atrial premature contraction being conducted through or around the AV node down a repolarized but relatively slow pathway. The fast pathway is thought to be in a refractory period following the previously normally timed atrial depolarization. If sufficiently slow conduction occurs, allowing recovery of the fast pathway, ventriculoatrial conduction up the fast pathway results in a sudden reentrant tachycardia.

The initiation and maintenance of this tachycardia depends on the refractory periods and conduction velocities within the slow and fast conduction pathways in the AV node. The timing of the arrival of the premature contraction is the critical factor in the initiation of the arrhythmia.

TREATMENT OF FETAL TACHYCARDIA

Sinus tachycardia is often encountered in the intrapartum period and usually reflects a drug effect, sympathetic fetal response to maternal infection, occult amnionitis, or, rarely, fetal hypoxia. The importance of identifying sinus tachycardia is not to institute a specific therapy, but to determine its cause and separate it from SVT (Fig. 7.1). Ventricular tachycardia, as defined by three or more consecutive premature ventricular systoles, is extremely rare in the fetus and its significance remains unknown. Ventricular fibrillation in the fetus has not been reported.

Treatment of fetal supraventricular tachycardia has been extensively reported. In utero pharmacologic therapy utilizing single drugs or various combinations of digoxin, calcium-channel blockers, beta-blockers, procainamide, and quinidine have all been reported with varying degrees of success (8). Once the diagnosis of SVT is made, with or without the associated signs of fetal cardiac failure, delivery of the mature fetus or in utero therapy of the immature fetus must be initiated. Fetal SVT requires urgent management at any gestational age. Digoxin has been the most commonly used drug for the initial treatment, and the combination of rapid digitalization and maintenance of the maternal digoxin level in the middle-to-upper therapeutic range with the addition of a calcium-channel blocker, such as verapamil, or beta-blocker, such as propranolol or atenolol, has been our most successful approach (Fig. 7.2 and 7.3). Quinidine is an alternative drug that, following adequate digitalization, can be of value in controlling fetal SVT. Unfortunately, 30% of patients cannot tolerate this drug because of severe nausea and vomiting. Digoxin should be initiated as a single agent with an intravenous loading dose of 1.0 mg (0.5 mg fol-

lowed by 0.25 mg at 6-hour intervals) while the patient is hospitalized and on continuous cardiac monitoring. The goal is to achieve a maternal blood level at the upper end of the therapeutic range. If there is no improvement in fetal rhythm after 2 days with a high therapeutic blood level of digoxin in the mother, a second agent or even third agent may be required. It is very important to consider that many of these additional antiarrhythmic agents increase both the serum level and bioavailability of digoxin. Consequently, the maternal digoxin dose should be reduced by at least 50% when using such agents as quinidine, verapamil, or amiodarone. When M-mode echocardiography reveals atrial flutter or fibrillation, one of the drugs of choice to control the associated rapid ventricular response due to AV node bypass

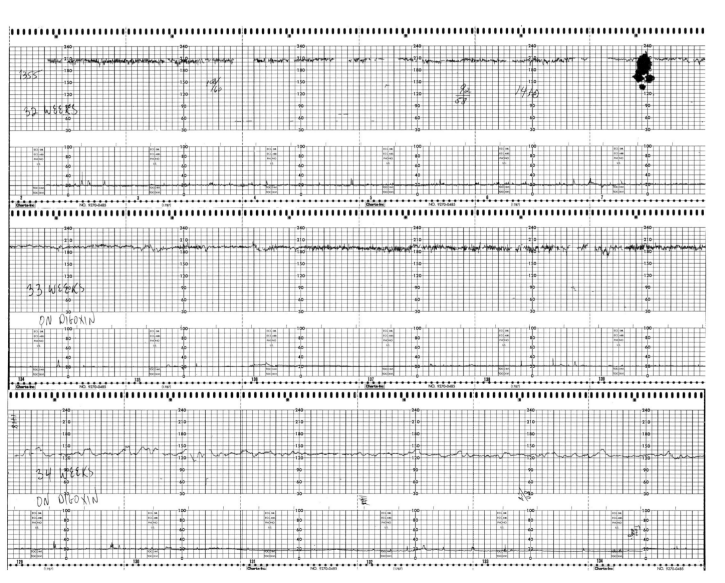

FIGURE 7.2. Sequential examples of fetal supraventricular tachycardia cardioverted in utero with digoxin treatment of the mother. The fetus was not hydropic during treatment.

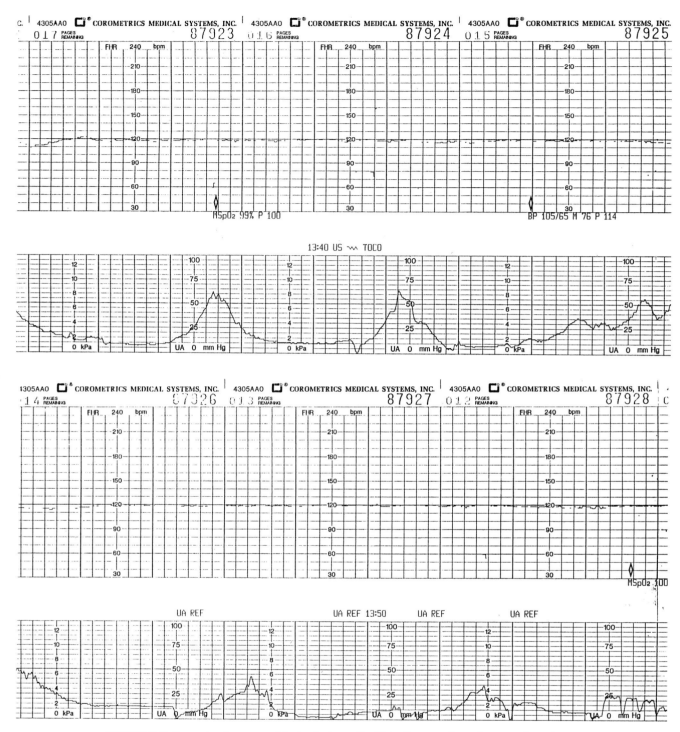

FIGURE 7.3. Example of supraventricular tachycardia. Note the complete absence of accelerations in the fetal heart rate (FHR). The actual FHR was 240 beats per minute with signal halving resulting from the monitor logic.

is procainamide, following the administration of digoxin, verapamil, or propranolol. The different types of fetal SVT can be controlled most frequently with digoxin and either verapamil or propranolol. When a combination of agents is indicated, the best choice is to combine the use of an agent that affects the fast pathway along with one that affects the slow pathway (Tables 7.1 and 7.2). With the exception of digoxin, cardiac antiarrhythmic drugs used to treat reentrant SVT also decrease automaticity with consequent lowering of the incidence of premature beats.

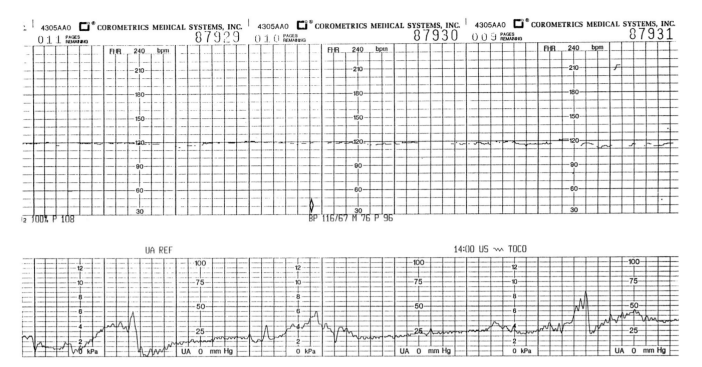

FIGURE 7.3. *(continued)*

TABLE 7.1. ANTIARRHYTHMIC DRUG CLASSES

Class	Repolarization	Indications	Drug
I A	Prolongs	Atrial flutter	Quinidine
		Atrial fibrillation	Procainamide
		SVT	Disopramide
		VT	
I B	Shortens	VT	Lidocaine
			Mexilitine
I C	Unchanged	VT	Flecainide
		SVT	Encainide
II	Unchanged	Atrial tachycardia	β-Blockers
		VT	
III	Markedly	VT	Amiodarone
	prolongs	Atrial flutter	Sotalol
		Atrial fibrillation	
		SVT	
IV	Unchanged	Reciprocating SVT	Verapamil
			Diltiazem
			Adenosine

SVT, supraventricular tachycardia; VT, ventricular tachycardia.
From Kleinman CS, Copel JA: Electrophysiological principles and fetal antiarrhythmic therapy. *Ultrasound Obstet Gynecol* 1:286–297, 1991, with permission.

TABLE 7.2. DEPRESSION OF AV NODAL CONDUCTION-FAST AND SLOW PATHWAYS

Antegrade (slow) limb	Retrograde (fast) limb
Digitalis	Class IA—Quinidine,
β-Blockers	Procainamide
Calcium-channel blockers	Class IC—Flecainide

CONGENITAL HEART BLOCK

Although most fetal arrhythmias are either extrasystoles or tachyarrhythmias, bradyarrhythmias due to complete heart block comprise approximately 10% of cases (9). The forms of heart block are first, second, and third degree (complete). Prolongation of the interval between the P and R waves (first degree AV block), usually secondary to impaired conduction in the AV junction proximal to the bundle of His, requires no treatment and has not been reported in the fetus. Second-degree or partial AV block, in which some but not all atrial impulses are conducted to the ventricles, is present in most fetuses with SVT. Second-degree AV block presents in two forms, Mobitz types I and II. In Mobitz type I block, the P-R interval increases progressively until complete blockage of an atrial impulse results in a dropped ventricular beat (Wenckebach type). This cycle is repeated, following anywhere from two to eight consecutive impulses with progressive lengthening of the P-R interval. In the fetus, Mobitz type I second-degree block is rarely either persistent or of any significance (10). Mobitz type II block occurs infrequently and is more serious. The delay is at a level below the AV junction and the P-R interval is normal or increased but fixed. This arrhythmia has dropped beats in a regular or irregular frequency and usually results from blockage in the bundle of His or trifascicular block. Mobitz type II second-degree block has been well described in the fetus (11). This form may precede development of complete heart block.

Complete, or third-degree, AV block has been the focus of most reports of fetal or neonatal heart block. Thought to be due to a failure of union of the AV node and His bundle in early fetal development, complete congenital heart block may also result from damage to the conducting system after it has been normally formed. It results in the fetus from blockage at the AV junction with, by definition, complete dissociation of the atria and the ventricles. The ventricular rate is usually between 40 and 60 BPM, and fetal hemodynamic compensation, presumably secondary to an increase in stroke volume, is frequently observed (Fig. 7.4). In the absence of significant underlying congenital heart disease, the neonate often does well, although a pacemaker may need to be placed very soon after delivery (12). However, this clinical condition offers a guarded prognosis for the newborn, whatever the actual cause may be. As many as 50% of infants with complete heart block have associated congenital cardiac malformations (10). Mothers of infants with congenital heart block in the absence of congenital heart disease are at increased risk for connective tissue disease, particularly systemic lupus erythematosus (SLE), either subclinical or overt (13). The maternal disease may be nonexistent, heralded by a serologic abnormality, or associated with current or subsequent development of severe connective tissue disease. Evaluation of the mother once

fetal congenital heart block is diagnosed is clearly indicated as only 50% of fetuses with bradycardia are born to women with a history of connective tissue disease (14).

The presence of specific antibodies to the soluble tissue ribonucleoprotein antigen Ro (SS-A) in the serum of mothers giving birth to infants with complete heart block has been described (15). There is immunofluorescent evidence of maternal anti-Ro immunoglobulin in the cardiac tissue of infants with congenital heart block. This finding suggests a transplacental passage of this immunoglobulin with direct effects in the fetal cardiac conduction system (16). This anti-Ro immunoglobulin can be measured in the serum of pregnant women with SLE, and if present, close fetal cardiac evaluation should be performed prospectively during pregnancy.

Treatment of congenital heart block depends on the coexistence of major cardiac abnormalities and fetal and neonatal tolerance of the fixed low heart rate. As mentioned, temporary or permanent pacemakers may need to be placed following delivery. Complete fetal heart block resulting in nonimmune hydrops from heart failure in utero occurs in approximately 25% of cases and is associated with high mortality. The mother may be exposed to unnecessary surgical risks when the arrhythmia is unknown and confused with a preterminal bradycardia in the intrapartum period (Fig. 7.5). In the fetus with complete heart block

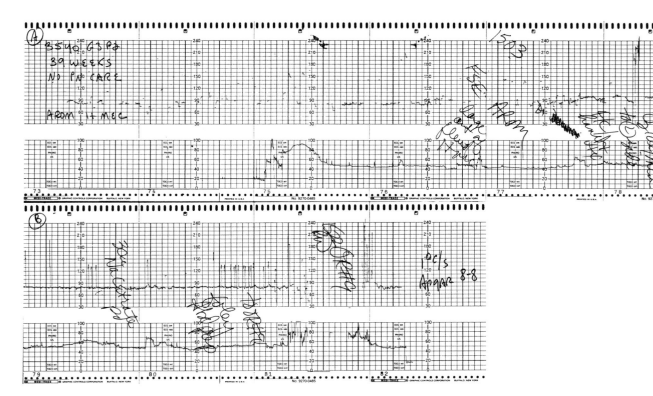

FIGURE 7.4. Example of emergency delivery for a patient presenting with a fetal heart rate of 80 beats per minute and no prenatal care. At delivery, the infant was discovered to have congenital heart block. The mother was antinuclear antigen negative and asymptomatic for any connective tissue disease.

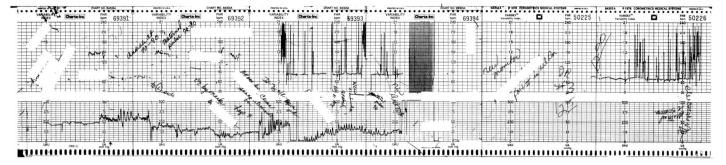

FIGURE 7.5. When complete heart block in the fetus is undiagnosed prior to entry into labor and delivery, it is not possible to determine the exact etiology of the abnormally slow fetal heart rate. The assumption that the heart rate was a prolonged fetal deceleration led to emergent cesarean section in this patient. At delivery, the infant was in no distress but maintained a heart rate of between 65 and 80 beats per minute. At discharge, he did not need a pacemaker, and the child has continued to do well. Workup of the mother diagnosed serologic evidence for systemic lupus erythematosus, although she has remained asymptomatic.

diagnosed before labor, the use of frequent intrapartum fetal pH determinations or continuous pulse oximetry of the fetus can result in a successful vaginal delivery. Our experience, however, has been that patients with fetal congenital heart block without congenital heart abnormalities incompatible with life are usually delivered via cesarean section because of the difficulty in monitoring these patients intrapartum. When intermittent, it is possible to allow these patients a trial of labor (Fig. 7.6).

Many forms of fetal therapy have been suggested in cases of complete fetal heart block (17). The treatment most often recommended is maternal administration of steroids, such as dexamethasone, in an effort to limit fetal inflammatory response to the transplacentally acquired maternal autoantibodies. Such treatment is associated with frequent and potentially severe maternal effects and there is no evidence that the antibody-mediated damage of the fetal conduction system is reversible. Other therapies include intravenous gamma globulin and maternal plasmapheresis, but these therapies are not proven in the prevention or reversal of fetal heart block. Various medications to increase the FHR have also been reported (i.e., ritodrine, terbutaline, and isoproterenol) with variable responses and no proven benefit.

Direct pacing of the fetal heart in cases of complete heart block with nonimmune hydrops has also been reported. Carpenter reported the first case of percutaneous transthoracic fetal heart pacing with successful capture but fetal death within 3 hours (18). More recently, Harrison performed open fetal surgery with placement of an epicardial pacing wire and pulse generator (19). Once again, fetal death occurred quickly despite successful pacing.

Close monitoring of the fetus diagnosed with complete heart block is recommended. This includes both maternal perceptions of fetal movement as well the use of real-time ultrasound to identify early development of cardiac decompensation. Such assessment includes observing early hydropic changes, ventricular size and function, and AV valve insufficiency. The exact role of either medical or surgical therapies for treatment of fetal heart block remains unclear. The mortality rate for newborns with complete heart block is approximately 25%. After the neonatal period, survival is close to 90% with most deaths related to pacemaker failure (20). The newborn with complete heart block in the absence of congenital heart disease frequently has neonatal lupus erythematosus often manifested by a distinctive skin rash due to antibody deposition on basal keratinocytes (14). Additional manifestations include anemia, thrombocytopenia, hepatosplenomegaly, hepatitis, myasthenia, or myopathy. This constellation of findings may appear to a greater or lesser degree and will disappear by 6 months of age.

MONITORING FETAL ARRHYTHMIAS

Accurate diagnosis of fetal arrhythmias is very difficult, if not impossible, using the FHR monitor alone. Monitors may have the logic system in operation at all times on the external mode and, therefore, heart rates above 200 BPM will often not even record. Figure 7.7 shows an expanded view of the recording of a fetal arrhythmia when the premature beat prompts a sudden rise and the following pause prompts a sudden drop in the rate, resulting in the characteristic vertical lines associated with the instantaneous FHR recording of fetal arrhythmias. Because electrical noise or maternal electrocardiograph (ECG) artifact can precipitate the same pattern, it is important to examine the raw fetal ECG tracing on the scope to differentiate between arrhythmia and artifact. Other examples of fetal arrhythmias and premature ventricle contractions are displayed in Figs. 7.8 through 7.10. Congenital heart block is shown in Fig. 7.11

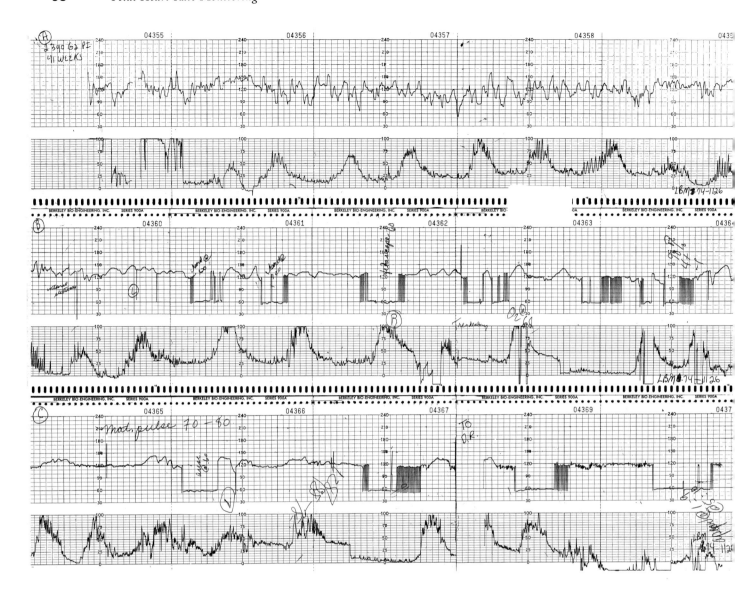

FIGURE 7.6. An interesting case of fetal heart block. Note that the **first panel,** recorded with a Doppler system containing excessive logic, shows an erratic pattern. The **middle and lower panels** are from a direct fetal scalp electrocardiograph (ECG). There are intermittent abrupt drops to 60 beats per minute (BPM) from the 120-BPM baseline. Where it says "heard at 120 BPM," the nurse was using a Doppler listening device and counting the atrial rate. With the third episode of 60 BPM, the nurse listened with a fetoscope (phone) and the rate of 60 BPM agreed with the ECG of 60 BPM, indicating the ventricular rate. Thus, a diagnosis of an intermittent 2-to-1 heart block was made.

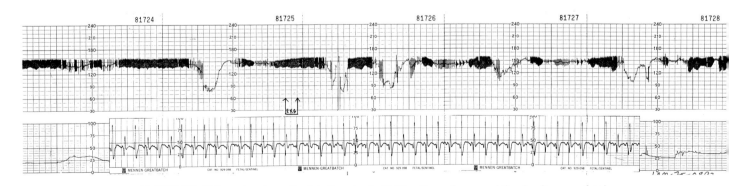

FIGURE 7.7. This tracing shows the fetal heart rate (FHR) pattern **above** and the simultaneous fetal electrocardiograph (ECG) **below.** The large vertical excursions on the FHR scale are caused by the fetal arrhythmia, which is shown on the fetal ECG tracing to be due to premature multifocal atrial contractions. Note the biphasic P waves.

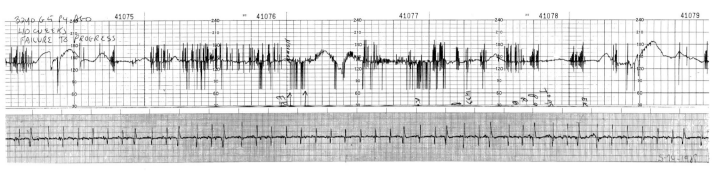

FIGURE 7.8. This tracing shows the fetal heart rate (FHR) patterns **above** and the simultaneous fetal echocardiograph (ECG) **below.** The large vertical excursions on the FHR scale are caused by the fetal arrhythmia, which is shown on the fetal ECG tracing to be due to premature ventricular contractions. Note the changing configuration of the fetal QRS complexes with each premature beat.

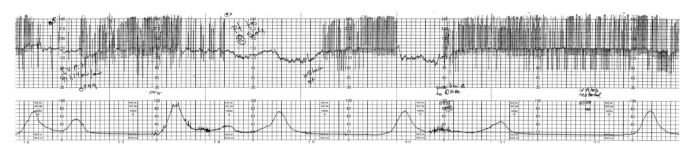

FIGURE 7.9. This tracing is an example of frequent multifocal premature ventricular contractions. Note the brief appearance of normal sinus rhythm following contractions.

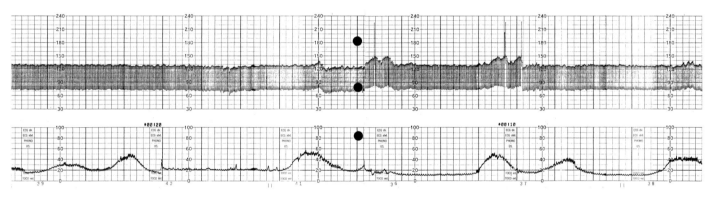

FIGURE 7.10. This is an example of frequent unifocal premature ventricular contractions. This was noted to be bigeminy on neonatal electrocardiography.

in a patient with antepartum diagnosis early in the third trimester.

Although when very frequent, continuous monitoring of FHR may be difficult, the clinical significance of these arrhythmias should be appreciated. Premature atrial and ventricular contractions usually have no clinical significance. Although there has been some association with other congenital abnormalities in the cardiac and other organ systems, this occurs infrequently. PACs and PVCs are not to be considered signs of fetal hypoxia and do not carry any significance as far as intervention. We do not

recommend a fetal echocardiograph for patients with an antepartum finding of FHR irregularity consistent with PACs or PVCs. However, frequent assessment of FHR to rule out evolution to SVT is recommended. Sometimes, a terminal FHR pattern will show some PACs or PVCs (21), but the significance of the pattern comes from the periodic and baseline FHR characteristics. Transient fetal cardiac standstill should be similarly managed. Position change, examination to rule out cord prolapse or rapid descent, and elevation of the presenting part are suggested maneuvers (22). Figure 7.12 displays an example

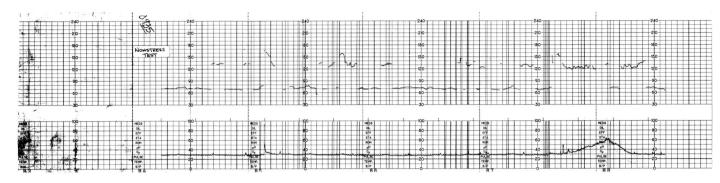

FIGURE 7.11. This is an example of intermittent congenital heart block detected during routine auscultation at the time of a prenatal visit. A nonstress test revealed areas of reactivity as well as a prolonged period of heart block. Ultrasound failed to reveal any structural cardiac defects or signs of cardiac failure. The patient was observed closely with no evidence of fetal deterioration. She was admitted in active labor at 35 weeks and delivered vaginally a normally grown, apparently healthy newborn. On postpartum day 3, because of frequent prolonged episodes of bradycardia and hypoxia, a pacemaker was placed in the neonate with excellent response. Workup of the mother was negative for any evidence of connective tissue disease.

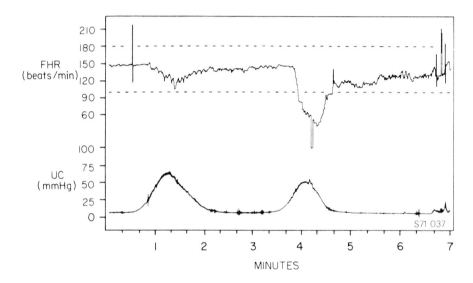

FIGURE 7.12. An example of a fetal heart rate (FHR)/uterine contraction tracing containing an episode of transient fetal cardiac arrest. At the 4-minute mark, during the course of severe variable deceleration, there was a transient fall of FHR to the zero level. Concomitant examination of the fetal electrocardiograph tracing proved the episode of transient fetal cardiac arrest. (From Yeh S, Zanini B, Petrie RH, et al.: Intrapartum fetal cardiac arrest: a preliminary observation. *Obstet Gynecol* 50: 571, 1977, with permission.)

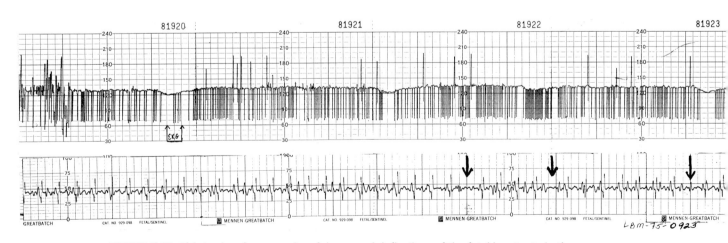

FIGURE 7.13. This tracing shows a series of downward deflections of the fetal heart rate in the **upper tracing**; the **lower tracing** of the simultaneous fetal electrocardiograph shows absent QRS complexes or dropped beats.

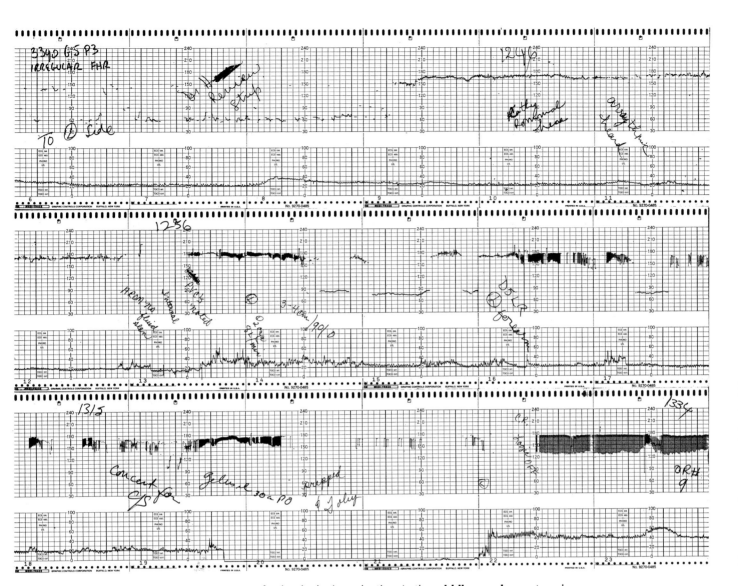

FIGURE 7.14. Intrapartum fetal arrhythmia evaluation. In the **middle panel,** an external monitor is recording a fetal heart rate of 80 to 90 BPM, most likely representing compensatory pauses of PVCs. In the **third panel**, when the logic is on, the monitor does not record because of the frequent premature beats with "abnormal" R-R intervals.

of transient fetal cardiac asystole mediated by vagal stimulations during a variable deceleration.

One will occasionally see a tracing with all downward deflections. This may be due to dropped beats (Figs. 7.13 and 7.14), a very low amplitude signal, or premature beats where the interval is too short to be counted (less than 250 milliseconds) and causes only the compensatory pause to be shown. In rare cases, PVCs occur every other beat, creating the bigeminal rhythm noted in Fig. 7.10.

The key to interpreting artifacts and arrhythmias is an understanding of fetal monitor instrumentation. The correct diagnosis and appropriate management can only be

achieved with careful application of the technologic advances in assessment of the fetal heart.

REFERENCES

1. Platt L, Manning F, Craigan G, et al.: Antenatal detection of fetal A-V dissociation utilizing real time B-mode ultrasound. *Obstet Gynecol* 53:595, 1979.
2. DeVore G, Siassi B, Platt L: Fetal echocardiography. III. The diagnosis of cardiac arrhythmias using real time directed M-mode ultrasound. *Am J Obstet Gynecol* 146:792, 1983.
3. Ron M, Adoni A, Hochner-Celnikier D, et al.: The significance

of baseline tachycardia in the post-term fetus. *Int J Gynaecol Obstet* 18:76, 1980.

4. Shenker L: Fetal cardiac arrhythmias. *Obstet Gynecol Surv* 34:561, 1979.

5. Heovall G: Congenital paroxysmal tachycardia: a report of three cases. *Acta Paediatr Scand* 62:550, 1973.

6. Klein A, Holzman I, Austin E: Fetal tachycardia to the development of hydrops-attempted pharmacologic cardioversion: case report. *Am J Obstet Gynecol* 134:347, 1979.

7. Kleinman CS, Copel JA: Electrophysiological principles and fetal antiarrhythmic therapy. *Ultrasound Obstet Gynecol* 1:286–297, 1991.

8. Kleinman CS, Copel JA, Weinstein EM, et al.: In utero diagnosis and treatment of supraventricular tachycardia. *Semin Perinatol* 9:113, 1985.

9. Kleinman CS, Hobbins JC, Joffe CC: Echocardiographic studies of the human fetus: prenatal diagnosis of congenital heart disease and cardiac dysrhythmias. *Pediatrics* 65:1059–1066, 1980.

10. Komaromy B, Gaal J, Lampe L: Fetal arrhythmia during pregnancy and labor. *Br J Obstet Gynaecol* 84:492, 1977.

11. Chan T, Potter RT, Liu L: Congenital intraventricular trifascicular block. *Am J Dis Child* 125:82, 1973.

12. Griffiths PS: Congenital heart block. *Circulation* 43:615, 1971.

13. Berube S, Lister G, Towes W, et al.: Congenital heart block and maternal systemic lupus erythematosus. *Am J Obstet Gynecol* 130:595, 1978.

14. McCauliffe DP. Neonatal lupus erythematosus: a transplacentally acquired autoimmune disorder. *Semin Dermatol* 14:47–53, 1995.

15. Scott JS, Maddison PH, Taylor PV, et al.: Connective tissue disease, antibodies to ribonucleoprotein and congenital heart block. *N Engl J Med* 309:209, 1983.

16. Litsey S, Noonan J, O'Connor W, et al.: Maternal connective tissue disease and congenital heart block. Demonstration of immunoglobulin cardiac tissue. *N Engl J Med* 312:98, 1985.

17. Schmidt KG, Ulmer HF, Silverman NH: Perinatal outcomes of fetal complete AV block: a multi-centered experience. *J Am Coll Cardiol* 17:1360–1366, 1991.

18. Carpenter RJ, Strasburger JF, Gorsen A Jr: Fetal ventricular pacing for hydrops secondary to complete AV block. *J Am Coll Cardiol* 8:1434–1436, 1986.

19. Harrison MR: Fetal surgery. *Western J Med* 159:341–349, 1993.

20. Vetter VL, Rashkind H: CHB and connective tissue disease. *N Engl J Med* 309:236–238, 1983.

21. Cetrulo C, Schifrin BS: Fetal heart rate patterns preceding death in utero. *Obstet Gynecol* 48:521, 1976.

22. Kates RB, Schifrin BS: Fetal cardiac asystole during labor. *Obstet Gynecol* 67:549, 1986.

8

FETAL ACID-BASE MONITORING

Although this text is primarily concerned with electronic fetal heart rate (FHR) monitoring, a discussion of fetal acid-base monitoring is included because it is sometimes used as an adjunct to electronic FHR monitoring. An understanding of aerobic and anaerobic metabolism will also give the reader a greater understanding of the significance of fetal acidosis in relation to fetal oxygenation.

In the absence of oxygen, the fetus will be restricted to anaerobic metabolism, with the production of lactic acid, and it is for this reason that fetal pH can be used as an indirect measure of fetal oxygenation. A brief review of glucose metabolism will serve to remind the reader that glucose is first broken down to lactic acid during the anaerobic phase of the carbohydrate metabolic pathway. There is only a minimal amount of energy produced at this point, but when lactic acid is converted to CO_2 in the presence of oxygen, there is a large amount of energy produced by this more efficient aerobic phase of glucose metabolism. When oxygen is absent, the lactic acid cannot be broken down and it accumulates, causing a retention of hydrogen ions, resulting in metabolic acidosis. In the presence of oxygen, the lactic acid is converted to CO_2, which is easily transferred across the placenta to the maternal circulation. When there is umbilical cord occlusion, however, the CO_2 being produced by the fetus cannot be transferred to the maternal circulation, with a resulting CO_2 accumulation in the fetal compartment. The excess CO_2 is hydrolyzed and carbonic acid (H_2CO_3) is formed. The increase in H_2CO_3 forces the equilibrium toward the dissociated H^+ and HCO_3^- components, resulting in fetal acidosis. Of course, this respiratory acidosis can be easily reversed when the umbilical cord occlusion is released and CO_2 is equilibrated across the placenta by the maternal circulation (Fig. 8.1).

During periods of metabolic acidosis resulting from fetal hypoxia with production of lactic acid, there is a decrease in the buffer base as the various components (bicarbonate, phosphates, hemoglobin, and protein) absorb the excess hydrogen ions being produced. The normal fetal base deficit is approximately 7 mEq/L, but when fetal metabolic acidosis occurs, it may exceed 10 or 15 mEq/L (1). The pCO_2 may be mildly increased and, of course, the fetal pH will be decreased.

Fetal respiratory acidosis is characterized by a high pCO_2. The normal fetal pCO_2 is usually 40 to 50 mm Hg. With prolonged umbilical cord occlusion, it may increase significantly, which will result in a respiratory acidosis characterized by very little change in the base deficit, a decrease in pH, and an increased pCO_2.

Fetal scalp pH values usually fall between the umbilical artery (lower pH) and the umbilical vein that has a higher pH because it is carrying freshly oxygenated and decarbonated blood from the placenta. In the previous edition of this book, fetal scalp blood pH values below 7.20 were considered a basis for expeditious delivery (2,3). More recent studies indicate that the lower range of umbilical arterial pH in normal pregnancies is in the range of 7.10 to 7.15 (4). In the past decade, there have been numerous publications that point to an umbilical arterial pH of 7.0 as being the threshold for pathologic fetal acidemia (4–14). In fact, today fetal scalp pH monitoring is not done in most institutions, but cord blood pH at delivery is frequently done. Therefore these values for umbilical artery pH assume more importance when determining the degree of hypoxia that may have preceded birth.

When a fetus is hypoxic, the resulting metabolic acidosis can really only be reversed by adequate fetal oxygenation, because we lack the ability to directly administer fixed base to the fetus the way we can to the neonate in the form of bicarbonate. The process for reversing fetal metabolic acidosis usually takes 20 or 30 minutes or longer depending on the degree of acidosis (15). Thus, if one were to recognize a remedial cause for hypoxic fetal metabolic acidosis, the trend of serial fetal pH values would be more important than the absolute value in assessing recovery. This concept of intrauterine resuscitation is important to consider because hasty intervention with an acidotic fetus may result in an acidotic neonate with compromised pulmonary blood flow due to the acidosis: The reoxygenation of this neonate may be more difficult than having allowed more time for intrauterine resuscitation. Of course, the validity of this concept is dependent on the remedial character of the fetal hypoxia. If the fetal hypoxia is not remedial, delay could be detrimental. Thus, if the cause of the fetal hypoxemia were an abruption, delay would be deleterious; but, if the cause

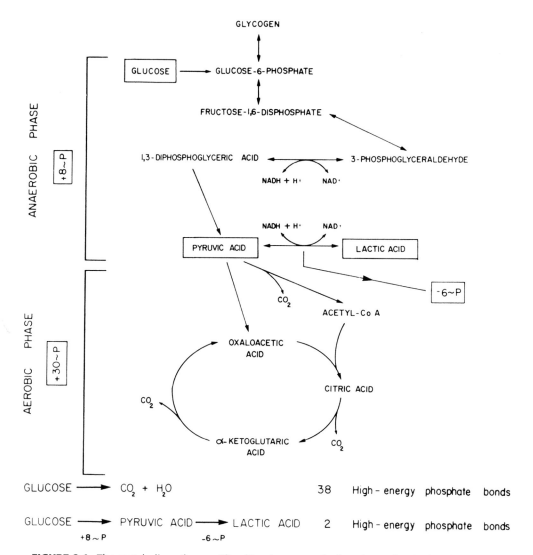

FIGURE 8.1. The metabolic pathway utilized in glucose catabolism shows that in the absence of oxygen (anaerobic phase), the end product is lactic acid, which will produce metabolic acidosis if not metabolized to CO_2 via aerobic metabolic pathways. (From Hon EH, Khazin AF: Biochemical studies of the fetus. I. The fetal pH monitoring system. *Obstet Gynecol* 33:220, 1968, with permission.)

were oxytocin hyperstimulation, delaying the intervention with discontinuation of the oxytocin, position change, and administration of oxygen could clearly benefit the fetus more than a cesarean section.

Fetal respiratory acidosis due to umbilical cord occlusion will clear very rapidly if the cord occlusion is released. The main significance of fetal respiratory acidosis is that, if one is not aware of its possibility, it may be misinterpreted as fetal metabolic acidosis and could lead to inappropriate intervention. Clinically, it is important to understand that if a fetal scalp sample is taken during or soon after a variable deceleration pattern in the FHR, a low fetal pH may be seen because of cord occlusion and respiratory acidosis (Fig. 8.2). For this reason, it is usually valuable to measure a pCO_2 and/or a base deficit on the scalp or umbilical cord blood to know the respiratory component.

At the time of the first fetal scalp blood sample, the clinician may also measure the maternal venous blood pH if significant maternal acid-base imbalance is suspected (15). Fetal scalp blood pH usually runs about 0.1 pH unit below the maternal pH; this guideline may be used in interpreting fetal scalp pH values in association with a significant maternal acidosis or alkalosis. Maternal metabolic acidosis may be seen in association with dehydration and exhaustion, especially during late labor. Maternal respiratory alkalosis has been reported in association with hyperventilation (16) and may be significant in patients instructed in breathing aids to labor where hyperventilation is prominent. A study by Bowen et al. (17) indicated that maternal-fetal pH differences were of more significance than absolute fetal scalp pH alone.

During late labor, caput formation and stasis of blood in the fetal scalp may produce local acidosis, resulting in a fetal

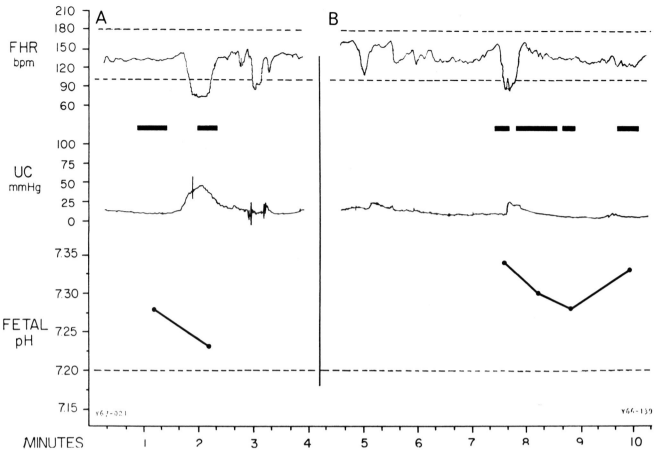

FIGURE 8.2. Fetal scalp blood pH changes during variable deceleration. Note the rapid fall and rise in pH associated with variable deceleration of the fetal heart rate. *UC*, uterine contraction. (From Hon EH, Khazin AF: Biochemical studies of the fetus. 1. The fetal pH monitoring systems. *Obstet Gynecol* 3 3:20, 1968, with permission.)

scalp blood pH below that of the central fetal circulation (18). There is no way to be certain that this is the case until after delivery, when a fetal scalp blood pH lower than the umbilical artery pH would clearly indicate a local cause of the fetal scalp blood acidosis.

EQUIPMENT NECESSARY FOR FETAL SCALP BLOOD SAMPLING

Before sampling fetal blood, the correct equipment must be available, and there must also be an assistant to help hold the patient in position, make notations on the monitor, connect the light source to the battery, accept the filled capillary tubes from the physician, and prepare them properly for the laboratory.

A sterile tray (now available with disposable items) should contain the following: (a) four or five 200-μL heparinized capillary tubes, (b) a conical endoscope with light source, (c) a 2-mm blade on a long handle, (d) silicone grease, (e) 10 or 15 sponges, and (f) a long-handled sponge

holder. The physician should wear sterile gloves and the patient should be prepped and draped in a sterile manner.

TECHNIQUE OF FETAL SCALP BLOOD SAMPLING

The optimum position of the patient for fetal scalp blood sampling is very important. This technique is difficult in early labor, and without proper patient positioning, it is impossible.

The lithotomy position with a patient in stirrups and the maternal buttocks extending over the edge of the table is preferred by most. This can be done in most convertible labor beds, but, if not available, it is easily accomplished in the delivery room. The lateral Sims' position is also satisfactory, requires less patient movement, and allows the patient to remain in the lateral position. When using the lateral Sims' position, it is important that the patient be well flexed at the hip with the lower leg extended. The upper leg should be flexed and held by an assistant with the patient's buttocks extending well over the edge of the bed to allow the person taking the scalp sample to be positioned below the level of the maternal vagina. With both lithotomy and Sims' techniques, the most important factor is for the scalp sampler to be able to angle the cone downward below the horizontal.

With the patient in position, the cone (with light source) is inserted into the posterior fornix under direct visualization. Once the cone is inserted past the anterior lip of the cervix, the cone is angled anteriorly into the cervix and the presenting part is visualized. A sponge is used to wipe the scalp surface clean and then silicone grease is applied to form a nonwettable surface that will allow the fetal scalp blood to form in easily accessible beads. A standard fetal scalp blade with a depth of 2 mm is then used with a quick "stab" to make a clean incision and blood will appear. A 200-μL heparinized capillary tube is then inserted to touch the drop of blood, and keeping the tube angled downward, the blood is allowed to flow by gravity. About one fourth of a tube of blood without bubbles is needed for a pH, but for complete fetal scalp blood gases (pH, pCO_2, pO_2, and base deficit) the tube should be about three-fourths full. After taking the sample, the capillary tube should be immediately handed to an assistant for proper sealing and mixing with a magnetic "flea." Pressure with a sponge should be kept on the scalp wound through the next two contractions and it should then be observed during another contraction to be sure the bleeding has stopped. Sometimes, more pressure is required, and other times (rarely), it may be necessary to put a skin clip on the wound to stop the bleeding. Once fetal scalp blood sampling has been done, continued observation of the patient must be carried out, as even what appears to be "heavy show" during labor may be significant fetal hemorrhage from the scalp puncture site [19].

INDICATIONS FOR FETAL SCALP BLOOD SAMPLING

Total agreement on the indications for fetal scalp blood sampling does not exist. Certainly, if an institution does not have 24-hour ready access to accurate microblood gas analysis with a 10- to 15-minute turnaround time, fetal scalp blood sampling should not be used. The ability to implement decisions for rapid operative intervention is also necessary to effectively use this technique.

Given the necessary logistical support, the indications for fetal scalp blood sampling should be limited to patients who are in labor with ruptured membranes and cervical dilatation sufficient to allow introduction of the cone (usually 2 to 3 cm) and with the fetal head at a station that is within 2 cm of the spines. Fetal scalp blood sampling for acid-base studies should be limited to patients who have electronic FHR tracings suggestive of hypoxia or to clarify a pattern of absent variability without decelerations or accel-

erations. The better one understands FHR monitoring, the less necessary fetal scalp blood sampling will be. On our service, fetal scalp sampling is used in the following situations.

1. A confusing FHR pattern is present with elements that suggest fetal hypoxia.
2. There is a sustained flat FHR without ominous periodic changes.
3. Uncorrectable late deceleration with good variability is present in a patient for whom vaginal delivery is anticipated within 60 to 90 minutes.

CORRELATION BETWEEN FETAL HEART RATE PATTERNS, FETAL pH, AND OUTCOME

Continuous electronic FHR monitoring provides the best "front-line screen" for intrapartum fetal surveillance because the technique is easy, can be done with intact membranes, and most importantly, because it gives continuous data. Fetal scalp blood sampling will only give information about the time the sampling occurred, cannot be done until labor is well under way with ruptured membranes, and is much more difficult than the application of the electronic monitoring device. For these reasons, electronic FHR monitoring is used as the primary means of surveillance, with fetal scalp blood pH sampling used as the backup technique as a comment on the electronically derived FHR pattern.

Early studies on the correlation between FHR patterns and fetal scalp blood pH revealed that there was at least a general correlation [3,12,15,20–24]. Kubli et al. [2] showed that it was indeed rare to have a fetal scalp blood pH value below 7.20 with an innocuous FHR pattern. However, many patterns of late deceleration and moderate-to-severe variable deceleration were often associated with fetal scalp blood pH values above 7.20. Furthermore, approximately 10% of fetal scalp blood pH samples obtained at the time of delivery were found to be below the values found in the umbilical artery [17]. This suggests that local factors in the fetal scalp may frequently be responsible for a falsely low fetal scalp blood pH value.

The correlation between fetal scalp blood pH measurement and neonatal Apgar score increases as the sample is taken closer to the time of birth. With samples taken within 5 minutes of delivery, Hon and Khazin [15] and Modanlou et al. [19] showed that the correlation between low pH and low Apgar scores at both 1 and 5 minutes was very high. However, there appears to be a rather poor correlation between fetal pH and Apgar scores between 7 and 10. This may be accounted for partially by local factors that may make the fetal pH low at the scalp when the central fetal circulation is normal, especially at the time of delivery when caput formation is the greatest.

Finally, it should be kept in mind that changes in fetal scalp blood pH develop only after significant anaerobic metabolism has occurred, whereas FHR changes of late deceleration may occur with early hypoxemia before metabolic acidosis has developed. This probably accounts for the higher correlation between low pH and low Apgar scores with scalp sampling (15) and the high correlation between normal FHR patterns and high Apgar scores with electronic FHR monitoring. Studies from the past 10 to 12 years indicate that unless fetal arterial cord blood pH is below 7.00, it is unlikely that asphyxia proximate to delivery can account for subsequent central nervous system damage.

INTERPRETATION OF UMBILICAL CORD pH AND BLOOD GASSES OBTAINED AT THE TIME OF DELIVERY

Today, fetal scalp blood sampling is seldom done and blood gas interpretation is most often done on umbilical arterial and venous samples obtained from a clamped cord segment obtained just after the fetus delivers. It is from this data that the critical level of pH on the umbilical artery appears to be 7.0, above which acute intrapartum events do not appear to cause central nervous system damage (4–8). Furthermore the pCO_2 and base deficit must be evaluated to determine the degree of the acidosis, which is metabolic as opposed to respiratory. With sudden acute events where umbilical flow through the placenta is decreased, such as with umbilical cord occlusion, there is a rapid increase in pCO_2 on the arterial side, and because of decreased flow through the placenta, the acidosis may be mostly due to CO_2 accumulation in the fetus. This respiratory acidosis occurs very rapidly, and similarly, if the umbilical flow through the placenta is restored, the respiratory acidosis clears rapidly due to the high diffusibility of CO_2 across the placenta. Because of this rapid correction of respiratory acidosis, there is characteristically a wide difference in both the pH and the pCO_2 between the umbilical artery and vein when cord occlusion is the cause of the umbilical arterial respiratory acidosis. Under conditions of fetal hypoxia due to uteroplacental insufficiency with adequate umbilical flow, the metabolic acidosis is the result of lactic acid accumulation because of the incomplete metabolism of glucose, which requires oxygen to convert lactic acid to carbon dioxide. This process occurs over time and develops much slower than respiratory acidosis due to acute umbilical arterial occlusion. Similarly, this metabolic acidosis takes longer to clear and there is a much smaller difference between the umbilical arterial and umbilical venous pH and an increase in the base deficit results because of the depletion of buffer base by the acid production resulting from anaerobic metabolism.

With these principles in mind, the significance of fetal acidosis can be better understood if one looks at pCO_2 and base deficit in both the umbilical artery and vein. For example, if there is a low pH in the umbilical artery associated with primarily an elevated pCO_2, it is unlikely to explain

neurologic damage occurring as a result of events proximate to delivery. Furthermore an associated large pH and pCO_2 difference between the artery and vein indicates that the umbilical arterial acidosis is not due to hypoxia unless there is also an increased base deficit which will be seen to be more equal between the artery and vein. Unfortunately, sometimes it is only possible to get umbilical venous blood, and in this case the base deficit still allows the clinician to evaluate the significance of the venous blood gases because if sufficient anaerobic metabolism had occurred to cause later CNS damage, the base deficit would be elevated in the vein as well, even though the pCO_2 in the umbilical vein does not reflect the umbilical arterial values. In cases of fetal umbilical arterial pHs below 7.0 due to acute intrapartum events, there is usually a mixed respiratory and metabolic acidosis, but if the base deficit is below 12 to 16 mmol/L, the likelihood of later cerebral palsy due to hypoxia proximate to birth is low (11).

FETAL SCALP AND ACOUSTIC STIMULATION AS A SUBSTITUTE FOR pH SAMPLING

In 1982, Clark and coworkers (25) reported on 200 patients who had fetal scalp blood sampling and noted that none were acidotic if there was a FHR acceleration associated with the fetal scalp blood sampling. In a subsequent prospective study, they found that no fetus with a fetal scalp blood pH below 7.19 demonstrated acceleration at the time of scalp sampling (26). In 1986, Rice and Benedetti (27) showed that 70 of 71 fetuses with acceleration had a pH above 7.20, whereas 7 of 32 with no acceleration had fetal scalp blood pH values below 7.20 (Figs. 8.3 and 8.4).

Smith et al. (28) recently reported on a similar correlation between fetal acceleration in response to sound stimulation with an artificial larynx. In their study of fetuses with abnormal FHR patterns, 30 of 64 fetuses that showed acceleration in response to sound had a pH above 7.25, while 18 of 34 that showed no acceleration with sound were acidotic.

These data on fetal scalp stimulation and fetal sound stimulation would indicate that fetuses that respond to either of these stimuli with FHR acceleration are very unlikely to have a simultaneous fetal scalp blood pH that is acidotic. If the fetus does not respond with acceleration to either of these stimuli, it would appear that approximately 50% will show acidosis on a simultaneously obtained fetal scalp blood sample. Because most hospitals with obstetrics units do not have fetal scalp sampling available (29), this approach would seem to be helpful when there is concern about the FHR pattern. In fact, even if one does have fetal scalp blood sampling available, it would not appear to be necessary in the fetus that responds to sound or scalp stimulation with FHR acceleration. In some institutions, fetal scalp stimulation and acoustic stimulation have virtually replaced fetal scalp blood sampling without an increase in

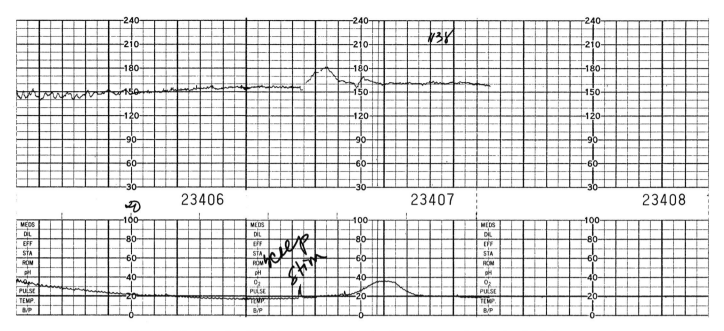

FIGURE 8.3. Example of fetal heart rate acceleration in response to fetal scalp stimulation.

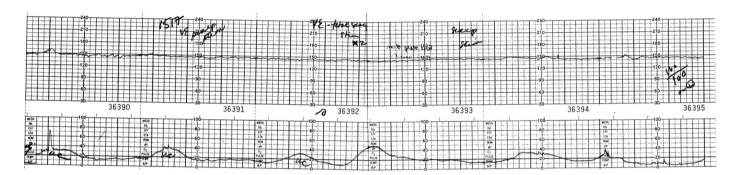

FIGURE 8.4. Example of no fetal heart rate acceleration in response to fetal scalp stimulation.

cesarean section rates for nonreassuring fetal status on the electronic fetal monitor recording (30). It is inappropriate to use scalp or vibroacoustic stimulation during a deceleration. The value of these techniques is when the stimulation occurs during a time when the FHR is at its baseline rate and the acceleration evoked is above the baseline.

CLINICAL INTERPRETATION OF FETAL SCALP pH VALUES

In patients with nonreassuring FHR patterns, if the fetal scalp blood pH is above 7.20, or if the fetus responds to scalp or sound stimulation with FHR acceleration, it is reasonable to continue to observe the patient. If the nonreassuring FHR pattern persists, however, one is then obliged to resample or repeat scalp or sound stimulation at appropriate intervals not to exceed 30 minutes, but sometimes less, depending on other findings and the evolution of the FHR pattern.

When using fetal scalp blood sampling, if the fetal scalp pH is above 7.20, in patients with nonreassuring FHR patterns, continued observation is appropriate. Because the level of pathologic fetal acidosis, consistent with possible damaging asphyxia, does not occur before the umbilical artery pH is below 7.0, when monitoring patients by fetal scalp pH with nonreassuring FHR patterns, strategies for intervention would involve avoidance of delivering a fetus with an umbilical arterial pH in the 7.0 or below range.

It is thus left for the clinician to use electronic FHR monitoring, fetal scalp blood sampling, and the response to fetal scalp or sound stimulation as complementary methods that are still only parts of the whole clinical picture to be appreciated in making appropriate decisions for intervention or nonintervention (Fig. 8.5).

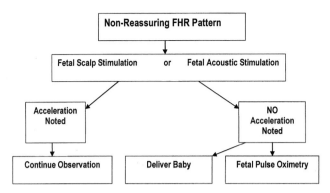

FIGURE 8.5. Algorithm for management of nonreassuring fetal heart rate patterns with fetal scalp stimulation and fetal scalp blood sampling.

In Chapter 10 a full discussion of fetal pulse oximetry will be presented as a possible means of evaluating nonreassuring FHR patterns.

REFERENCES

1. Hon EH, Khazin AF: Observations on fetal pH and fetal biochemistry. I. Base deficit. *Am J Obstet Gynecol* 105:721, 1969.
2. Kubli F, Hon E, Khazin A, et al.: Observations on heart rate and pH in the human fetus during labor. *Am J Obstet Gynecol* 104:1190, 1969.
3. Saling E, Schneider D: Biochemical supervision of the foetus during labour. *J Obstet Gynaecol Br Commonw* 74:799, 1967.
4. Gilstrap LC, Leveno KJ, Burris J, et al.: Diagnosis of birth asphyxia on the basis of fetal pH, Apgar score, and newborn cerebral dysfunction. *Am J Obstet Gynecol* 161:825–830, 1989.
5. Goldaber KG, Gilstrap LC, Leveno KJ, et al.: Pathologic fetal acidemia. *Obstet Gynecol* 78:1103–1107, 1991.
6. Andres RL, Saade G, Gilstrap LC, et al.: Association between umbilical blood gas parameters and neonatal morbidity and death in neonates with pathologic fetal acidemia. *Am J Obstet Gynecol* 181: 867–871, 1999.
7. Winkler CL, Hauth JC, Tucker JM, et al.: Neonatal complications at term as related to the degree of umbilical artery acidemia. *Am J Obstet Gynecol* 164:637–641, 1991.
8. Goodwin TM, Belai I, Hernandez P, et al.: Asphyxial complications in the term newborn with severe umbilical acidemia. *Am J Obstet Gynecol* 162:1506–1512, 1992.
9. van den Berg PP, Nelson WLDM, Jongsma HW, et al.: Neonatal complications in newborns with an umbilical artery pH < 7.00. *Am J Obstet Gynecol* 175:1152–1157, 1996.
10. Sehdev HM, Stamilio DM, Macones GA, et al.: Predictive factors for neonatal morbidity in neonates with an umbilical cord pH less than 7.00. *Am J Obstet Gynecol* 177:1030–1034, 1997.
11. Low JA, Lindsay BG, Derrick EJ: Threshold of metabolic acidosis associated with newborn complications. *Am J Obstet Gynecol* 177:1391–1394, 1997.
12. Low JA, Panagiotopoulos C, Derrick EJ: Newborn complications after intrapartum asphyxia with metabolic acidosis in the preterm fetus. *Am J Obstet Gynecol* 172:805–810, 1995.
13. Low JA: Intrapartum fetal asphyxia: definition, diagnosis and classification. *Am J Obstet Gynecol* 176:957, 1997.
14. King TA, Jackson GL, Josey S, et al.: The effect of profound umbilical artery acidemia in term neonates admitted to the newborn nursery. *J Pediatr* 132:624–629, 1998.
15. Hon EH, Khazin AF: Biochemical studies of the fetus. I. The fetal pH monitoring system. *Obstet Gynecol* 33:219, 1968.
16. Miller F, Petrie R, Arce J, et al.: Hyperventilation during labor. *Am J Obstet Gynecol* 120:489, 1974.
17. Bowen L, Kochenour N, Rehm N, et al.: Maternal-fetal pH difference and fetal scalp pH as predictors of neonatal outcome. *Obstet Gynecol* 67:487, 1986.
18. Kubli, F: Influence of labor on fetal acid-base balance. *Clin Obstet Gynecol* 11:155, 1968.
19. Modanlou H, Smith E, Paul RH, et al.: Complications of fetal blood sampling during labor. *Clin Pediatr* 12:603, 1973.
20. Modanlou H, Yeh SY, Hon H, et al.: Fetal and neonatal biochemistry and Apgar scores. *Am J Obstet Gynecol* 117:942, 1973.
21. Wood C, Lumbley J, Renou P: A clinical assessment of foetal diagnostic methods. *J Obstet Br Commonw* 74:823, 1967.
22. Tejani N, Mann L, Bhakthavathsalan A, et al.: Correlation of fetal heart rate-uterine contraction patterns with fetal scalp blood pH. *Obstet Gynecol* 46:392, 1975.
23. Hon EH, Khazin AF: Biochemical studies of the fetus. II. Fetal pH and Apgar scores. *Obstet Gynecol* 33:237, 1969.
24. Schifrin B, Dame L: Fetal heart rate patterns prediction of Apgar score. *JAMA* 219:322, 1973.
25. Clark S, Gimovsky M, Miller F: Fetal heart rate response to fetal scalp blood sampling. *Am J Obstet Gynecol* 144:706, 1982.
26. Clark S, Gimovsky M, Miller F: The scalp stimulation test: A clinical alternative to fetal scalp pH blood sampling. *Am J Obstet Gynecol* 148:274, 1984.
27. Rice PE, Benedetti TJ: Fetal heart rate acceleration with fetal blood sampling. *Obstet Gynecol* 68:469, 1986.
28. Smith C, Nguyen H, Phelan J, et al.: Intrapartum assessment of fetal well-being: a comparison of fetal acoustic stimulation and acid base determinations. *Am J Obstet Gynecol* 155:726, 1986.
29. Clark S, Paul R: Intrapartum fetal surveillance: the role of fetal scalp blood sampling. *Am J Obstet Gynecol* 153:717, 1985.
30. Goodwin TM, Milner-Masterson L, Paul RH: Elimination of fetal scalp blood sampling on a large clinical service. *Obstet Gynecol* 83:971–974, 1994.

CLINICAL MANAGEMENT OF NONREASSURING FETAL HEART RATE PATTERNS

The general premise of electronic fetal heart rate (FHR) monitoring is that when the FHR pattern is normal or "reassuring," then the likelihood of a hypoxic, acidotic fetus is highly unlikely. The opposite is, however, often not the case; that is, when the FHR is suggestive of hypoxia and/or acidosis the fetus is more often vigorous and not acidotic at birth. Therefore the term previously used, "fetal distress," was inaccurate. This has generally been replaced by the term "nonreassuring fetal status," which is to say that all of the data available for assessing the fetus in labor do not provide reassurance that the fetus is not hypoxic and acidotic. If the term fetal distress is used, one must realize its limitations. There is no agreed definition of fetal distress because the term has various meanings for different people. Although not interchangeable, the terms fetal distress, fetal asphyxia, and asphyxial trauma are often freely substituted and erroneously equated. This confusion creates many problems for obstetricians, particularly in the increasingly litigious climate of our society. *Dorland's Medical Dictionary* defines asphyxia as a "lack of oxygen and respired air resulting in impending or actual cessation of life." Its Greek origin, "a stopping of the pulse," gives the definition of birth asphyxia an imprecise meaning at best. In the past, asphyxia has been the assumed cause of depressed newborns with low Apgar scores. In the fetus, asphyxia refers to a lack of oxygen resulting in metabolic acidosis (1). Asphyxial trauma suggests cellular damage, primarily to the central nervous system (CNS), subsequent to antepartum or intrapartum compromise. Neither fetal distress nor asphyxia is necessarily associated with cellular death leading to fetal morbidity or mortality (2). In fact, the correlation between a nonreassuring FHR and ultimate outcome is usually poor.

The American College of Obstetricians and Gynecologists carefully reviewed the relationship between FHR patterns, Apgar scores, umbilical cord gases, newborn course, and subsequent outcome. It was determined that birth asphyxia will only correlate with subsequent neurologic damage when the following criteria are met:

1. Profound umbilical artery metabolic or mixed acidemia (pH <7.00, base deficit >20).

2. Five-minute Apgar of 0 to 3.
3. Neonatal neurologic sequelae such as seizures, coma, and hypotonia.
4. Multiorgan system dysfunction such as the cardiovascular, gastrointestinal, hematologic, renal, and/or pulmonary systems (3).

Obtaining an umbilical artery blood gas assessment is critical in establishing this condition (4). We do not recommend routinely obtaining a blood specimen pH assessment on all deliveries as often (about 5% to 10%) an abnormal cord pH will be found in a baby with normal Apgar scores. These babies rarely have complications known to be correlated with acidosis or other problems in the newborn period. Hence we do not find that a cord pH is helpful in a newborn with normal Apgar scores. We do recommend obtaining a specimen of umbilical arterial blood for pH, pCO_2, and base deficit (or excess) in the following situations: all depressed newborns; nonreassuring FHR pattern immediately before delivery, especially when operative delivery has been performed for that indication; heavy meconium staining; babies with anomalies or other situations where the baby is likely to go to the neonatal intensive care unit, and very premature infants (≤32 weeks).

Ideally, the goal of FHR monitoring is to detect fetal hypoxia at its earliest stage and to attempt to prevent asphyxic damage resulting from prolonged and severe hypoxia. The progression of normoxia to hypoxia to metabolic acidosis to asphyxic damage and ultimately death always occurs in that order (Fig. 9.1). When the FHR pattern suggests hypoxia, all measures short of operative delivery (hydration, position change, supplemental oxygen, decreasing/discontinuing oxytocin, etc.) should be used to try to reverse the situation. If the hypoxic pattern cannot be reversed, then the ideal goal is to deliver the baby expeditiously when a metabolic acidosis occurs but before damage results. If delivery is done only when the fetus is hypoxic but not acidotic, then far too many unnecessary operative deliveries will be done, for the majority of hypoxic babies will never become acidotic and will be vigorous at birth and have normal outcomes.

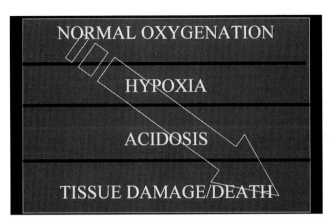

FIGURE 9.1. Model for declining fetal oxygenation with progressive development of hypoxia, metabolic acidosis, damage, and death.

Reassuring FHR patterns include those with accelerations, normal baseline rate, and normal variability. Early decelerations and mild variable decelerations are associated with normal Apgar scores, no acidosis at birth, and normal perinatal outcome. Nonreassuring patterns include the more severe forms of variable deceleration, persistent late decelerations, prolonged decelerations, and various atypical or preterminal patterns. Such nonreassuring patterns are usually associated with normal Apgar scores, but low Apgar scores, when they occur, are usually associated with these patterns (5).

A most important concept that must be realized in evaluating and managing abnormal FHR patterns is the issue of the normal progression of these changes when they are due to hypoxia. For example, tachycardia can be a result of

hypoxia (see Fig. 6.20), but only when there are associated decelerations suggestive of hypoxia. That is to say in the laboring patient persistent late, moderate-to-severe variable or prolonged decelerations are the first indicators of hypoxia and virtually always precede tachycardia if the increase in heart rate is due to hypoxia. Similarly, loss of variability or disappearance of accelerations will not be the first sign of hypoxia and does not require further evaluation or intervention unless associated decelerations suggest a progressive hypoxia. The only exception to this can be the fetus who has tachycardia, absent or decreased variability, and/or no accelerations when the monitor is first placed on the patient. In this situation, one cannot be sure that no hypoxic deceleration pattern preceded these findings.

LATE DECELERATIONS

Late decelerations are found in association with uteroplacental insufficiency and imply some degree of fetal hypoxia (6). A decrease in pO_2 detected by the fetal brain is the only trigger for late decelerations. In their mildest form, late decelerations are associated with normal or increased FHR variability. The pattern is characteristically described as uniform, appearing consistently from one contraction to the next and with the depth of the deceleration often corresponding to the magnitude of each contraction. This rule probably is more applicable once fetal hypoxia is established, but in the earliest phases of developing fetal hypoxia, the pattern may be seen occurring only intermittently (Fig. 9.2). While it would seem prudent to take measures to optimize uterine blood flow at

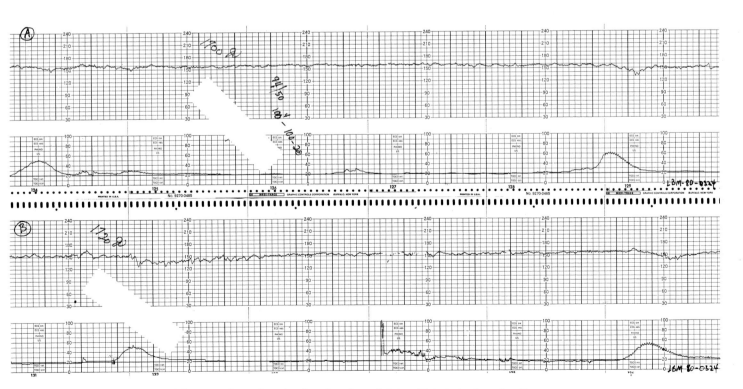

FIGURE 9.2. Intermittent late decelerations in early labor. Note lack of accelerations.

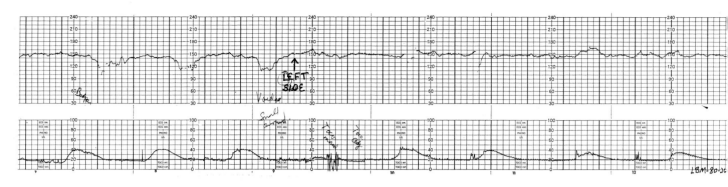

FIGURE 9.3. Late decelerations corrected by turning patient on her side.

this stage, intermittent late decelerations with good or increased FHR variability require close watching and may not become any more severe. In this situation, the patient should be laboring in the lateral position, she should be well hydrated, oxytocin should be decreased or discontinued if contractions seem excessive, and she should be receiving oxygen (Fig. 9.3). If the late decelerations have occurred in association with decreased maternal blood pressure following conduction anesthesia or following the administration of an antihypertensive agent in a patient with hypertension, appropriate measures should be taken to restore blood pressure and placental perfusion (Table 9.1).

TABLE 9.1. MEDICAL MANAGEMENT OF LATE DECELERATION

1. Place patient on side.
2. Administer O_2 (100%) by tight face mask.
3. Discontinue oxytocin.
4. Correct any hypotension.
   (a) Appropriate position change.
   (b) IV hydration with appropriate fluid.
   (c) Reserve pharmacologic pressor treatment (ephedrine) for severe or unresponsive hypotension due to conduction anesthesia.

IV, intravenous.

If persistent late decelerations develop despite maximizing uterine blood flow, the physician is obligated to be sure that a metabolic acidosis has not yet developed. The simplest and most straightforward way of ruling out acidosis is to look for spontaneous accelerations (Fig. 9.4), or in their absence attempt to elicit an acceleration with acoustic or scalp stimulation (Fig. 9.5A). In the presence of a nonreassuring FHR pattern, the presence of accelerations, whether spontaneous or elicited, rules out acidosis. The absence of any acceleration is associated with an approximate 50% chance of acidosis. When no acceleration is elicited, alternatives include continuous fetal pulse oximetry monitoring (Fig. 9.5B) or intermittent scalp pH (Fig. 9.6). As long as the late decelerations persist, this process of ruling out acidosis must be repeated every 20 to 30 minutes. The presence of repeated accelerations or a normal fetal oxygen saturation using oximetry allows the clinician to follow the late decelerations indefinitely as long as the labor is progressing satisfactorily. If one is using scalp pH, realistically this plan for repeating scalp pH every ½ hour can only be continued for a limited time. Therefore, intermittent scalp pH sampling is usually limited to the patient where delivery is expected in a few hours or less. Sometimes, fetal scalp blood sampling may be used for a longer period when there is a great risk to the mother from operative intervention and the clinician is willing to embark on a longer period of serial scalp sampling. If

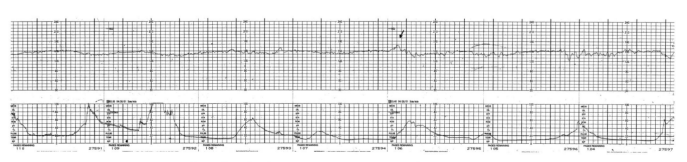

FIGURE 9.4. Persistent late decelerations. Note the presence of a spontaneous acceleration at **panel 27595** *(arrow).* The presence of the acceleration virtually eliminates, at this point in time, any likelihood of a metabolic acidosis.

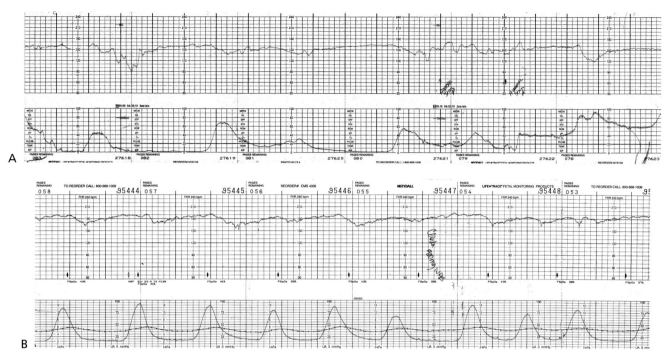

FIGURE 9.5. A,B: Both cases illustrate persistent late decelerations. In **A,** the clinician is reassured of the absence of a metabolic acidosis with an acceleration following acoustic stimulation. In **B,** reassurance is attained using fetal pulse oximetry, which reveals a continuous fetal oxygen saturation above 30%.

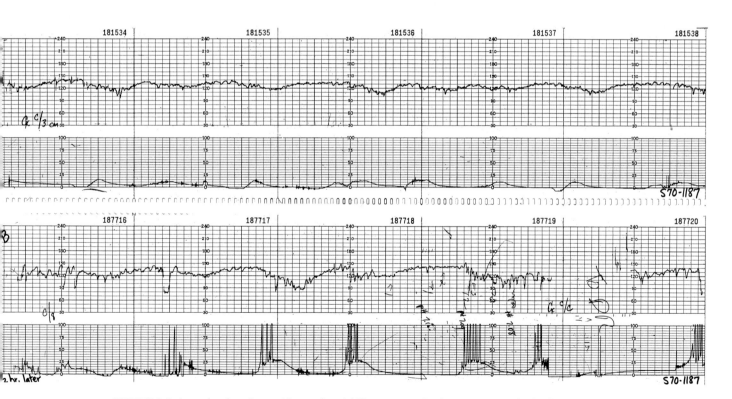

FIGURE 9.6. Late decelerations with good variability are seen in the **upper panel.** The **lower panel** is 1½ hours later, showing a continuation of late deceleration with good variability. The pH taken at this time was 7.08, suggesting that earlier intervention might have been advisable.

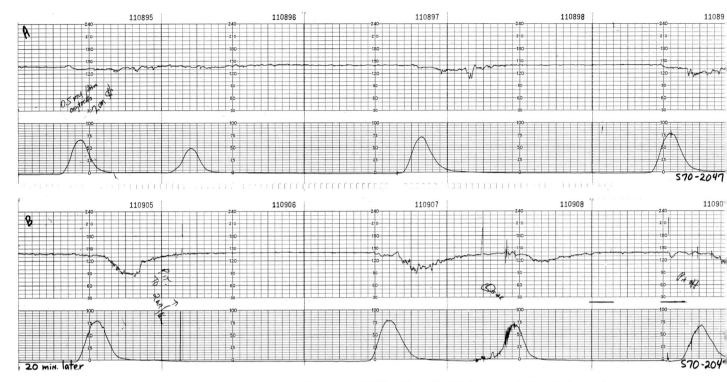

FIGURE 9.7. Late deceleration with poor variability. (From Paul R, Freeman R: *Selected records of intrapartum fetal monitoring with self instruction.* USC Publishers, Los Angeles, 1971, with permission.)

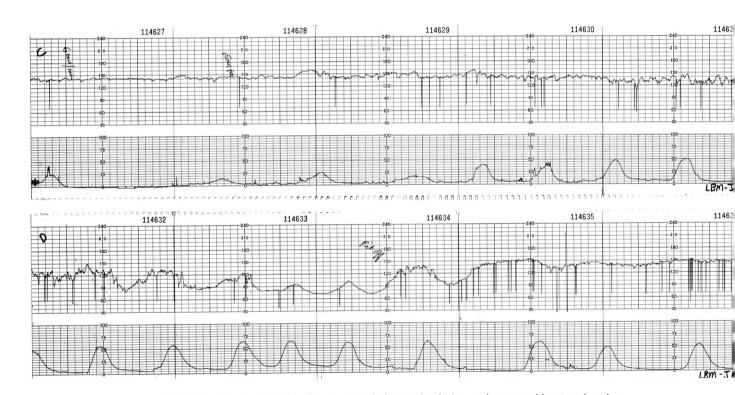

FIGURE 9.8. Late deceleration due to oxytocin hyperstimulation and corrected by stopping the oxytocin infusion when it says "Pit off" in **section 114634**. (From Paul R, Freeman R: *Selected records of intrapartum fetal monitoring with self instruction.* USC Publishers, Los Angeles, 1971, with permission.)

opting to use serial fetal scalp blood sampling, operative delivery can be avoided as long as the pH stays above 7.25. If there is a downward trend below 7.25 or if the value is less than 7.20, scalp sampling should be abandoned and delivery effected by the most expeditious means. However, it should be remembered that these guidelines are fairly conservative and individualization of intervention based on the rapidity of the trend, the stage of labor, the trend and severity of the FHR pattern, and the entire clinical picture of the patient can and should be taken into account. When accelerations alone are relied on to ensure the absence of acidosis in the setting of irreversible persistent late decelerations, the absence of accelerations for more than 30 minutes will usually require operative delivery.

The discussion thus far has concerned the management of late deceleration in association with good variability. An FHR pattern of persistent late decelerations with complete absence of variability is much more ominous and almost always associated with fetal acidosis (Fig. 9.7). When encountered in the antepartum or intrapartum period, our approach is to discontinue uterine stimulation and expedite delivery. This is most often via cesarean section. These patients are unable to tolerate labor without continuing late decelerations (7).

One frequent cause of late decelerations is excessive stimulation of contractions with oxytocin. Frequently, discontinuation of oxytocin results in improvement of the FHR (Fig. 9.8). The careful reinstitution of oxytocin at a lower rate often results in continued labor progress without continued late decelerations.

One situation that arises not infrequently, we often call fetal intolerance to labor. When the late decelerations are persistent and oxytocin is discontinued, the decelerations will often resolve; however, in this setting the labor may stop progressing. If the late decelerations reappear, but the fetus is reactive (or oximetry is reassuring), the clinician may choose to document the fact that he/she chooses to continue the oxytocin despite the late decelerations as long as there is no evidence of acidosis as this is the only way to have a chance of labor progressing to delivery.

VARIABLE DECELERATIONS

Variable decelerations are most frequently the result of umbilical cord compression. It is the most common periodic change observed in laboring patients, being present in over 50% of them at one time or another. The pattern is characterized by abrupt decreases in FHR to levels as low as 50 beats per minute (BPM). The pattern varies from one moment to the next and may be influenced by such simple things as maternal position changes. While the pattern is the most profound appearing of the periodic FHR changes, the vast majority of the time it cannot be considered nonreassuring, because, unless the cord occlusion is frequent, prolonged, and severe, there is no increased risk of low Apgar scores, fetal metabolic acidosis, or other significant neonatal morbidity. The problem with variable decelerations is that they may suddenly get much more severe. These decelerations are much less predictable from one minute to the next than late decelerations, which tend to follow a slowly deteriorating course, allowing their development to be watched over time. Also, because variable decelerations can change from one contraction to the next, it is hard to know what to expect in the near future. This makes the management of this pattern especially difficult, particularly when working in a setting without the capability to move rapidly to operative delivery.

We have found that it is much easier to define the limits of reassuring variable decelerations than it is to give absolute criteria for when variable deceleration represents sufficient evidence of hypoxia to demand operative intervention. The following four criteria may be used as a guide to the limits of reassuring variable deceleration (Fig. 9.9):

1. The FHR decelerations last no more than 40 to 60 seconds on a repetitive basis.
2. The return of the FHR to the baseline is abrupt. There is no persistent "late component" manifested by a slow return or a late deceleration after the return.
3. The baseline FHR is not increasing.
4. The FHR variability is not decreasing.

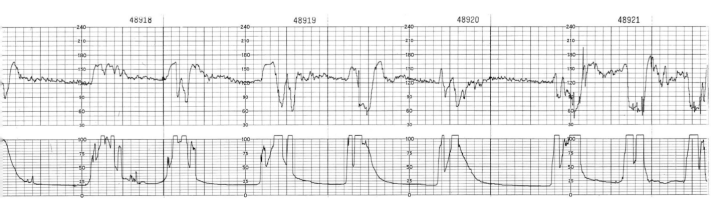

FIGURE 9.9. Reassuring variable decelerations.

While severe variable decelerations, increasing baseline heart rate, and loss of variability in the face of progressive variable decelerations are reasonably reliable indicators of progressively severe cord compression and developing hypoxia, this may not be the case with a slow return to baseline. As described in the chapter on the physiology of FHR patterns, there may be two and possibly three potential causes of a slow return to baseline. First, progressively severe cord compression may result in sufficient residual fetal hypoxia as to result in this pattern (see Fig. 6.21). The other primary mechanism is a combination of late and variable decelerations caused by two different mechanisms: cord compression and placental insufficiency. Finally, there may be a third, more benign cause, perhaps due to slower than usual release of the cord compression. In a recent review of variable decelerations with slow return to baseline in patients who were also being monitored with pulse oximetry, we found that when these patterns were preceded by severe variable or persistent late decelerations, there was indeed an increased likelihood of significant hypoxia. However when such patterns were preceded by neither, there was no more likelihood of hypoxia than in patients with mild variable decelerations (8). Thus slow return to baseline may not always be considered a nonreassuring pattern.

When criteria for nonreassuring variable decelerations are met and the pattern persists, the ability to effect immediate delivery is crucial. Increasing baseline, loss of variabil-

ity, and/or delayed return to baseline can evolve in a short time with variable decelerations (Figs. 9.10 and 9.11). Similar to late decelerations, when variable decelerations meet any of the previous criteria as a nonreassuring pattern, one must either be reassured of the absence of acidosis, using the presence of spontaneous or elicited accelerations, scalp pH, or fetal pulse oximetry, or move expeditiously to delivery.

It is useful from a management perspective to categorize variable decelerations based on their most likely cause (Table 9.2). Variable decelerations due to oligohydramnios usually appear relatively early in labor and these are best reversed using amnioinfusion. Probably the most common cause of variable decelerations are nuchal cords. Nuchal cords probably cause decelerations, not due to compression, but due to the cord tightening, becoming stretched as the fetal head descends into the pelvis. Because in most labors, the rapid phase of descent usually begins between 8 and 10 cm of dilation, it is most common for nuchal cords to manifest variable decelerations at this stage (Fig. 9.12). These patterns are not likely to benefit from amnioinfusion or maternal repositioning. If the pattern becomes nonreassuring, the patient will often benefit by having her push less frequently, giving the fetus more time to recover from the cord compression between contractions (Fig. 9.13). A rare cause of variable or prolonged deceleration is umbilical cord prolapse. When significant variable or prolonged decelera-

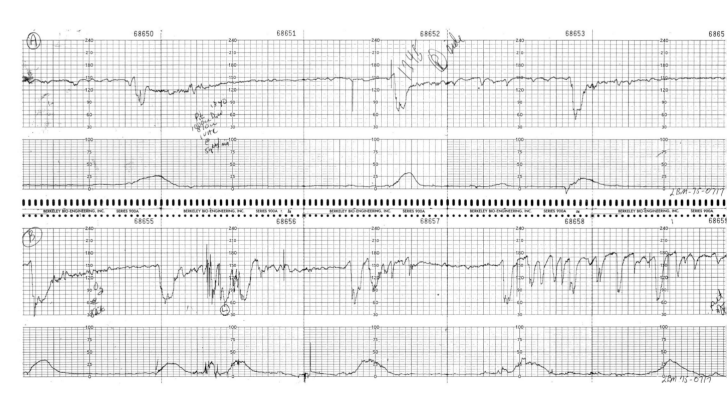

FIGURE 9.10. Variable deceleration with a rising baseline and slow return to baseline. This is a nonreassuring pattern.

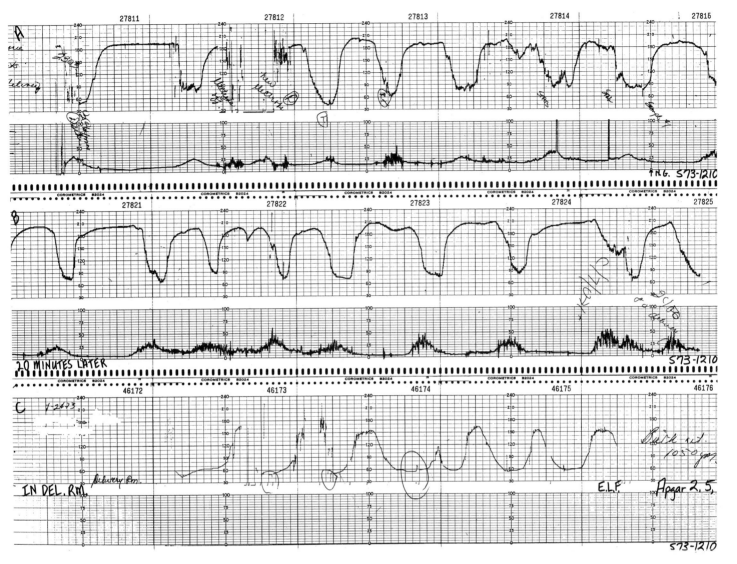

FIGURE 9.11. Variable deceleration with tachycardia and loss of fetal heart rate variability. This pattern is nonreassuring. (From Paul R. Petrie R: *Fetal intensive care current concepts.* USC Publishers, Los Angeles, 1973, with permission.)

TABLE 9.2. MANAGEMENT CLASSIFICATION OF VARIABLE DECELERATIONS

Etiology of Cord Compression	Typical Appearance	Treatment
Nuchal cord	8–10 cm dilation	May consider altering pushing efforts to allow more recovery between contractions
Oligohydramnios	Early in labor	Amnioinfusion
Cord prolapse	Sudden onset, often at the time of membrane rupture	Elevation of presenting part, immediate cesarean section

Unusual cord compression
    Short cords
    Other cord entanglement
    True knots
	Variable timing and shape	Repositioning

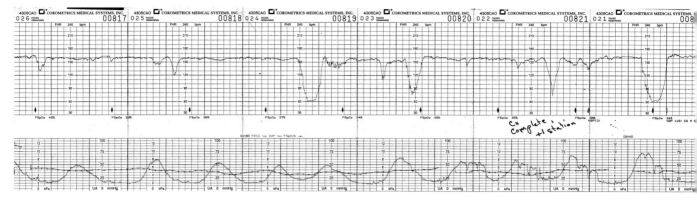

FIGURE 9.12. The new onset of variable decelerations occurring late in labor often heralds the transition to the second stage of labor. As seen in this patient, shortly after the appearance of the first deep variable deceleration, she begins spontaneously pushing and is found to be completely dilated.

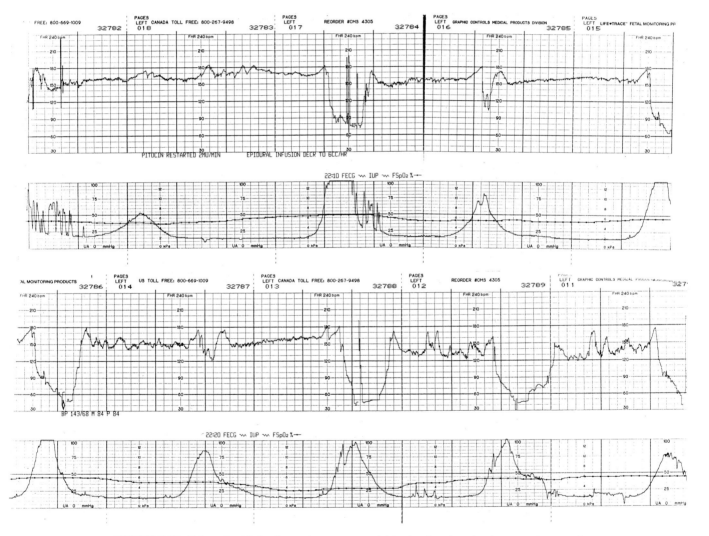

FIGURE 9.13. This patient is having rather severe variable decelerations in the second state of labor. Note that the depth and duration of the deceleration diminishes when the patient is not pushing. This is an effective method to allow additional recovery when significant variable decelerations are occurring in the second stage of labor.

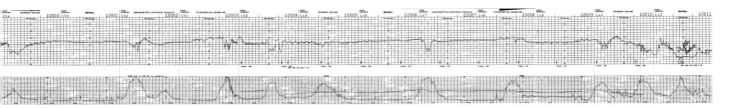

FIGURE 9.14. These variable decelerations are typical of "unusual cords." Their frequency, depth, duration, and shape are inconsistent and they do not bear a regular relationship to contractions. At delivery the umbilical cord was noted to be quite short (11 inches).

tions suddenly appear, this etiology should be considered and a pelvic examination performed immediately because cord prolapse virtually always requires elevation of the presenting part and immediate cesarean section. Finally, there is a group in which no good treatment other than perhaps repositioning may help relieve the cord compression. This group includes cord entanglement other than nuchal cords, such as around a fetal extremity or body, a true knot in the cord, or a short cord. The presentation of these may occur at any time during labor and their appearance may be quite variable (Fig. 9.14).

Generally speaking, persistent and uncorrectable nonreassuring variable decelerations in early labor are best managed with cesarean section delivery unless persistent evidence of absence of acidosis (e.g., accelerations) can be found. On the other hand, during the second stage of labor, it is very common to see variable decelerations with mater-

nal pushing. With continued pushing, these decelerations may become nonreassuring (Fig. 9.15). However, if progress is being made with descent of the presenting part, and the baseline heart rate level and variability remain unchanged, it is better to allow labor to progress than to attempt a difficult midpelvic delivery. It is common to see variable decelerations lasting more than a minute at 2- to 3-minute intervals during the second stage of labor. Other than position change and attempting to have the mother not push with each contraction, we continue to monitor and allow labor to continue as long as the baseline rate is not increasing and the baseline variability remains.

The role for scalp pH in the management of variable decelerations is somewhat problematic. The timing of the sample has a direct influence on the pH result for patients with recurrent variable decelerations. Specimens obtained at or immediately following the nadir of the deceleration

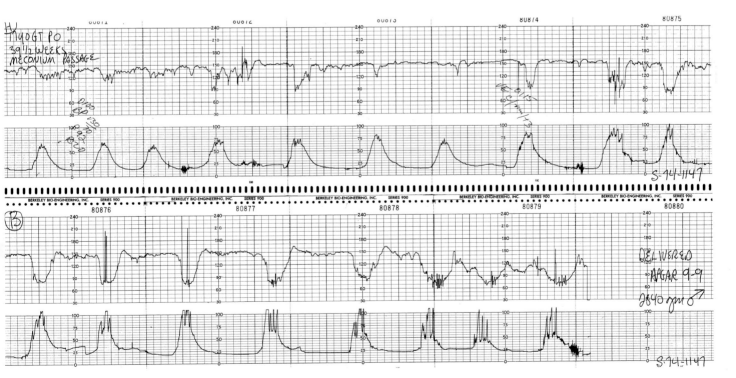

FIGURE 9.15. Variable deceleration of progressive severity occurring at the end of the second stage of labor.

TABLE 9.3. MEDICAL MANAGEMENT OF SEVERE VARIABLE DECELERATIONS

1. Change position to where FHR pattern is the most improved. Often Trendelenburg is helpful.
2. Discontinue oxytocin if running.
3. Check for cord prolapse or imminent delivery by vaginal examination.
4. Administer 100% O_2 by tight face mask.
5. Consider therapeutic amnioinfusion.

FHR, fetal heart rate.

may show transiently low pH due to CO_2 retention and may not reflect a metabolic acidosis. A capillary tube nearly full of fetal blood (>70 μL) is required to also obtain a pCO_2 and determine if the acidosis is metabolic or respiratory. Further, the very nature of variable decelerations is such that even a normal pH result is of little prognostic value if the FHR tracing continues to worsen.

The clinical guideline for management of patients with variable decelerations is, then, to be reassured if the pattern does not exceed the previously stated criteria for nonreassuring variable decelerations and to treat the patient expectantly. If these criteria are exceeded, the general rule is that the closer one estimates vaginal delivery to be, the higher will be the threshold for intervention (Table 9.3). Using this policy on our clinical service has allowed us to safely avoid

intervention in the vast majority of patients with variable decelerations without apparent jeopardy to the fetus. With the introduction of both prophylactic and therapeutic amnioinfusion, the frequency of variable decelerations should be decreased, often making management decisions much easier. Variable decelerations are responsible for most unnecessary cesarean sections performed when the physician is not experienced with fetal monitoring, and they must have been a major reason for operative intervention when only auscultatory FHR monitoring was available.

MANAGEMENT OF PROLONGED DECELERATIONS

Prolonged decelerations lasting several minutes and occurring as more or less isolated events will be observed either in association with identifiable causes or without apparent etiology. If there is no known cause, prolonged decelerations may represent umbilical cord compression of a severe degree or may represent a catastrophic event such as a sudden abruption or a ruptured uterus. The following is a list of known causes of prolonged decelerations that may be identified and managed during the intrapartum period.

1. Hypertonic or prolonged contractions (spontaneous or oxytocin-induced) (Fig. 9.16).

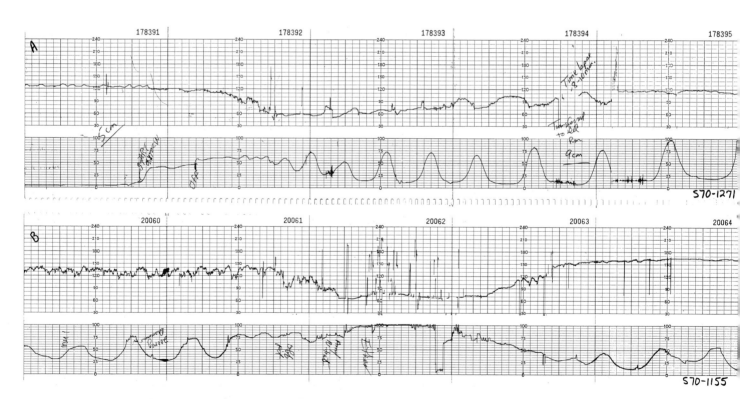

FIGURE 9.16. The **upper panel** demonstrates a tetanic contraction with severe prolonged fetal heart rate (FHR) deceleration after institution of oxytocin. The **lower panel** represents a tetanic contraction with a severe prolonged FHR deceleration after intravenous dimenhydrinate (Dramamine). (From Paul R, Freeman R: *Selected records of intrapartum fetal monitoring with self instruction.* USC Publishers, Los Angeles, 1971, with permission.)

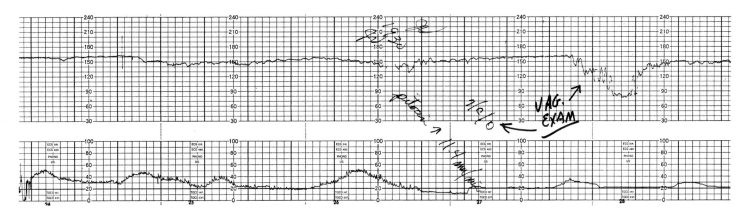

FIGURE 9.17. A prolonged deceleration associated with a vaginal examination.

2. Vaginal examination (Fig. 9.17).
3. Application of internal fetal scalp electrode.
4. Fetal scalp blood sampling.
5. Prolapsed umbilical cord (Fig. 9.18).
6. Maternal seizure.
7. Epidural or spinal block (Fig. 9.19).
8. Supine hypotension.
9. CNS anomalies.
10. Prolonged umbilical cord compression, often associated with rapid descent of the fetus.
11. Maternal respiratory arrest (high spinal, intravenous [IV] narcotic) or cardiac decompensation.
12. Uterine rupture (Fig. 9.20).
13. Abruptio placentae (Fig. 9.21).

When late or prolonged decelerations occur in patients soon after receiving a conduction anesthetic, initial management should be directed at correcting the maternal hypotension by positioning the patient either in the lateral position or, even more effectively, by leaving her supine,

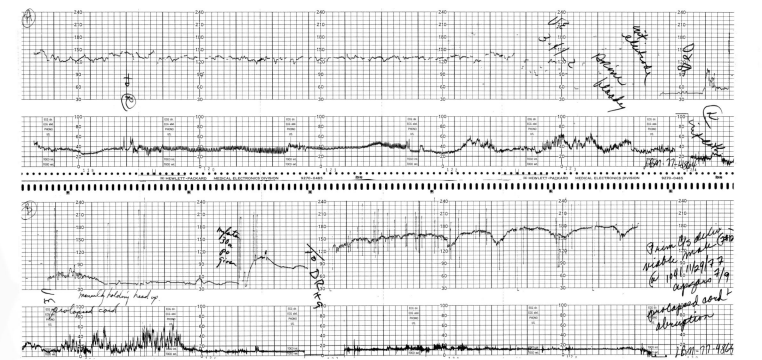

FIGURE 9.18. Toward the end of the **upper panel**, the membranes are ruptured and a fetal scalp electrode is applied because of severe vaginal bleeding. The fetal heart rate (FHR) is noted to be 40 beats per minute (BPM) following the previous 130-BPM rate from the previous Doppler recording. Reexamination at the beginning of the **lower panel** reveals a prolapsed umbilical cord. After elevating the presenting part, the FHR shows a marked tachycardia just before a cesarean section revealed an abruption. The Apgar scores were 7 and 9 at 1 and 5 minutes, respectively.

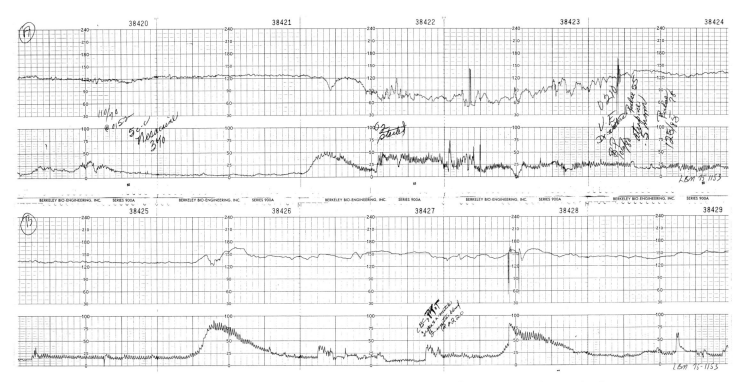

FIGURE 9.19. A prolonged fetal heart rate (FHR) deceleration after activation of an epidural block. During the deceleration, the mother's blood pressure was not low but her pulse rate was only 55, so the anesthesiologist administered 0.5 mg of atropine intravenously. Note the subsequent increase in the FHR and the loss of short-term variability.

instituting sustained left uterine displacement, and raising her legs in the air. These measures will give the patient an "auto-transfusion" of several hundred milliliters of blood. In addition, the patient should receive a rapid infusion of IV fluids (preferably she would have been prehydrated before the block) and be started on oxygen inhalation. In addition, attention should be given to uterine tone because this may be increased with uterine ischemia. With tetanic contractions and prolonged FHR decelerations, consideration should be given to acute tocolysis with a beta agonist such as terbutaline. In the event that these measures do not

restore the blood pressure and the FHR, the use of ephedrine is indicated. Because this drug has both alpha and beta adrenergic effects, it restores blood pressure and is the least likely agent to reduce uterine blood flow (9).

The clinical response to prolonged decelerations in general should follow the following sequence. First, take your time in responding. The few minutes that you do not overreact will result most of the time in two favorable events: first the deceleration will usually spontaneously recover and second you are less likely to unnecessarily frighten the patient. If the deceleration should persist for

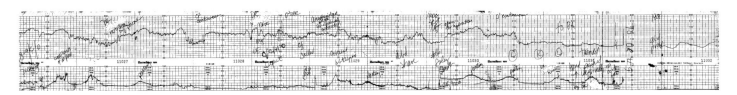

FIGURE 9.20. This is a gravida 2, para 1 with a previous low transverse cesarean section in spontaneous labor at term. Upon reaching 9 cm dilation, the fetus began having variable decelerations. Because of her complaint of the onset of severe lower abdominal pain in conjunction with these decelerations, the physician became concerned over the possibility of a uterine rupture and decided upon cesarean section. In the process, the variable decelerations progressed to an ominous prolonged deceleration. An urgent cesarean section was performed and a large uterine rupture was found. The fetus had Apgar scores of 1 at 1 minute, 4 at 5 minutes, and 7 at 10 minutes, with an umbilical cord arterial pH of 6.90, pCO_2 90, BE −14 and venous pH of 7.10, pCO_2 50, BE −9. This mixed metabolic and respiratory acidosis is characteristic of uterine rupture. The baby ultimately survived without apparent neurologic damage.

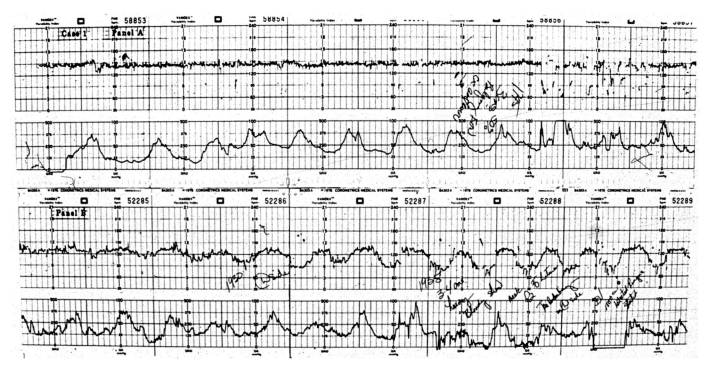

FIGURE 9.21. This patient presents in active labor at term. Other than being in an unusual amount of pain, she had no other historical factors that alert the clinician to a problem. However, on the monitor it is apparent that she is having frequent (tachysystolic) contractions. In the lower panel, late decelerations appear, and in the latter half of that panel, the patient begins having vaginal bleeding. A forceps delivery yielded a baby with Apgar scores of 4 at 1 minute and 7 at 5 minutes, and a large abruptio placentae was revealed when the placenta was delivered. Abruption may present either with prolonged decelerations or persistent later decelerations that may evolve into a prolonged deceleration depending on the severity of the abruption and the degree of uterine hyperactivity.

more than a few minutes (2 to 4 minutes, depending on rate and variability), the next step, especially if this is the first prolonged deceleration, is to perform a vaginal examination. This will reveal if either rapid descent and impending delivery or a prolapsed cord as the etiology. Obviously these are the two most critical issues to identify immediately. The next step is to carefully review the clinical status of the patient and the fetal monitor for possible explanations, going through a mental checklist as outlined in the list at the beginning of this section. The most positive possibility is that a treatable etiology will be identified and the FHR will return to normal. Bleeding and uterine tachysystole or tetany associated with prolonged deceleration may represent abruption and require immediate delivery, as may evidence of uterine rupture.

If a treatable cause, as described in the earlier paragraphs of this section, is not identified and the deceleration persists, the next step, usually now after 5 to 7 minutes, is to move the patient to the operating or delivery room and mobilize the nursing and anesthesia team. Upon arrival to the operating or delivery room, the monitor should be immediately reconnected. If the FHR is still low, then immediate operative delivery is probably now indicated.

The rapidity with which this must be accomplished depends on a number of variables including what the FHR looked like before the onset of the deceleration; whether there is any suggestion of abruption or uterine rupture, which are the most rapidly progressing insults; the depth and duration of the deceleration; how much variability is lost during the deceleration; and whether the FHR appears to be returning to baseline periodically or just stays down. Often following recovery of the prolonged deceleration, if the insult is sufficient, a period of tachycardia and loss of variability and even late decelerations will follow (Fig. 9.18). If the insult is resolved, there is no need for immediate intervention. If the decision is made to proceed to delivery anyway, allowing for intrauterine resuscitation before abdominal or vaginal delivery will in many cases be in the best interest of both the mother and her fetus. How long this will take will vary with the etiology and duration of the insult and the status of the baby before the insult, but often 20 to 40 minutes will elapse before the rate and variability return to normal.

The other common management dilemma with this pattern is with recurrent prolonged decelerations. These are usually due to prolonged cord compression. If they

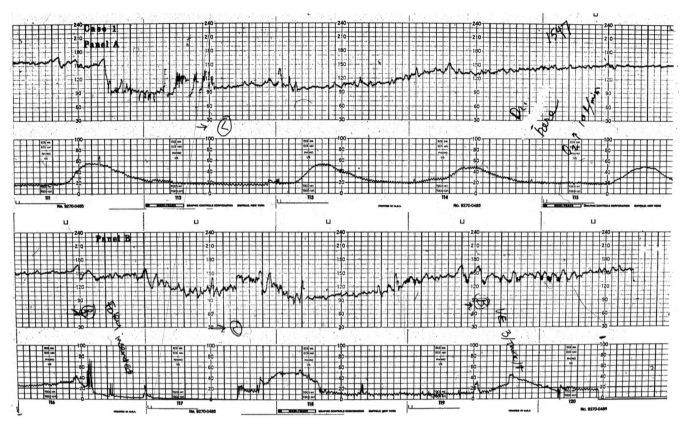

FIGURE 9.22. Recurrent prolonged decelerations are seen in this fetal heart rate (FHR) tracing in early labor. While variability remains normal and there are no signs that the fetus may be becoming acidotic, this remains a concerning pattern as there is a substantial likelihood that the FHR may again go down and not recover or recover as well.

occur in the earlier part of labor and are associated with oligohydramnios, they may resolve with amnioinfusion. If not, they are one of the most difficult patterns to manage. Unlike other patterns, where the basic premise with a nonreassuring pattern is to rule out acidosis, the situation here is quite different. The concern is that the next deceleration will not return to baseline and the clinician will be faced with the urgency of the prolonged deceleration that does not remit as described in the previous paragraph. Thus one must integrate how often they are occurring, how long they stay down below baseline, whether variability is lost during the deceleration, what the pattern looks like when the deceleration resolves, whether meconium is present, and how long before the patient is expected to deliver. In addition, consideration must be given to the individual facility's response time. So early in labor, in a nulliparous patient after several prolonged decelerations, one may choose to intervene operatively fully aware that the fetus is most likely not acidotic nor depressed. The decision is a complex one, and there is never a single right answer as one can never truly have a crystal ball in such situations (Fig. 9.22).

INTERVENTIONS FOR NONREASSURING FETAL STATUS

The ideal intervention for fetal hypoxia is a cause-specific, noninvasive one that permanently reverses the problem. While not always possible this should certainly be the goal. Obviously, the first step in achieving this goal is to recognize the cause of the abnormal FHR pattern. A thorough knowledge of the pathophysiology of FHR changes coupled with a careful clinical patient evaluation and a knowledge of common causes of specific FHR changes will maximize the opportunity for this goal to be achieved. In addition to cause-specific types of interventions, virtually all cases of hypoxia should theoretically also benefit by more generic interventions that have the potential to maximize oxygen delivery and placental exchange.

Nonsurgical Interventions

Oxygen Administration

One of the most obvious ways of maximizing oxygen delivery to the fetus is to give additional oxygen to the mother.

While diffusion across the membrane is driven by pO_2 as opposed to oxygen content, and while maternal pO_2 can be raised substantially with mask oxygen, it is not well-demonstrated that fetal pO_2 is increased substantially by routine maternal oxygen administration. Recent evidence, while still preliminary, from fetuses being monitored with pulse oximetry, does not substantiate a significant rise in fetal SpO_2 using a regular face mask (10). A tight-fitting non-rebreathing mask does appear to increase fetal SpO_2, at least somewhat (10). While this is the state of current knowledge, routine oxygen administration via face mask has become such standard practice with nonreassuring FHR patterns that it is difficult to recommend otherwise until further studies are available to substantiate these preliminary data.

Lateral Positioning

The ideal is for all patients to labor in the lateral recumbent position, at least from the standpoint of maximizing uterine perfusion. The reasons for this are, at least theoretically, twofold. In being inactive and recumbent, the body is required to deliver the least amount of blood flow to other muscles. In either lateral position, there is no compression by the uterus on the vena cava or aorta, thus maximizing cardiac return and cardiac output.

Hydration

Most patients in labor are either restricted or prohibited from taking oral fluids for fear of a requirement of an urgent operative delivery in the presence of a full stomach. If not fluid restricted, individuals involved in sustained exercise, and possibly by inference in active labor, do not voluntarily ingest adequate amounts of fluid and become relatively dehydrated due to this phenomena called "autodehydration." Recent evidence would suggest that the usual amount of intravenous fluid of 125 cc/hour is a gross underestimate of the replacement required in labor (11). Thus by increasing fluid administration, there is potential to maximize intravascular volume and thus uterine perfusion.

Oxytocin

In a patient with a nonreassuring pattern, the more time there is between contractions, the more time there is to maximally perfuse the placenta and deliver oxygen. In patients receiving oxytocin, there is potential to improve oxygenation by decreasing or discontinuing oxytocin. Often, however this becomes a difficult situation, as many patients will stop progressing in labor in terms of continued dilation, descent, or both, if the oxytocin is discontinued. Once the nonreassuring pattern improves or resolves, it is often necessary to restart or increase the oxytocin. If the

nonreassuring pattern then returns, the clinician has a significant dilemma. At this point, it may be appropriate to continue the oxytocin despite the nonreassuring decelerations, especially if there are accelerations or other means of documenting the absence of acidosis (e.g., oxygen saturation). Written documentation, explaining the necessity and appropriateness of continuing oxytocin in this situation is especially important. The situation with patients in whom persistent nonreassuring patterns develop, especially with loss of accelerations or absence of other reassurance, and who require discontinuation of oxytocin, but then fail to progress because adequate contractions cannot be sustained, is often referred to as "fetal intolerance to labor."

Tocolytic Therapy for Abnormal Fetal Heart Rate Patterns

Although first reported by Caldeyro-Barcia et al. in 1969, the use of tocolytic therapy as an approach to treatment of fetal distress has not been widely pursued (12). In the initial case reported, continuous intravenous infusion of a beta-mimetic agent (metaproterenol) was used, and sequential scalp pH samples were drawn. Once pH recovered to greater than 7.30, the patient was delivered by cesarean section of a vigorous baby. Other drugs reported to be used successfully in relieving acute fetal distress include hexoprenaline (13), terbutaline (14–16), ritodrine (17), and magnesium sulfate (18). Improvement in both FHR pattern and fetal pH was seen in the majority of treated patients. In many of these cases, delivery is still by cesarean section, although vaginal delivery following acute tocolytic therapy for fetal distress has occurred as well.

Although adverse fetal effects have not been reported from these various efforts at pharmacologic in utero resuscitation, there are certain maternal conditions in which they should not be used. Because beta-sympathetic agonists will increase maternal pulse, stroke volume, systolic blood pressure, and blood glucose, and decrease diastolic blood pressure and serum potassium, their use is contraindicated in women with cardiac disease, arrhythmias, hypertension, hemorrhage, diabetes (relative contraindication), severe hypertension, or hyperthyroidism. FHR patterns that are consistent with a diagnosis of acute fetal distress and increased uterine activity and that are not responsive to position change and cessation of oxytocin infusion may be treated with a subcutaneous injection of 0.125 to 0.250 mg of terbutaline. There are several specific circumstances where tocolytic agents may be used in the setting of a nonreassuring FHR pattern. Most commonly, when a prolonged deceleration is seen in a patient with a tetanic or prolonged deceleration not on oxytocin; or if the pattern does not respond to positioning alone after several minutes and the contraction continues, tocolytic administration will usually resolve the problem (Fig. 9.23). In a setting of recurrent prolonged or severe variable decelerations where there

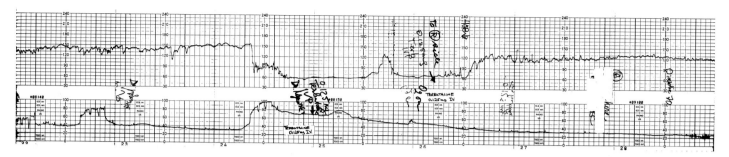

FIGURE 9.23. Tetanic contractions may result from excessive oxytocin administration or may occur spontaneously. In this example, the patient is in spontaneous labor at term. A prolonged deceleration is seen associated with a tetanic uterine contraction. Beta-agonist therapy is administered twice (terbutaline, 0.125 mg intravenously) with subsequent fetal heart rate return to baseline. The patient delivered a healthy baby 3 hours later.

is spontaneous hyperstimulation or an otherwise dysfunctional hypertonic uterine contraction pattern, tocolytic administration may result in decreased contractions, resolution of the FHR pattern, and the patient may still progress in labor (Fig. 9.24). Finally, tocolytics have been shown to improve Apgar scores when given while preparing for cesarean section. This is especially helpful when there is a delay anticipated once the decision for operative intervention has been made.

Amnioinfusion

Variable decelerations are the most frequent and, in many ways, the most difficult FHR abnormality to manage. Vari-

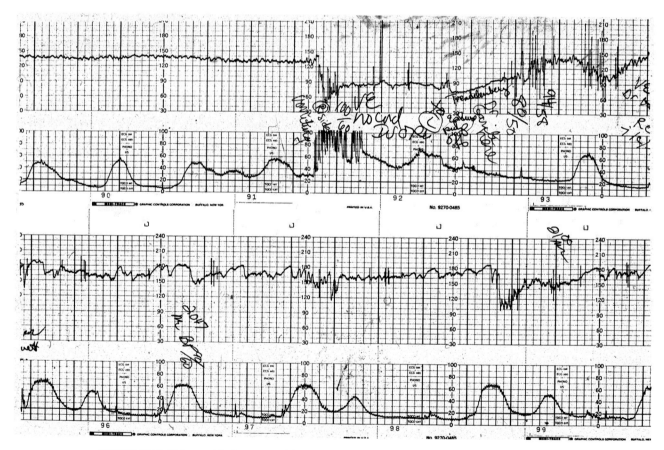

FIGURE 9.24. This gravida 2, para 1 with a previous cesarean section is at term in spontaneous labor. She is having recurrent prolonged decelerations as seen in the **upper panel** associated with spontaneous prolonged contractions (not on oxytocin). Terbutaline was administered allowing a more spaced out contraction pattern that subsequently resulted in a spontaneous vaginal delivery of a vigorous newborn.

able decelerations indicate umbilical cord compression and may rapidly progress to fetal distress. In addition, they are a source of patient, nurse, and physician distress that may lead to inappropriate intervention on behalf of an otherwise well-oxygenated fetus. During the first half of the first stage of labor, variable decelerations are most commonly seen in association with oligohydramnios either in a postterm or growth-retarded gestation or following rupture of membranes. Indeed, in patients with preterm premature rupture of membranes, the risk for developing intrapartum fetal distress is increased, with the most common pattern being nonreassuring variable decelerations (19). Vintzileos has shown that the frequency and severity of variable decelerations vary directly with the severity of oligohydramnios (20) in the setting of premature rupture of membranes. Gabbe showed in fetal monkeys that removing amniotic fluid resulted in variable decelerations, and when the fluid was restored the decelerations resolved (21).

Miyazaki and Taylor first reported on the acute use of saline amnioinfusion in the treatment of variable or prolonged decelerations (22). Rapid infusion of normal saline through the intrauterine pressure catheter was effective in relieving the majority of repetitive variable or prolonged decelerations without apparent adverse maternal or fetal risk (Fig. 9.17). This was followed by a confirmatory prospective study from the same institution (23). Several subsequent randomized trials of therapeutic amnioinfusion have confirmed the benefits in reducing cesarean section for fetal distress and in improving Apgar scores and/or cord pH values (24–26). Thus in patients in whom variable and/or prolonged decelerations appear in early labor and are most likely due to oligohydramnios, and especially when there is progression toward nonreassuring elements, the use of amnioinfusion will often result in the improvement or resolution of this concerning pattern (Fig. 9.25).

Nageotte et al. prophylactically infused warm saline intrapartum in women in early labor with preterm premature rupture of membranes and documented oligohydramnios (24). In this prospective randomized study, preterm patients with premature rupture of membranes receiving prophylactic amnioinfusion experienced fewer decelerations in both the first and second stages of labor, had higher mean umbilical artery and vein pH, and had a clear trend toward a decreased cesarean section rate for fetal distress when compared with control patients. What has not been established yet is whether in some situations, amnioinfusion should be started prophylactically when there is an unusually high risk for the development of variable decelerations from oligohydramnios, such as preterm premature rupture of membranes. Theoretically, using amnioinfusion before the onset of the decelerations in certain fetuses, such as very premature ones or those with intrauterine growth restriction who will progress to acidosis and depression much more rapidly with cord compression, will prevent the rapid evolution of hypoxia and acidosis. No studies are available as of yet to compare therapeutic as opposed to prophylactic amnioinfusion.

OPERATIVE INTERVENTION FOR NONREASSURING FETAL STATUS

When the fetus is determined to have a persistently nonreassuring FHR pattern and backup methods (scalp pH, accelerations, pulse oximetry) cannot provide reassurance that the fetus is not acidotic, operative intervention is indicated to expeditiously deliver the baby to avoid further deterioration. Several questions arise when the decision has been made for intervention for nonreassuring fetal status. What is the best choice, operative vaginal delivery or cesarean section? How much time do we have to perform the delivery? What anesthetic should be used? What is the prognosis of the baby? And finally are there situations where the baby is too damaged or otherwise not likely to benefit from this intervention?

Choosing operative vaginal delivery or cesarean section is not difficult if the patient is in early labor. For the patient near or at complete dilation, this becomes a question of judgment. Which route is more likely to create the more rapid delivery while at the same time result in the least com-

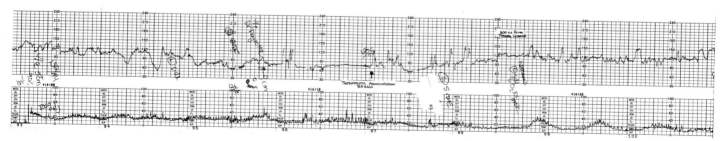

FIGURE 9.25. Prolonged decelerations in active labor may be unaccompanied by uterine hypertonus. Presumably due to continuous compression of the umbilical cord, various maneuvers are recommended: position change, cervical examination for cord prolapse, administration of oxygen, and rapid hydration. Acute amnioinfusion is another potentially therapeutic modality that can be used, particularly when cord entrapment is suspected. In this example, the fetus was having recurrent moderate-to-severe variable decelerations without evidence of uterine hypertonus.

plications for mother and baby? When the clinician is unsure whether an attempt at operative vaginal delivery will succeed, the question is even more difficult. This decision will depend not only on the variables that predict success of operative vaginal delivery (station, clinical pelvimetry, size of the baby, skill of the clinician, etc.) but also on the severity of the FHR pattern and whether there is time to find out whether an operative vaginal delivery will succeed. The time for intervention also is a question of judgment. Except for the situation of a prolonged deceleration to less than 70 BPM with loss of variability that will not recover that requires the most rapid intervention safely possible, most other situations require judgment and integration of the entire clinical picture of mother and baby. The question of how much time is available to perform operative intervention in the face of a nonreassuring FHR pattern is a complex one, muddied not only by the unpredictability of the nonreassuring pattern, but by the medical-legal pressures that have occurred as a result of EFM. The American College of Obstetricians and Gynecologists recommends that "all hospitals have the capability of performing a cesarean delivery within 30 minutes of the decision to operate," but that "not all indications for a cesarean delivery will require a 30 minute response time" (27). The examples they give of those situations that mandate an expeditious delivery include hemorrhage from placenta previa, abruptio placentae, prolapse of the umbilical cord, and ruptured uterus. In some situations (e.g., sustained prolonged deceleration to < 70 BPM with loss of variability) 30 minutes may be too long to avoid damage; in others, this 30-minute dictum may be too restrictive and result in suboptimal anesthetic choices and compromised preoperative preparation. Thus, a judgment based on the severity of the FHR pattern and the overall clinical status of mother and baby must be integrated into this difficult decision.

ADDITIONAL ISSUES IN THE MANAGEMENT OF NONREASSURING FETAL HEART RATE PATTERNS

Meconium

The presence of meconium is an extremely confusing issue in evaluating the fetus in labor. The quandary arises from the fact that while a hypoxic insult eliciting a significant vagal response from the fetus often results in the passage of meconium from the fetal gut, passage of meconium can also occur in the absence of any significant or sustained hypoxia. The meconium is not only a potential sign of fetal hypoxia but is also a potential toxin if the fetus aspirates this particulate matter with a gasping breath in utero or when it takes its first breaths following birth. The thickness of the meconium is also a reflection of the amount of amniotic fluid. Thick meconium virtually always reflects some degree of oligohydramnios. Thus there may be a vicious cycle in such

a situation. Oligohydramnios often leads to cord compression; the vagal response to cord compression may also lead to further passage of meconium, but also when it is sustained or prolonged may lead to fetal gasping increasing the likelihood that meconium aspiration can occur before birth. Furthermore, because oligohydramnios may be an indicator of failing placental function, meconium may also be the indicator that the fetus is at risk for placental insufficiency as well. In general, meconium should alert the clinician to the potential for oligohydramnios, umbilical cord compression, placental insufficiency, and meconium aspiration. Fortunately, a reassuring FHR tracing remains reliable and patients with meconium can be treated expectantly. But in the presence of meconium, especially thick meconium, the risk factors associated with meconium should be entered in the equation when managing relatively nonreassuring patterns as should all clinical variables. The vast majority of patients with meconium have no evidence of ongoing hypoxia and meconium is not a predictor of CNS damage.

Amnioinfusion also has been proposed, in several prospective randomized trials, to be used to avoid the fetal/neonatal pulmonary problems in the presence of meconium (28). The evidence for efficacy is in general good. But clear evidence that this modality avoids a full-blown meconium aspiration syndrome is lacking, because the complication is relatively infrequent, and some of these complications will be avoided with good perineal and neonatal suctioning. The theory behind this use of amnioinfusion is that it dilutes the meconium by increasing fluid volume and that by avoiding fetal gasping, which can occur with significant hypoxic episodes (i.e., sustained cord compression), it avoids the meconium aspiration that can occur prior to delivery. Surveys of university hospitals suggest that amnioinfusion is used for both variable decelerations and meconium in the vast majority of institutions (29). When meconium is present, with delivery of the fetal head, immediate deep suctioning of the nasopharynx and oropharynx using a bulb syringe and a DeLee suction trap should be performed. Most obstetric units will call for a neonatal resuscitation team in the presence of thicker degrees of meconium passage. Once delivery is completed, the pediatrician or obstetrician can inspect the cords with a laryngoscope, and if meconium is present endotracheal intubation and tracheal suctioning should be performed until meconium is cleared. It should be reemphasized that meconium suctioning and vocal cord inspection will affect the Apgar score, which will not be reliable, and in this circumstance umbilical cord gases should be obtained. Documentation of all these maneuvers should be made in the delivery record. This aggressive approach has been demonstrated to markedly decrease the incidence of meconium aspiration with its attendant morbidity and mortality (30). In utero meconium aspiration secondary to fetal gasping in response to severe antenatal stress with stillbirth or neonatal death, although rare, has been documented, and obviously may have occurred before fetal monitoring was initiated (31,32). Thus it is probable that all cases of meconium aspiration will not be avoided with the present approach.

Preterminal Patterns

The dying fetus may not have a classic FHR fetal distress pattern. However, before death, loss of variability is virtually always present. In addition, most fetuses will have a period of profound bradycardia as a terminal event. Periodic changes may resemble variable deceleration but the patterns are very rounded and "blunted" (Fig. 9.26). Tachycardia may or may not precede fetal death. Rarely, sinusoidal patterns have been seen in terminal fetuses. Although the baseline FHR in the terminal fetus is usually unstable and characterized by a blunted slow wandering, some terminal fetuses will have an absolutely fixed heart rate that appears to have been drawn with a ruler. Intermittent premature beats are frequently seen, and a rapid beat-to-beat alternating atrial pacemaker has been reported in a severely hypoxic fetus just preceding death (Fig. 9.27). Finally, one must be aware that these "preterminal" patterns may be seen in fetuses with major congenital anomalies (Fig. 9.28) (33).

The implications for intervention become very difficult when dealing with one of these profoundly severe patterns because some interventions have occurred with salvage of apparently normal neonates. However, too often, the neonate is either severely damaged or does not survive. It is impossible based on FHR patterns, however, to be sure that prompt intervention will not improve the fetal outcome. Thus these patterns should be treated as other urgent nonreassuring patterns and immediate operative intervention should be undertaken.

Scalp and Acoustic Stimulation Tests

As has been mentioned often in this chapter, in both the antepartum and intrapartum periods, acceleration of the FHR (increase of FHR by 15 BPM lasting 15 seconds) is a reliable sign of fetal well-being. More specifically, accelerations in labor, in the face of a nonreassuring FHR pattern, have been shown to be a reliable sign of the absence of acidosis. Accelerations in response to fetal movement, or manual, visual, or auditory stimuli all provide virtually the same assurance. Clark et al. originally described and subsequently prospectively demonstrated a strong positive correlation between acceleration of FHR in response to scalp stimulation and normal scalp pH (i.e., pH > 7.19). (Fig. 9.29) (34,35). In performing scalp stimulation, if acceleration of the FHR results, a normal fetal pH can be assumed. If no acceleration occurs, however, an abnormal pH is not necessarily present. Indeed, the majority of patients not responding to scalp stimulation still had a pH greater than 7.20. Subsequent studies

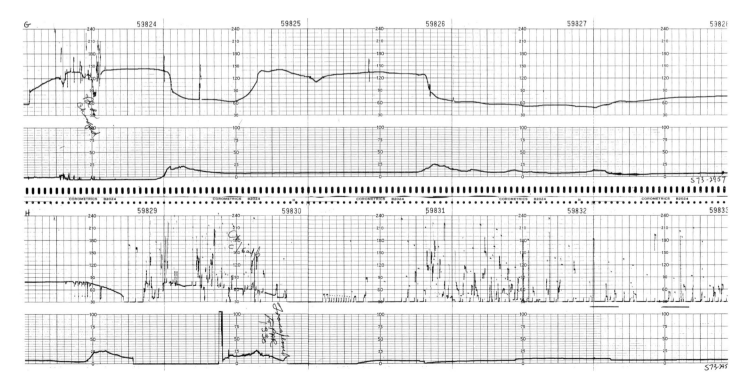

FIGURE 9.26. A terminal fetal heart rate pattern with "blunted" variable decelerations.

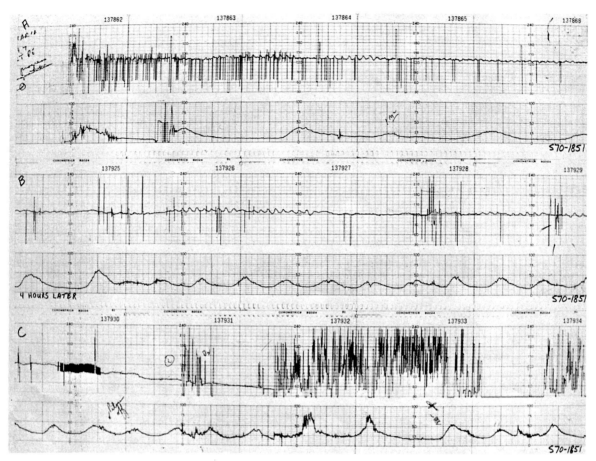

FIGURE 9.27. This tracing represents a terminal fetus. Note the absent short-term variability and intermittent sinusoidal pattern. Just before the final terminal bradycardia, there is an apparent arrhythmia.

showed virtually identical predictive ability using a vibroacoustic stimulator placed on the maternal abdomen, similar to that described with antepartum testing (36). This simple test modality is a valuable tool for intrapartum evaluation of the fetus with an abnormal heart rate, and it markedly decreases the need for inappropriate delivery or scalp pH determination. It has the advantage over quantifying FHR variability of being more objective and hence not subject to variance in interpretation among nurses and doctors.

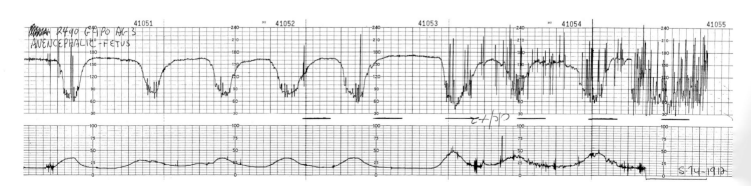

FIGURE 9.28. This pattern shows absent fetal heart rate variability, "blunted" variable deceleration, and fetal tachycardia. This was an anencephalic fetus with fetal death occurring at the end of the tracing, just before delivery.

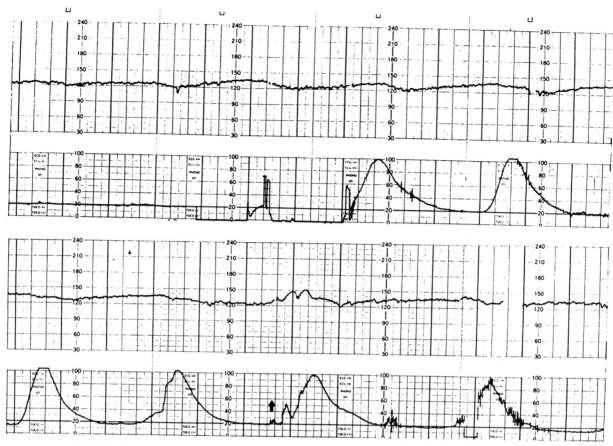

FIGURE 9.29. Decreased variability and late decelerations are present. Scalp stimulation (*arrow*) is accompanied by an acceleration of the fetal heart rate. Scalp pH is normal. (From Clark S, Gimovsky M, Miller F: The scalp stimulation test: a clinical alternative to fetal scalp blood sampling. *Am J Obstet Gynecol* 148:274, 1984, with permission.)

Case 1

This case illustrates a nonreactive FHR leading to a suspected intrapartum diagnosis of a fetal CNS abnormality (Fig. 9.30). In the first panel, the patient is having her initial contraction stress test because of a gestation of 41½ weeks. Pregnancy was uncomplicated and an ultrasound was reported as normal at 17 weeks' gestation. In Fig. 9.30, the patient is having a breast stimulation contraction stress test that is nonreactive, but no late decelerations are seen. Because of the gestational age, the patient was admitted for induction of labor and repeat ultrasound. Figure 9.30, B and C, shows an intrapartum tracing with a persistent lack of reactivity and a possible wandering baseline. However, no late or variable decelerations are seen. Real-time ultrasound revealed massive hydrocephaly with a biparietal diameter of 13.5 cm. Because of the size of the fetal head, the patient underwent a primary cesarean section. She delivered a 4,950-g female with Apgar scores of 2 and 3 at 1 and 5 minutes, with normal umbilical artery and vein pH

values. A computed tomography scan confirmed massive hydrocephaly, and the infant died 18 hours after delivery. This is a good example of a nonreactive tracing not resulting from asphyxia but rather from a major CNS abnormality. The lack of late decelerations with a persistently nonreactive tracing raises the suspicion of previous neurologic injury, major CNS abnormality, or maternal use of depressive or narcotic drugs. Intrapartum use of ultrasound may be helpful in identifying possible CNS abnormality or injury.

Case 2

This case illustrates an unusual FHR pattern with a wandering baseline. The patient entered the hospital at 40 weeks' gestation for a labor check. Pregnancy had been without complication. Figure 9.31A shows the FHR tracing during the time of evaluation for early labor. Note the smooth changes in baseline FHR without reactivity. These

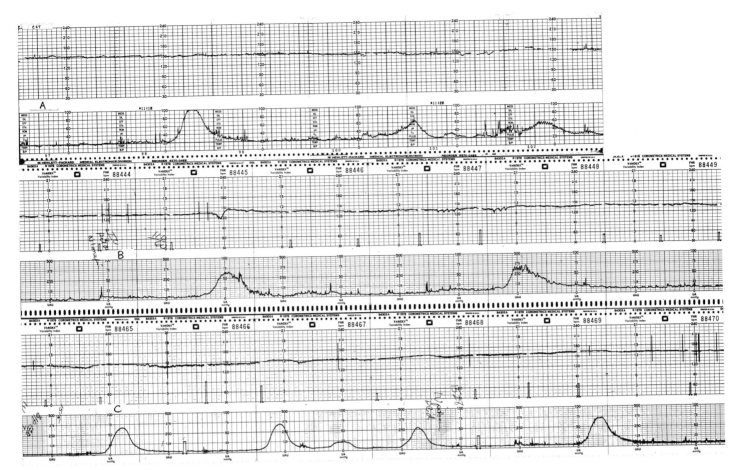

FIGURE 9.30. Case 1.

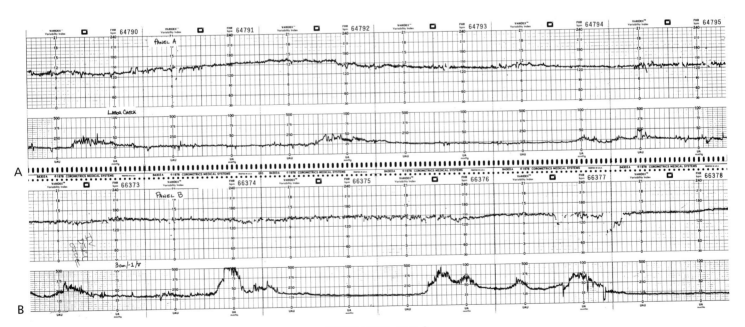

FIGURE 9.31. Case 2.

were interpreted as prolonged accelerations and the patient was discharged home. Figure 9.31B shows the FHR 15 hours later when the patient returned in active labor. Persistent late decelerations were noted and a cesarean section performed under general anesthesia resulted in the delivery of a 6-lb, 8-oz female. Apgar scores were 1 and 2 at 1 and 5 minutes, respectively. The infant began having seizures within 2 hours of delivery, but had no respiratory distress. Problems with feeding and seizure control persisted for 2 weeks before the infant was discharged home. A computed tomography scan obtained before discharge revealed a 2-cm diameter cystic mass in the right parietal area of the brain. At 1 year of age, the infant has achieved normal milestones with the exception of limited use of the left arm.

This most likely represents a case of a previous in utero asphyxial event. Although the initial evaluation was incorrect in interpreting the wandering baseline as accelerations, it is such an unusual pattern that it is easy to understand the

misinterpretation. It was not until labor occurred that further hypoxia was present, as demonstrated by late decelerations. It is doubtful that earlier intervention would have had any significant impact on ultimate neurologic outcome, but it is difficult to establish that all the damage resulted from a preexisting condition.

Case 3

This case illustrates the FHR-uterine contraction pattern while a patient's uterus is rupturing. The patient entered into labor at 40 weeks' gestation with a known previous cesarean section. She was monitored with a scalp electrode and uterine pressure catheter. She was fully effaced, 6 cm dilated, and at 0 station when monitoring began. In Fig. 9.32A, there is a mild tachycardia of 160 BPM with good variability and mild variable decelerations, and at the end of Fig. 9.32A, there is a fetal tachycardia of 180 BPM. Figure

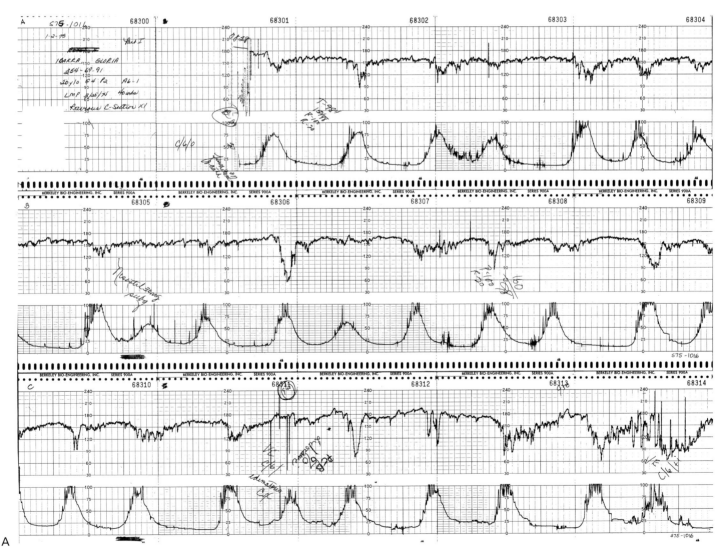

FIGURE 9.32. A,B: Case 3. *(Continued on next page)*

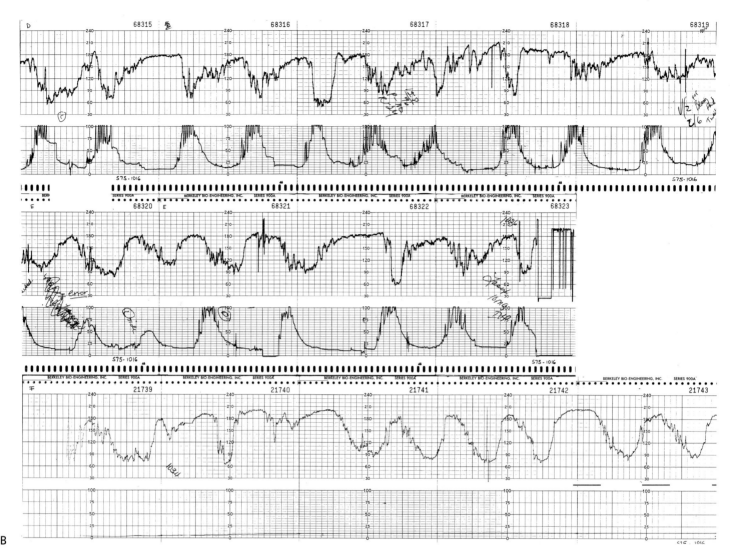

FIGURE 9.32. *(continued)*

9.32B shows further progression of the late component mixed with moderate variable deceleration. A decision to perform a cesarean section was made in the last panel of Fig. 9.32B, and the uterine catheter was removed. The severe decelerations can be seen to merge during the last half of Fig. 9.32 B, and the baseline FHR continued to increase. A cesarean section was performed soon after the end of this tracing, and a ruptured lower segment transverse incision was encountered. The fetus weighed 3,840 g and was moderately depressed but did well. The uterus was repaired.

This case indicates that there was no evidence of a loss of uterine pressure, even though the rupture was probably present during monitoring. The fetus probably fills the defect and keeps the uterine cavity effectively a closed space. Severe variable and/or prolonged decelerations appear to be the most sensitive warning sign of such catastrophes, and in this case, earlier intervention probably would have been wiser. Clearly, if one is to allow labor after a previous

cesarean section, it would be wise to electronically monitor the labor.

Case 4

This case illustrates the effect of decreasing maternal blood pressure on the FHR and fetal pH (Fig. 9.33). The patient was a severe preeclamptic with blood pressure 172/120 mm Hg after full treatment with $MgSO_4$. The tracing in the upper panel shows a normal FHR-uterine contraction tracing with good variability and a baseline rate of approximately 135 BPM. There are no periodic decelerations. The middle panel shows the FHR tracing after the maternal blood pressure was dropped to 140/104 mm Hg with a parenterally administered antihypertensive drug. Note the decrease in variability, the increase in baseline FHR to approximately 160 BPM, and the presence of late decelerations. At the beginning of the bottom panel, oxygen is started, the baseline

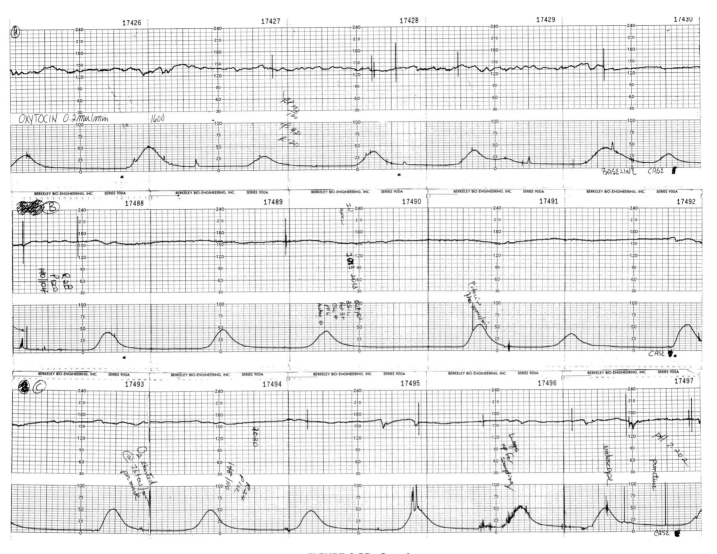

FIGURE 9.33. Case 4.

FHR remains elevated, and late decelerations are still present. At the end of the bottom tracing, a fetal scalp pH was 7.20, indicating moderate fetal acidosis. The FHR pattern persisted and the patient was delivered by cesarean section of a baby with normal Apgar scores.

This case illustrates that even though blood pressure lowering may be indicated for maternal reasons, one must be careful to watch the fetal response. Even though the maternal pressure was still increased after the diazoxide treatment, the decrease from 172/120 to 140/104 mm Hg represented relative hypotension from the fetal standpoint.

Case 5

This case illustrates the evolution of FHR changes to fetal death (Fig. 9.34). The patient was at 34 weeks' gestation with amnionitis and meconium staining. This is a case from many years ago but illustrates the natural course when no

intervention occurred because of a perceived maternal risk of cesarean section in the face of an infected uterus and a fetus of only 34 weeks' gestation.

Figure 9.34A shows fetal tachycardia, possibly due to the maternal fever, with late decelerations beginning in the lower panel. The variability is moderately decreased by the end of the lower panel. Figure 9.34B shows persistence of late deceleration with progressive loss of variability and progressively shorter latent periods between the onset of the contractions and the onset of the late decelerations. Figure 9.34C shows continuation of late decelerations, tachycardia, and no variability.

At the end of the middle panel, rather deep decelerations are seen that progress to a disorganized pattern in the lower panel and fetal death, which occurs at the end of the lower panel. This tracing represents 3 hours of monitoring, and it would be reasonable to expect that fetal salvage could have occurred with earlier intervention.

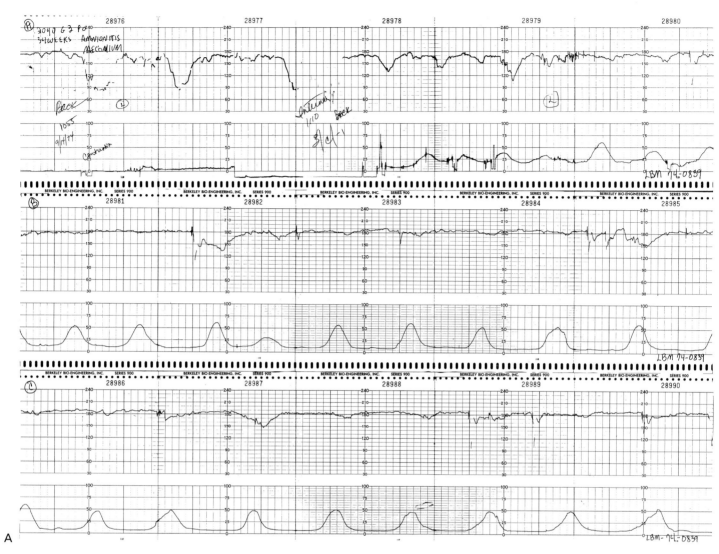

FIGURE 9.34. A–C: Case 5.

Case 6

This case illustrates the value of FHR monitoring during the initial evaluation of severe preeclampsia (Fig. 9.35). It also shows the difficulty sometimes encountered in detecting uterine activity from a small uterus. The patient was a severe preeclamptic admitted at 28 weeks' gestation with increased liver enzyme levels and thrombocytopenia. It was decided to effect delivery for maternal indications. Oxytocin was started and she was monitored with Doppler and external tocodynamometer. The upper panel of Fig. 9.35 reveals no evidence of uterine activity despite several attempts to adjust the tocodynamometer. The FHR is smooth and there are several decelerations

characteristic in shape for late deceleration. The patient was moderately obese and the uterus measured only 22 cm, but good dates with sonographic confirmation revealed a 28 weeks' gestation with probable fetal growth restriction and oligohydramnios accounting for the small uterus. The FHR pattern was thought to represent late decelerations with decreased or absent variability, and a cesarean section was performed that resulted in a moderately depressed 740-g growth-retarded neonate that did well in the nursery. Even though contractions cannot always be recorded, the FHR changes should be observed closely, and, if the clinical picture fits as in this case, the clinician should be willing to interpret such changes as ominous.

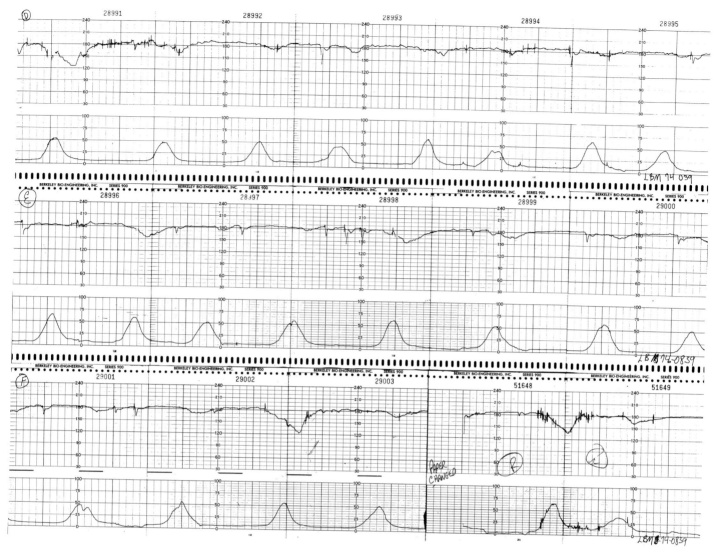

FIGURE 9.34. *(continued)*

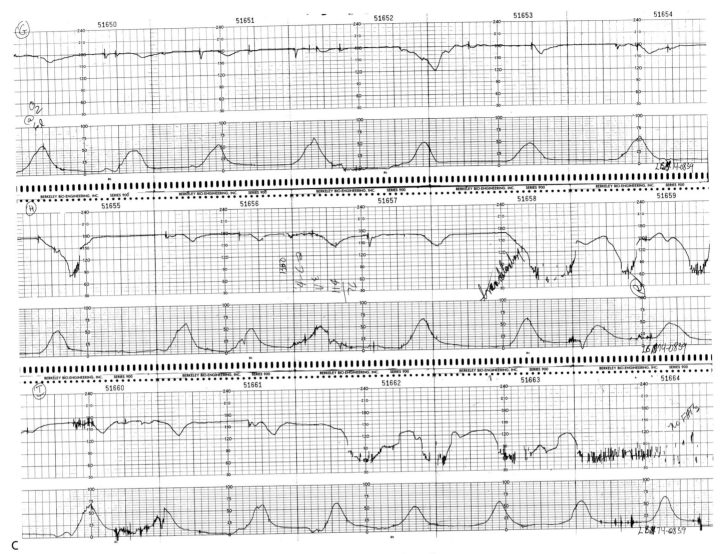

FIGURE 9.34. *(continued)*

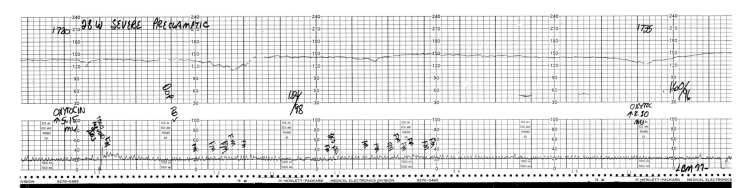

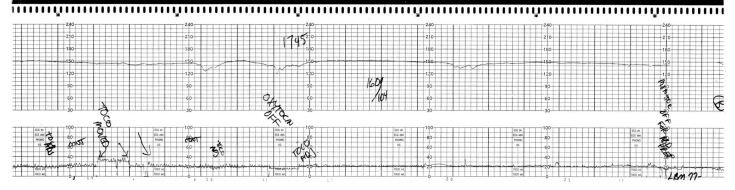

FIGURE 9.35. Case 6.

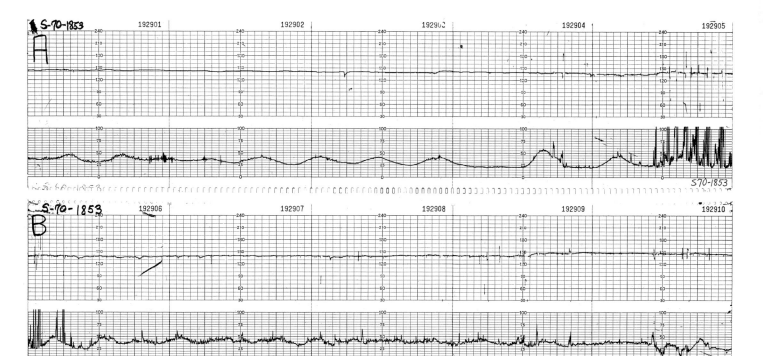

FIGURE 9.36. Case 7.

Case 7

This case represents an example of complete loss of variability without periodic changes (Fig. 9.36). The neonate was severely depressed but had a normal umbilical cord pH. Complete absence of variability without periodic changes may represent an already damaged fetus who is not currently hypoxic or who may have suffered brain damage from a previous insult. It also may represent a CNS malformation. This is one of the most difficult patterns to manage. An ultrasound is warranted to rule out major CNS anomalies, and a drug screen may reveal CNS depressant drugs. In the absence of another explanation, there are several alternatives. In early labor a biophysical profile may be helpful, later in labor, one or two normal scalp pH values may rule out significant hypoxia and acidosis. Alternatively, fetal pulse oximetry may be useful in ruling out ongoing hypoxia. If any of these tests are normal, it is likely that the cause is not ongoing hypoxia and immediate delivery is not likely to be helpful, but it does not rule out a previous asphyxic insult.

Case 8

This case illustrates lack of variability and evolution of atypical variable decelerations during labor in a patient with marked metabolic alteration. The patient was a 27-year-old

gravida 4 para 1 insulin-dependent diabetic (class D) with ketoacidosis and pregnancy-induced hypertension at 33 weeks' gestation. The patient was comatose with an arterial pH of 7.22 and a blood glucose concentration of 474 mg%. She had not taken insulin for 3 days because of persistent vomiting. As seen in Fig. 9.37A, FHR is nonreactive but without late decelerations. Figure 9.37B (45 to 50) shows the appearance of blunted variable decelerations with overshoot. Her cervix was 6 cm dilated and insulin was being infused continuously. Figure 9.37C shows deeper atypical variable decelerations with cervical dilatation of 8 to 9 cm. Figure 9.37D (84 to 89) is in the delivery room, where the patient spontaneously delivered a 3,010-g male with Apgar scores of 0 at 1 minute, 0 at 5 minutes, and 2 at 10 minutes. Cord

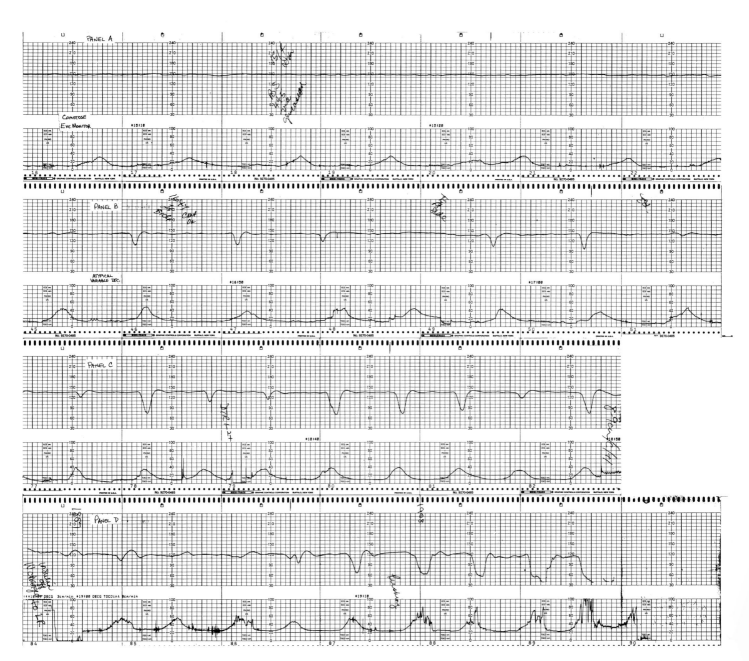

FIGURE 9.37. Case 8.

umbilical vein pH was 7.03 and umbilical artery pH was 6.96. The infant died in the nursery at 1 hour of age.

This is an example of preterminal FHR evolving in a very ill laboring woman without the option of cesarean section delivery because of the mother's compromised state. It is unclear what condition this infant was in on admission of the mother but at no point was there a reassuring FHR.

Case 9

This case demonstrates markedly increased variability of a highly atypical nature. The patient was a 22-year-old gravida 1 at 41 weeks' gestation admitted in early labor (Fig. 9.38A). Note the "sawtooth" pattern. This should be distinguished from the more common pattern of marked increased variability, often referred to as a "saltatory" pattern, which usually is not associated with significant hypoxia or acidosis. This continues intermittently over the next 2 hours (Fig. 9.38B and C) and then becomes continuous (Fig. 9. 38D). Therefore, a primary cesarean section was performed with delivery of a depressed newborn with Apgar scores of 2 and 3 at 1 and 5 minutes. Umbilical cord pH was 6.92 (umbilical artery) and 6.96 (umbilical vein). The infant was hypotonic for 24 hours but

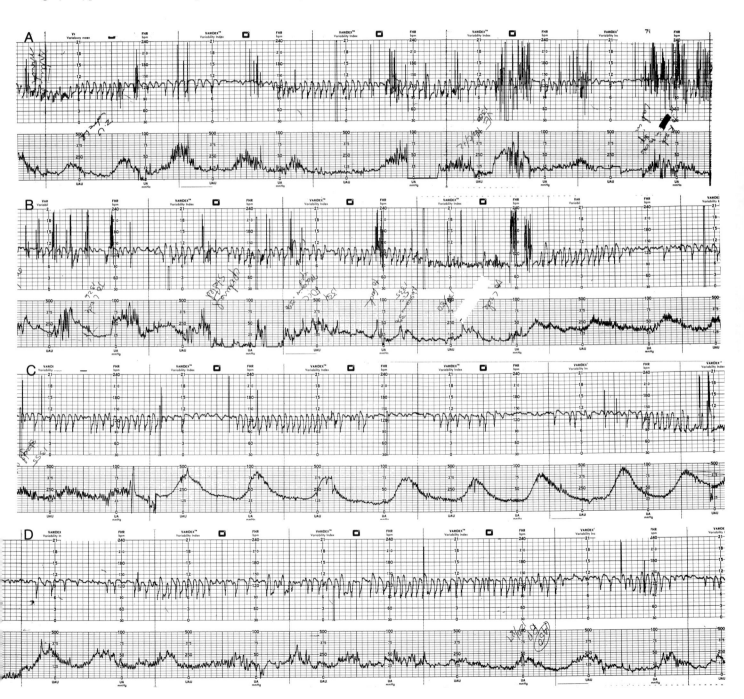

FIGURE 9.38. A–D: Case 9.

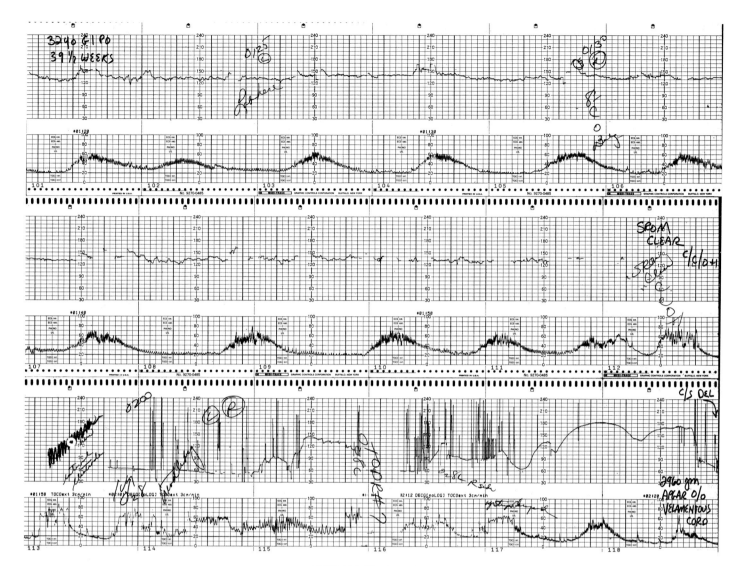

FIGURE 9.39. Case 10.

showed no other signs of complications due to asphyxia. After 6 days he was discharged home and appears normal at 2 years of age.

Case 10

There is sudden decompensation of FHR following spontaneous rupture of membranes (Fig. 9.39). Only 12 minutes passed between decision and delivery, yet a stillbirth resulted. Examination of the placenta and membranes confirmed a velamentous umbilical cord insertion and ruptured vasa previa. This is a classic example of a fortunately very rare vasa previa with fetal exsanguination secondary to inadvertent laceration of an umbilical vessel within the fetal membranes.

SUMMARY

The management of nonreassuring heart rate patterns in labor is a complex process that must be viewed in the context of both the limitations of the modality and the goal of erring on the side of avoiding fetal death and damage (Table 9.4). Generally this means that in many circumstances one will intervene operatively for presumed fetal distress only to deliver a vigorous baby without evidence of acidosis. The likelihood of a metabolic acidosis overall in labor is approximately 1% to 2%. Although there is a very high correlation between reassuring FHR patterns and normal Apgar scores, there is a poor correlation between nonreassuring patterns and low Apgar scores. Fewer than half of patients with nonreassuring FHR patterns will have newborns with 5-minute

TABLE 9.4. MANAGEMENT OF NONREASSURING FETAL HEART RATE PATTERNS: A PROPOSED PROTOCOL

The following algorithm for management of nonreassuring patterns is proposed.
1. When a pattern suggests the early development of hypoxia or is already nonreassuring:
   a. Identify when possible the cause of the problem (e.g., hypotension from an epidural)
   b. Correct the cause (e.g., fluids and ephedrine to correct the hypotension)
   c. Give measures to maximize placental oxygen delivery and exchange: oxygen by face mask, lateral positioning, hydration, consider decreasing or discontinuing oxytocin
2. If the pattern becomes or remains nonreassuring and the previous measures have been completed:
   a. Attempt to provide other measures of reassurance to rule out metabolic acidosis
      Accelerations—spontaneous or elicited
      Scalp pH
      Fetal pulse oximetry
   b. If reassurance using one of the above methods can be provided, and the pattern persists, continuous or intermittent (every 30 min) evidence of absence of acidosis must be ascertained.
   c. If reassurance of the absence of acidosis cannot be provided, deliver expeditiously by the safest and most reasonable means (operative vaginal or cesarean section).
      Patterns that qualify as nonreassuring and cannot be corrected and therefore warrant evidence of the absence of metabolic acidosis include:
      Persistent late decelerations (>50% of contractions)
      Nonreassuring variable decelerations
      Progressively severe
      With developing tachycardia and loss of variability
      With developing slow return to baseline
      Sinusoidal tracing
      Recurrent prolonged decelerations
      The patient comes in with a pattern of absent variability but without explanatory decelerations
      An unusual or confusing pattern that does not fit into one of the categories defined above but does not have elements of a reassuring pattern

FHR, fetal heart rate.

Apgar scores below 7. However, because we do not yet know where the point of permanent sequelae to intrapartum fetal hypoxia lies, the best approach should be one in which the endpoint is for the best outcome rather than for the highest correlation, provided the incidence of intervention is not excessive. In the presence of most nonreassuring FHR patterns, the clinician should, whenever possible find additional ways to find reassurance for the absence of a metabolic acidosis. Using modalities for this purpose, such as scalp and acoustic stimulation, scalp pH, or fetal pulse oximetry, will safely result in reducing unnecessary interventions.

On the opposite side of this coin, occasionally a depressed baby will be delivered following a reassuring FHR pattern. The following is a list of those factors that can explain low Apgar scores with a normal or reassuring FHR pattern:

1. Birth trauma (breech, midforceps, shoulder dystocia).
2. Drugs (general anesthesia with prolonged induction delivery time).
3. Infection (chorioamnionitis, TORCH, group B streptococcus).
4. Meconium aspiration.
5. Congenital malformations.
6. Extreme prematurity.
7. Fetal hemorrhage from an anterior placenta at cesarean section.
8. Upper airway obstruction in the newborn.

Sometimes we have seen instances in which a physician indicated that the FHR pattern was completely normal, none of the above factors were present, and there was an unexplained low Apgar score. In this situation it is common to find either that the FHR pattern was a poor quality external tracing without sufficient clarity to define the FHR pattern or that there were shallow unrecognized late decelerations present of a subtle nature and missed by the clinician. Finally, a common cause for poor correlation with outcome is that the monitoring is stopped when the patient is moved to the delivery room and 45 to 60 minutes pass before delivery, during which time there is no further monitoring of FHR.

Only by understanding the limitations of our present tools for intrapartum fetal evaluation and keeping in perspective the goals of avoiding damage as a result of intrapartum hypoxia and acidosis can one achieve the optimum balance between a good perinatal outcome and a minimum of unnecessary operative intervention.

REFERENCES

1. Freeman JM (ed): Prenatal and perinatal factors associated with brain disorders. Report to NICH. NIH Publication no. 85-1149, 1985.
2. Dennis J, Johnson A, Mutch L, et al.: Acid-base status at birth and neurodevelopmental outcome at four and one-half years. *Am J Obstet Gynecol* 161:213, 1989.
3. Gilstrap LC, Leveno KJ, Burris J, et al.: Diagnosis of birth asphyxia on the basis of fetal pH, Apgar, score, and newborn cerebral dysfunction. *Am J Obstet Gynecol* 161:825, 1989.
4. Thorp JA, Sampson JE, Parisi VM, et al.: Routine umbilical cord blood gas determinations? *Am J Obstet Gynecol* 161:600, 1989.
5. Schifrin B, Dame L: Fetal heart rate pattern of Apgar score. *JAMA* 219:322, 1973.
6. Martin CB, De Haan J, Wilot BVP, et al.: Mechanisms of late decelerations in the fetal heart rate. A study with autonomic blocking agents in fetal lambs. *Eur J Obstet Gynecol Reprod Biol* 9:361, 1979.
7. Braly P, Freeman R: The significance of fetal heart rate reactivity with a positive oxytocin challenge test. *Obstet Gynecol* 50:689, 1977.
8. Henigsman S, Garite T, Patillo C, et al.: Fetal pulse oximetry defines which variable decelerations with slow return to baseline are associated with hypoxia. *Am J Obstet Gynecol* 185:S131, 2001.
9. Greiss FC Jr, Crandell DL: Therapy for hypotension induced by spinal anesthesia during pregnancy. *JAMA* 191:793, 1965.
10. Dildy GA, Clark S, Loucks C: Intrapartum fetal pulse oximetry; The effects of maternal hyperoxia on fetal oxygen saturation. *Am J Obstet Gynecol* 171:1120, 1994.
11. Garite TJ, Weeks J, Peters-Phair K, et al.: A randomized controlled trial of the effect of increased intravenous hydration on the course of labor in nulliparas. *Am J Obstet Gynecol* 183:1544, 2000.
12. Caldeyro-Barcia R, Magana JM, Castillo JB, et al.: A new approach to the treatment of acute intrapartum fetal distress. In: *Perinatal factors affecting human development.* Scientific Publication no. 185. Washington, DC, Pan-American Health Organization, 1969:248–253.
13. Lipshitz J: Use of B2 sympathomimetic drug as a temporizing measure in the treatment of acute fetal distress. *Am J Obstet Gynecol* 129:31, 1977.
14. Tejani N, Verma Ul, Chatterjee S, et al.: Terbutaline in the management of acute intrapartum fetal acidosis. *J Reprod Med* 28:857, 1983.
15. Arias F: Intrauterine resuscitation with terbutaline a method for the management of acute intrapartum fetal distress. *Am J Obstet Gynecol* 131:39, 1977.
16. Patriarcho MS, Viechnicki BN, Hutchinson TA: A study on intrauterine fetal resuscitation with terbutaline. *Am J Obstet Gynecol* 157: 383, 1987.
17. Mendez-Bauer C, Shekarloo A, Cook V, et al.: Treatment of acute intrapartum fetal distress by beta Z sympathomimetics. *Am J Obstet Gynecol* 156:638, 1987.
18. Reece EA, Chervenak FA, Romero R: Magnesium sulfate in the management of acute intrapartum fetal distress. *Am J Obstet Gynecol* 148:104, 1984.
19. Moberg L, Garite TJ, Freeman RK: Fetal heart rate patterns and fetal distress in patients with preterm premature rupture of the membranes. *Obstet Gynecol* 64:68, 1984.
20. Vintzileos AM, Campbell WA, Nochimson DJ, et al.: Degree of oligohydramnios and pregnancy outcome in patients with premature rupture of membranes. *Obstet Gynecol* 66:165, 1985.
21. Gabbe SG, Ettinger BB, Freeman RK, et al: Umbilical cord compression associated with amniotomy. *Am J Obstet Gynecol* 126:353, 1976.
22. Miyazaki F, Taylor N: Saline amnioinfusion for relief of variable or prolonged decelerations. *Am J Obstet Gynecol* 14:670, 1983.
23. Miyazaki F, Nevarez F: Saline amnioinfusion for relief of repetitive variable decelerations: a prospective randomized study. *Am J Obstet Gynecol* 153:301, 1985.
24. Nageotte MP, Freeman RK, Garite TJ, et al.: Prophylactic intrapartum amnioinfusion in patients with preterm premature rupture of membranes. *Am J Obstet Gynecol* 153:557, 1985.
25. Strong TH, Hetzler G, Sarno AP, et al.: Prophylactic intrapartum amnioinfusion: a randomized clinical trial. *Am J Obstet Gynecol* 162:1370, 1990.
26. MacGregor SN, Banzhaf WC, Silver RK, et al.: A prospective, randomized evaluation of intrapartum amnioinfusion: fetal acid-base status and cesarean delivery. *J Reprod Med* 36:69, 1991.
27. American Academy of Pediatrics and American College of Obstetricians and Gynecologists: *Guidelines for perinatal care.* 4th ed, Washington DC, p 112, 1997.
28. Pierce J, Gaudier FL, Sanchez-Ramos L: Intrapartum amnioinfusion for meconium-stained fluid: meta-analysis of prospective trials. *Obstet Gynecol* 95:1051, 2000.
29. Wenstrom K, Andrews WW, Maher JE: Anmioinfusion survey: prevalence, protocols and complications. *Obstet Gynecol* 86:572, 1995.
30. Carson BS, Losey RW, Bowes WA, et al.: Combined obstetric and pediatric approach to prevent meconium aspiration syndrome. *Am J Obstet Gynecol* 126:172, 1976.
31. Manning FA, Schreiber J, Turkel SB: Fatal meconium aspiration "in utero:" a case report. *Am J Obstet Gynecol* 132:111, 1978.
32. Tuberville DF, McCaffree, Block MF, et al.: In utero distal pulmonary meconium aspiration. *South Med J* 72:535, 1979.
33. Garite TJ, Linzey EM, Freeman RK, et al.: Fetal heart rate patterns and fetal distress in fetuses with congenital anomalies. *Obstet Gynecol* 53: 716, 1979.
34. Clark S, Gimovsky M, Miller FC: Fetal heart rate response to scalp blood sampling. *Am J Obstet Gynecol* 144:706, 1982.
35. Clark S, Gimovsky M, Miller F: The scalp stimulation test: a clinical alternative to fetal scalp blood sampling. *Am J Obstet Gynecol* 148:274, 1984.
36. Smith CV, Nguyen HN, Phelan JP, et al: Intrapartum assessment of fetal well-being: a comparison of fetal acoustic stimulation with acid-base determinations. *Am J Obstet Gynecol* 155:726, 1986.

FETAL PULSE OXIMETRY

THE NEED FOR INTRAPARTUM FETAL EVALUATION

The benefits and negative consequences of intrapartum electronic fetal monitoring (EFM) are chronicled extensively elsewhere in this book. But to summarize for the purpose of this chapter, it is clear that the vast majority of fetal damage and death, which occurs as a result of *intrapartum* events, is due to asphyxia. Therefore, the primary purpose of intrapartum fetal evaluation is to detect fetal hypoxia, identify those fetuses destined for that hypoxia to lead to metabolic acidosis and the resultant tissue damage, and allow the clinician to intervene before that damage occurs.

EFM is generally agreed to be a sensitive device, meaning that virtually all babies with significant hypoxia, or hypoxia progressing to metabolic acidosis, will have a nonreassuring fetal heart rate (FHR) pattern. Conversely, however, since we are monitoring the responses of the fetal heart rate to input from the fetal brain, there are many alterations in the FHR that result from other stimuli and resultant central nervous system (CNS) responses besides hypoxia and acidosis. Furthermore, such changes are very common, and studies have shown that more than 30% of all patients in labor have periods of nonreassuring FHR patterns that cause concern among caregivers (1) and that lead to oxygen administration and other nonsurgical interventions, leading to what many have called the "medicalization" of normal labors. Finally, the monitor has created an expectation of perfect outcome, and, with perinatal complications or with children with neurologic handicaps, lawsuits are commonly filed, alleging perinatal asphyxia as the cause, even when events in the newborn period do not suggest this etiology. Because FHR patterns are difficult to interpret and agree upon, even by experts, this leads to confusion for juries in such cases, and large monetary awards are common.

Some of these problems with EFM can be overcome with the liberal use of fetal scalp pH. However, this method of determining which FHR patterns require immediate intervention and which do not has never had widespread acceptance by clinicians because of technical difficulties and the requirement for frequently repeating the test if the nonreassuring FHR pattern continues. Thus, there is a compelling need for a more specific, more accurate, easier to interpret, and easier to use method to monitor the fetus in labor. Devices such as continuous pH monitoring, electrocardiograph waveform analysis, continuous pO_2 monitoring, and pulse oximetry have been proposed as alternatives that could potentially fulfill these needs. To date, only fetal pulse oximetry has been developed to a point to provide an alternative for monitoring fetal oxygenation in labor.

PULSE OXIMETRY

Since the early 1980s, monitoring of oxygen saturation using pulse oximetry has been available for "air breathing" adults and children, and is now used in virtually every operating room and intensive care unit. By 1985, its use had become so pervasive that 95% of all patients in operating rooms in the United States were monitored with this device. In the state of Massachusetts in 1985, all hypoxia-related deaths were eliminated with use of pulse oximetry. And within a few years as a result of these factors, the malpractice premiums for anesthesiologists had been cut in half (2).

Oxygen is present in the blood in two forms. In the plasma, oxygen is dissolved and unbound (Fig. 10.1). This form accounts for approximately 1% of total blood oxygen and it is the portion responsible for all oxygen diffusion. Dissolved oxygen is measured as partial pressure, or pO_2. The remaining 99% of oxygen in blood is bound to hemoglobin. This form is measured as oxygen saturation *in vitro* by co-oximetry and *in vivo* by pulse oximetry and are both expressed as percent saturation. The percent saturation is the percentage of hemoglobin binding sites occupied by oxygen molecules (saturated hemoglobin) divided by the total number of binding sites (satu-

$$\% \text{ Oxygen Saturation} = \frac{\text{Oxyhemoglobin}}{(\text{Oxyhemoglobin} + \text{Deoxyhemoglobin})}$$

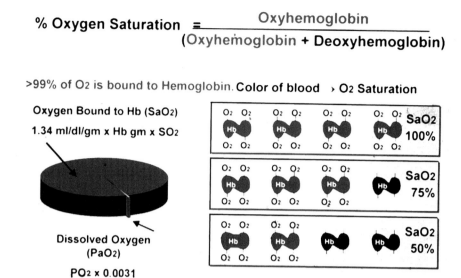

FIGURE 10.1. Both *in vivo* and *in vitro* measurement of pulse oximetry depends on calculating the relative number of oxygen binding sites on the hemoglobin molecule occupied by oxygen and dividing that by the total number of binding sites (deoxygenated and oxygenated hemoglobin).

rated + unsaturated hemoglobin). The measurement of oxygen saturation using pulse oximetry involves two principles. The first is that red and near-infrared light are alternately shined into tissue and the absorption of the transmitted or reflected light is measured. Deoxyhemoglobin absorbs red light better and oxyhemoglobin infrared; thus using standard curves, the oximeter is able to calculate the relative amounts of saturated and unsaturated hemoglobin and determine percent oxygen satura-

tion. To determine the light absorbed by arterial blood as opposed to venous blood and surrounding tissues, the oxygen saturation is determined at the peak of the pulse wave (equal to light absorbed by arterial and venous blood and surrounding tissue) and the nadir of the pulse wave (light absorbed only by venous blood and tissue) (Fig. 10.2). By subtracting the amount of light absorbed at the nadir from that absorbed at the peak, the amount remaining is that absorbed by arterial blood.

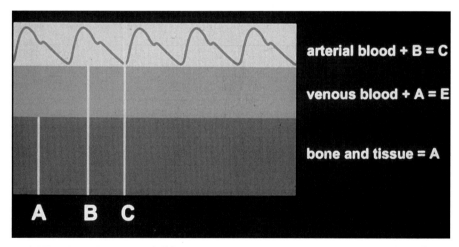

FIGURE 10.2. This figure illustrates how the pulse wave is used to separate the light absorption of arterial blood from that of venous blood and surrounding tissue.

FETAL PULSE OXIMETRY

Early Development

Why then, with the obvious need for an alternative to EFM, the obvious benefit of pulse oximetry in adults and children, and the fact that pulse oximetry actually measures what we are concerned about (oxygenation) and provides an objective number with which to interpret this end point, has it taken so long for the development of pulse oximetry for the fetus? The answer lies in the technologic difficulties, which have been encountered in trying to apply this device to the more inaccessible and physiologically different fetus. During labor, the only site that we have easy access to is usually the fetal scalp. The cervix must be sufficiently dilated and the membranes ruptured to have access. The scalp is covered by hair, and often mucous, blood, vernix, meconium, and vaginal secretions, all of which can interfere with light transmission and photodetection. The amplitude of the fetal pulse wave is small due to a low fetal pulse pressure, hindering accurate calculation of arterial saturation. In addition, when the scalp is used, there is often stasis within the developing caput, hindering access to the fetal pulse wave. The level of fetal oxygen saturation is normally only approximately 55%, and conventional oximeters do not work well at these low levels as they are optimally calibrated to work at levels in the range of 90% to 100%. Finally, fetal hemoglobin is different from that of the adult, altering light absorption characteristics. All of these complex factors and interactions have hindered the development of fetal pulse oximetry. Early efforts at trying to overcome these problems led to the testing of a number of rather creative sensors. Suction cups, glue, and clips were tried (Fig. 10.3). Scalp electrodes with photoemitters and the photodetector placed at the tip of the spiral and base of the electrode were the dominant method tried for many years. None of these devices overcame the hurdles created by the scalp, the interfering fluids, and the caput.

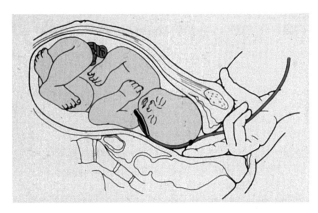

FIGURE 10.4. Picture of a pulse oximeter probe inserted transcervically to ultimately lodge against the fetal cheek. The catheter is inserted much like an intrauterine pressure catheter. The sensor is held against the fetal cheek by the pressure provided from the uterine wall and pelvic sidewall.

Recently a completely different approach to sensor placement was introduced that eliminated many of these hurdles. This device is inserted transcervically, much like an intrauterine pressure catheter, to ultimately lodge against the fetal cheek (Fig. 10.4). On the surface of the device are three gold electrodes to determine adequate electrical contact, a photoemitter, and a photodetector (Fig. 10.5). The sensor is connected to a fetal pulse oximeter (model N400, Nellcor/Tyco Inc., Pleasanton, CA) (Fig. 10.6) that processes the signal and calculates and displays the oxygen

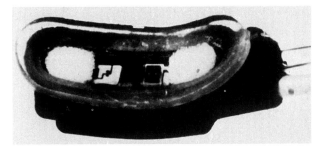

FIGURE 10.3. An early attempt at a suction cup device to attach the photoemitter and sensor to the fetal presenting part.

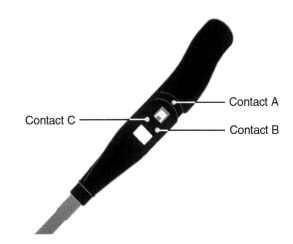

Contact C —
Contact A —
Contact B —

FIGURE 10.5. A photograph of the surface of the fetal pulse oximetry probe. On the surface of the device are three gold electrodes to monitor adequate electrical contact, a photoemitter, and a photodetector.

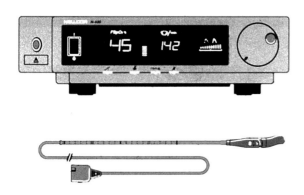

FIGURE 10.6. This is a fetal oxygen saturation monitor and sensor produced by Nellcor/Tyco and Company, Pleasanton, California. This monitor is similar to adult and pediatric pulse oximeter monitors often seen in the operating room and in the intensive care unit. However, the computer processor is quite different being calibrated and re-engineered to process fetal pulse oximetry signals. The monitor displays simultaneously fetal oxygen saturation, pulse wave amplitude, fetal heart rate, and electrical impedance measuring the contact of the probe.

saturation. The pulse oximeter is connected to a conventional FHR monitor that displays the signal on the lower (contraction) channel of the fetal monitor tracing. This provides a continuous tracing of fetal oxygen saturation (FSpO$_2$) that can be correlated with heart rate changes and uterine contractions (Fig. 10.7). Because moment-to-moment display of fetal oxygen saturation provides a very noisy tracing, the saturation is averaged over approximately 45 seconds, and the display of changes in oxygen saturation will lag by this interval.

The Concept of the Critical Threshold

A concept that is essential to the utility of fetal oxygen saturation monitoring is termed the "critical threshold." As a fetus becomes hypoxic, if that hypoxia is severe enough and lasts long enough, the fetus will generate energy with anaerobic metabolism, which leads to the production of organic acids. These organic acids are harmful to the fetus and can result in tissue and organ damage and ultimately death. The goal of intrapartum monitoring is to intervene

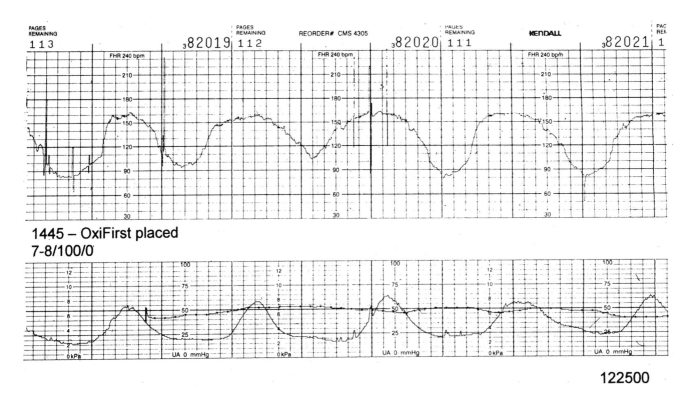

1445 – OxiFirst placed
7-8/100/0

122500

FIGURE 10.7. This fetal heart rate tracing with a typical heart rate on the upper channel and contraction tracing on the lower channel and is also continuously displaying the fetal oxygen saturation on the lower channel superimposed on the contractions.

early in the development of metabolic acidosis and avoid the consequent complications. Because fetuses often become hypoxic for short periods, revert to normal, and will never become acidotic, intervening with hypoxia but without acidosis will lead to far too many operations without benefit. Alternatively, waiting until the acidosis has persisted and progressed can lead to damaged babies. Therefore the challenge was to determine if there was a critical threshold of fetal hypoxia below which and if sustained for a defined duration would likely be associated with a metabolic acidosis and above which there would be virtually no risk of acidosis.

Animal Data

Animal studies in sheep, goats, and primates have confirmed that the fetus will not become hypoxic unless the oxygen saturation falls below 30% (3,4). As the fetus reaches this level, the pH begins to fall and levels of lactic acid begin to rise. When the oxygen level rises above 30%, the acidosis can be reversed and the pH rises toward normal (Fig. 10.8). Nijland's study also confirmed an excellent correlation between the N400 fetal pulse oximeter and oxygen saturation measured *in vitro* by co-oximetry, validating the accuracy of the device (3).

Human Studies

Many human studies have been performed using the N400 device (1,5–14). Several of these studies have demonstrated normal oxygen saturation values for the human fetus in labor, validated the 30% critical threshold, and compared outcomes of fetuses with normal and abnormal values (1,7–9). Normal fetal oxygen saturation in labor has been evaluated in a large number of patients.

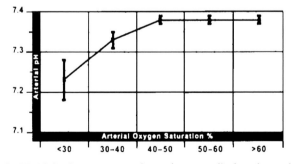

FIGURE 10.8. Oxygen saturation values are displayed correlating with fetal arterial pH. It can be seen that as the oxygen saturation drops below 30%, a metabolic acidosis begins to develop.

The normal values (± two standard deviations) range from 30% to 70% and approximately 3% of normal fetuses have values of less than 30% (5). Scalp and umbilical cord pH values have been compared to oxygen saturation in fetuses with nonreassuring FHR patterns in labor. Both types of studies have confirmed that in fetuses with oxygen saturation values that do not fall below a level of 30% for longer than 10 minutes have a very low risk of fetal metabolic acidosis. Kuhnert et al. in 1998 sampled 46 term fetuses with nonreassuring FHR patterns and correlated the pH with simultaneous $FSpO_2$ (7). The data revealed an 81% sensitivity and a 100% specificity for a scalp pH less than 7.20. The three fetuses with a low pH and a normal $FSpO_2$ all had mild acidosis (7.17 to 7.19) and normal outcomes. These authors further reported that only a $FSpO_2$ less than 30% for more than 10 minutes correlated with fetal acidosis. Scalp pH may not be the perfect gold standard, because both false-positive and false-negative values may be in the range of 5% to 10%. Carbonne and coworkers compared scalp pH with $FSpO_2$ for predicting acidosis by umbilical arterial pH; both showed nearly identical sensitivities and specificities (8). Alternatively Dildy et al. reviewed 1,101 paired umbilical artery pH values with umbilical artery oxygen saturation measured in vitro (SaO_2); they found insignificant fetal acidosis with an oxygen saturation greater than 30% (9). Additional studies have also shown a significant association between $FSpO_2$ and neonatal outcome that is quite comparable to the association with cord pH values (10). Thus it appears, using this concept of the critical threshold, that in the presence of a nonreassuring FHR pattern, fetal pulse oximetry is equivalent to scalp pH in evaluating the question of whether the hypoxia has progressed to a metabolic acidosis. Furthermore, an $FSpO_2$ value below 30% must be present continuously for some minutes before there is a likelihood of significant fetal acidosis.

Another way of validating fetal pulse oximetry is to show that FHR patterns known to correlate with hypoxia in animals show similar correlation to drops in oxygen saturation in humans measured with fetal pulse oximetry. Conversely, we should see that those patterns, which accurately document the absence of fetal hypoxia in animals, virtually always have normal oxygen saturation with human fetal pulse oximetry. Indeed, Lee et al. validated the relationship between FHR patterns and their association with hypoxia and/or acidosis in humans using fetal pulse oximetry with virtually unanimous consistency between their findings and what has previously been shown in animals (11).

Thus it appears that a reasonable body of evidence documents that fetal pulse oximetry accurately reflects fetal oxygen saturation in labor, and using a critical threshold of 30%, this device can be used in patients with nonreassuring FHR patterns to determine the presence or absence of sufficient hypoxia to know whether or not a metabolic acidosis is developing.

FETAL PULSE OXIMETRY IN CLINICAL PRACTICE

Several concepts are important to appreciate if fetal pulse oximetry is to be used in the evaluation of fetal oxygenation in labor. First, the fetus with a normal/reassuring FHR pattern is virtually always normally oxygenated. Given at least a 3% rate of falsely low FSpO$_2$ (fetal oxygen saturation) values in normal fetuses, one must either choose not to use fetal pulse oximetry in such situations (Fig. 10.9) or to be willing to accept that such values in the setting of a reassuring FHR are not most likely in

error and be willing not to become concerned and intervene. This would not be different than performing a scalp pH in the setting of a normal FHR pattern. Second, the concept of using FSpO$_2$ values as, in essence, a continuous scalp pH is essential to the appropriate application and understanding of the fetal pulse oximetry monitoring in the fetus with a nonreassuring FHR in labor. In available studies, as previously described, an FSpO$_2$ value continuously above 30% is highly reassuring/consistent with a fetus who does not have a metabolic acidosis. Thus in the presence of a nonreassuring FHR, where one would normally require the secondary reassurance of a scalp pH or elicited accelerations (reactivity), a continuously normal FSpO$_2$ provides the same reassurance of the absence of acidosis. Typical examples of such situations include persistent late decelerations where the fetus is no longer reactive (Fig. 10.10) or repetitive severe variable decelera-

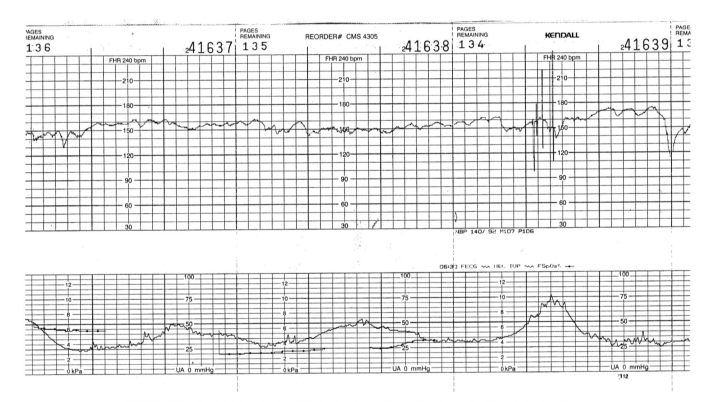

FIGURE 10.9. The fetal heart rate (FHR) tracing is reactive without any significant decelerations. This patient is being monitored with fetal pulse oximetry, which initially shows a normal saturation of 45%, but for a period of approximately 2½ minutes a low oxygen saturation of approximately 20% to 25% is displayed. In a few cases, a reassuring heart rate tracing will be associated with an apparently falsely low oxygen saturation. This is why it is important to react to interpret the picture as nonreassuring only when both the FHR and the oxygen saturation reveal nonreassuring values.

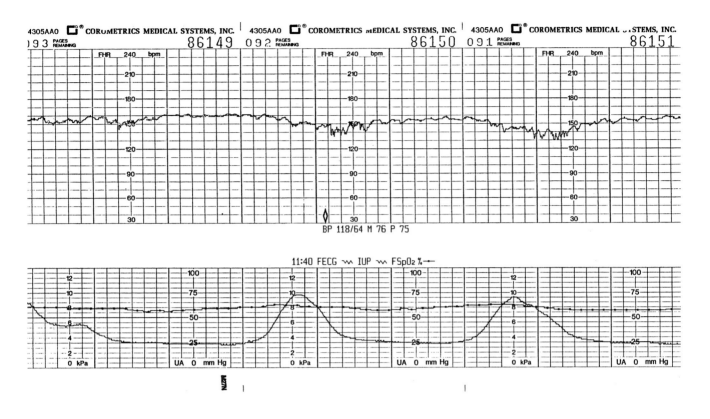

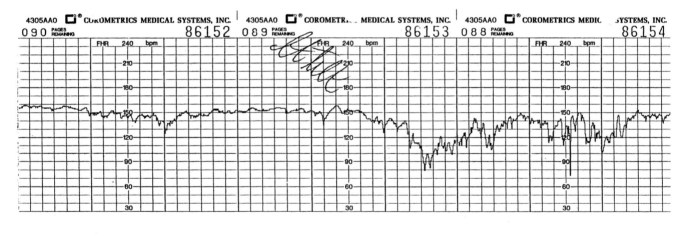

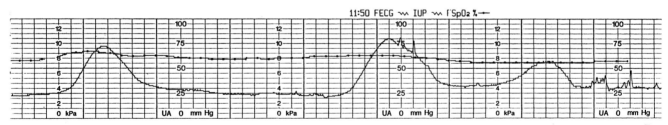

FIGURE 10.10. This fetus is having persistent late decelerations, a classical nonreassuring deceleration pattern. Although the variability is average, there are no accelerations and one cannot be absolutely reassured of the absence of a metabolic acidosis. The continuously normal fetal oxygen saturation tracing, with values in this case of 50% to 60%, however, does provide a reassurance of the absence of acidosis. *(Continued on next page)*

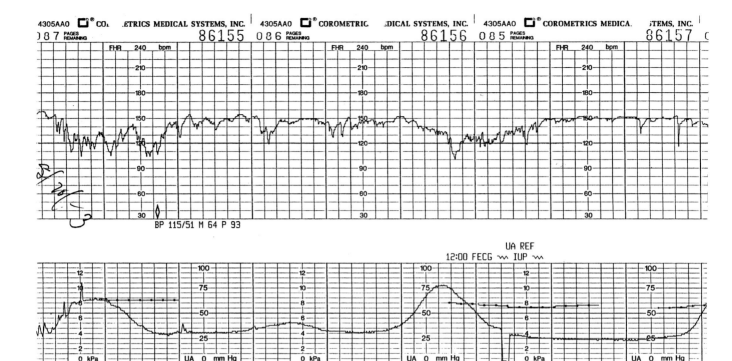

FIGURE 10.10. *(continued)*

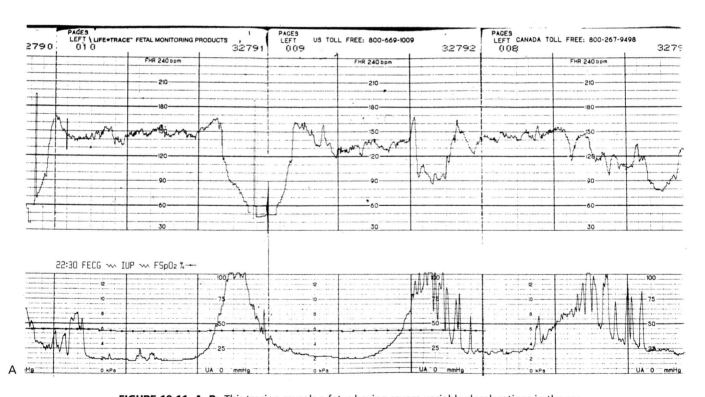

FIGURE 10.11. A, B: This tracing reveals a fetus having severe variable decelerations in the second stage of labor. The variable decelerations are descending as low as 50 beats per minute and lasting up to 1 minute. Given the depth and duration of the decelerations, these would qualify as nonreassuring variable decelerations.

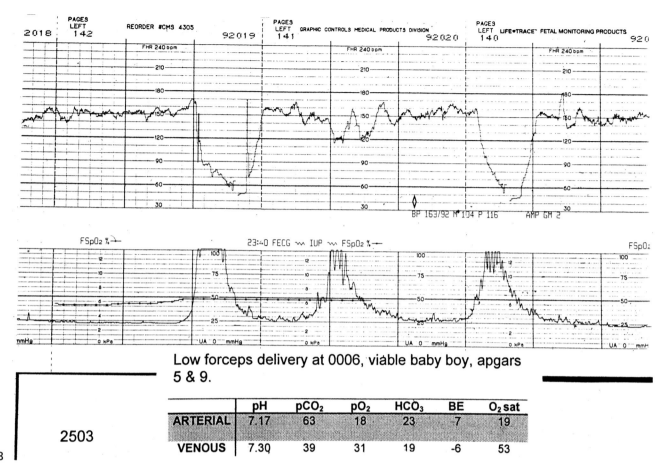

Low forceps delivery at 0006, viable baby boy, apgars 5 & 9.

2503

	pH	pCO₂	pO₂	HCO₃	BE	O₂ sat
ARTERIAL	7.17	63	18	23	-7	19
VENOUS	7.30	39	31	19	-6	53

FIGURE 10.11. *(continued)* In the absence of acceleration, there is no clear-cut way to rule out fetal acidosis with the heart rate alone. However, with an oxygen saturation tracing as seen in this case with values of 40% to 50%, one can be assured of the absence of metabolic acidosis. This baby delivers approximately 30 minutes after the end of **panel B** and has Apgar scores of 5 at 1 minute and 9 at 5 minutes with cord pH values as shown, consistent with mild respiratory but no metabolic acidosis.

tions (Fig. 10.11) with secondary signs of hypoxia (e.g., tachycardia or loss of variability), with loss of accelerations, or with slow return of the deceleration to baseline (Fig. 10.12). Occasionally, recurrent prolonged decelerations or bradycardias that develop in the second stage of labor will also be situations where fetal pulse oximetry monitoring can provide reassurance (Fig. 10.13); however, these often appear suddenly, and when they do not and cannot be made to return to baseline, it is generally unwise to take the time to insert a pulse oximeter because

the patient must be moved expeditiously to delivery. This is especially true when the patient exhibits a particularly profound deceleration (e.g., <70 beats per minute [BPM]), has sudden loss of variability, and/or does not show signs of returning to baseline, despite conservative resuscitative values. Another particularly useful situation where the concept of a reassuring FSpO₂ value can provide valuable and reliable reassurance is when there is a confusing FHR pattern that does not fit the typical pattern of hypoxia nor is typically reassuring (Fig. 10.14). Also patients with difficult

(text continues on page 160)

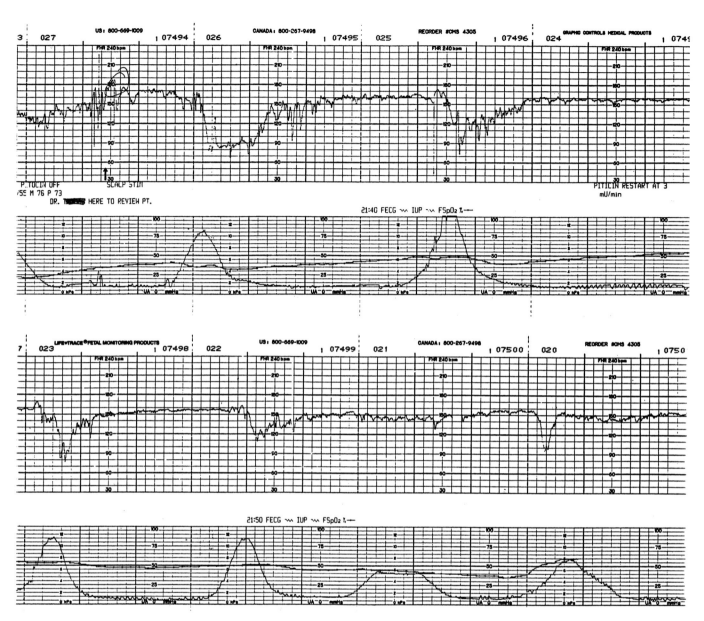

FIGURE 10.12. Variable decelerations with slow return to baseline are often difficult to interpret. It is, in general, a nonreassuring pattern, which requires additional reassurance to rule out acidosis. Although the variability in this heart rate tracing is normal and an acceleration is ultimately seen, the pulse oximetry tracing with normal saturations rising to above 30% with all contractions provides reassurance of the absence of metabolic acidosis at the present time. This patient subsequently delivered a vigorous newborn vaginally.

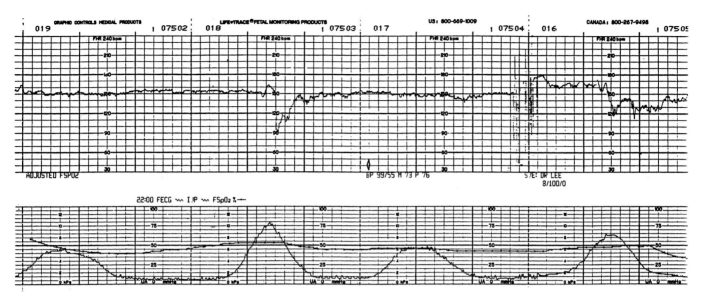

FIGURE 10.12. *(continued)*

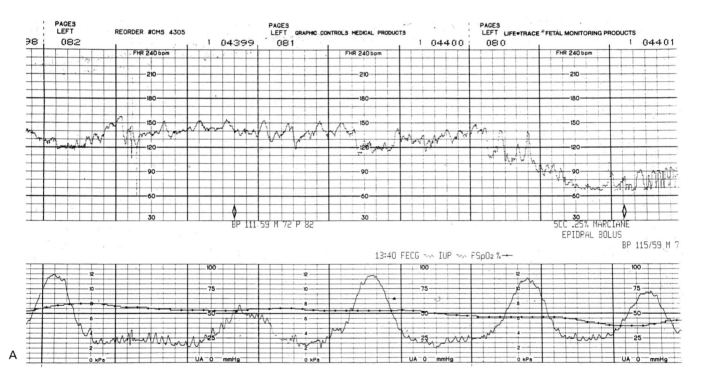

FIGURE 10.13. A–C: This illustrates a case of a 27-year-old gravida 2 para 1 who is in active labor and progressing well. The patient has a sudden prolonged deceleration down to 60 beats per minute (BPM) lasting 6 minutes and returning to baseline but subsequently in **panel C** going down to 90 BPM and remaining down. It is often difficult not to intervene operatively in such cases given the persistent prolonged deceleration. In most cases, either the fetal heart rate will return to normal and/or the patient will deliver a vigorous newborn. The oxygen saturation, which in this case is persistently above 30%, provides reassurance that no urgent intervention is absolutely required. *(Continued on next page)*

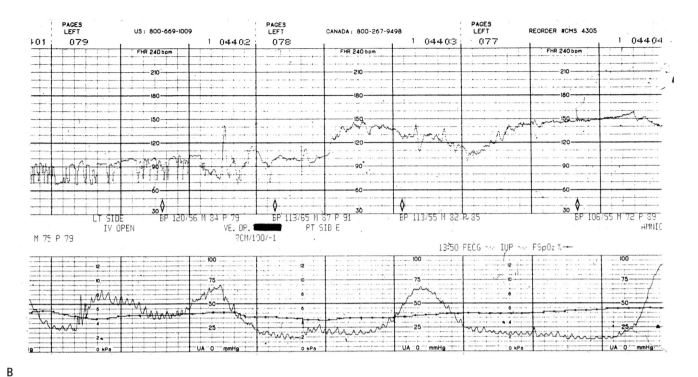

B

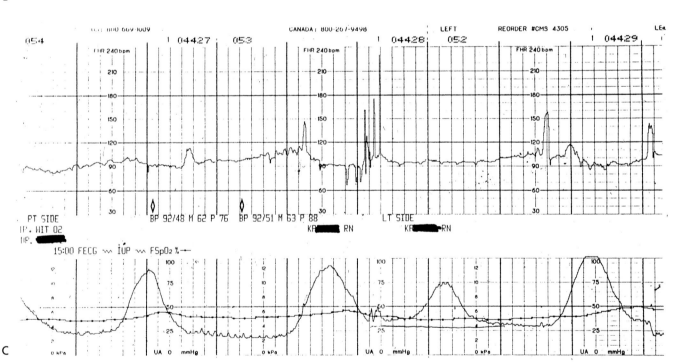

C

FIGURE 10.13. *(continued)* This patient also subsequently delivered a baby with Apgar scores of 9 and 9 approximately 2 hours after the end of **panel C** and the deceleration had returned to baseline.

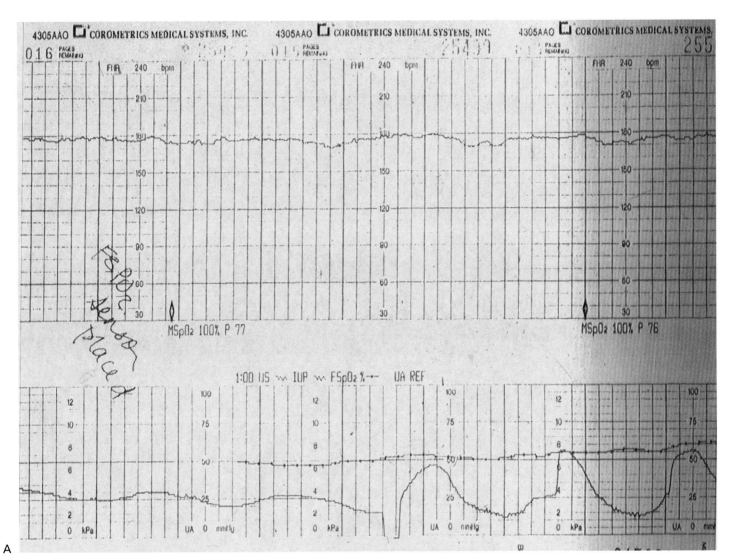

A

FIGURE 10.14. This tracing illustrates the kind of case where fetal pulse oximetry may prove to be the most useful of all. The patient presents with a fetal tachycardia in the range of 170 to 180 beats per minute. There are initially associated decelerations that may be late decelerations, but ultimately the pattern evolves to one of decreased variability and unusual decelerations that are difficult to classify. One would certainly find nothing about this fetal heart rate tracing that is reassuring. However, it is also not easy to classify as a typical pattern of persistent late variable or prolonged decelerations or other pattern that is clearly interpretable. *(Continued on next page)*

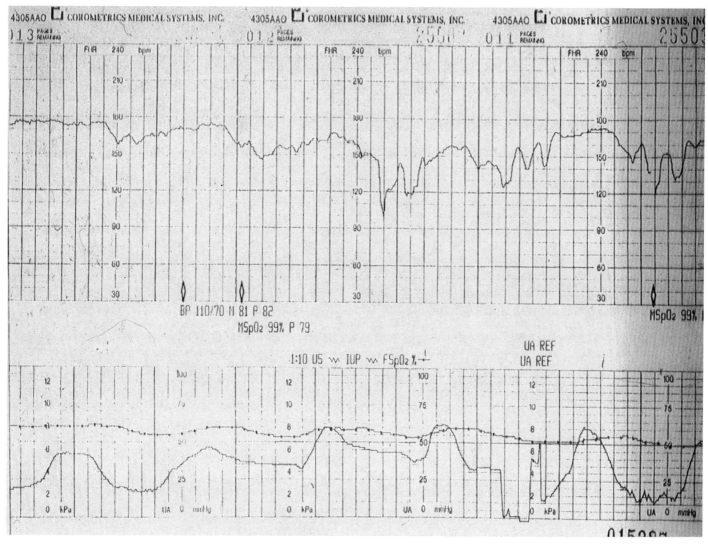

B

FIGURE 10.14. *(continued)* The use of fetal pulse oximetry in such a case can often provide enough reassurance that intervention is not needed, as occurred in this case where the oxygen saturation persistently ranges from 45% to 60% and is continuously reassuring.

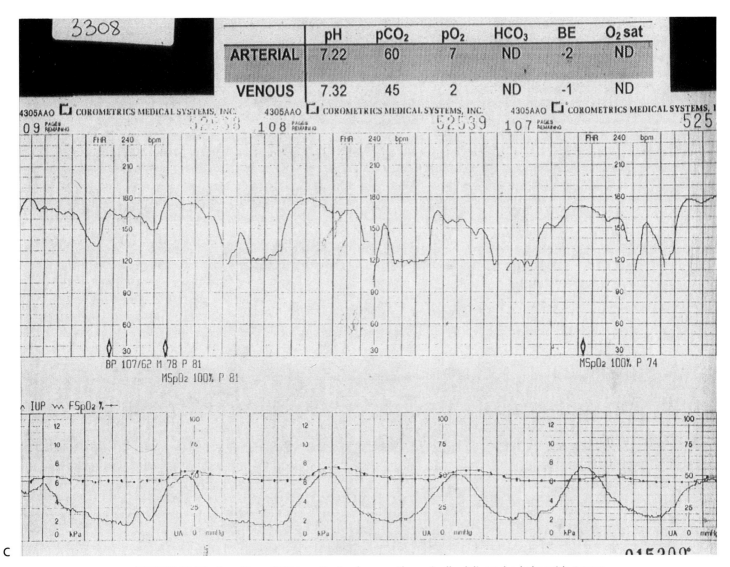

	pH	pCO$_2$	pO$_2$	HCO$_3$	BE	O$_2$ sat
ARTERIAL	7.22	60	7	ND	-2	ND
VENOUS	7.32	45	2	ND	-1	ND

FIGURE 10.14. *(continued)* This patient subsequently vaginally delivered a baby with Apgar scores of 7 at 1 minute and 9 at 5 minutes and cord pH, illustrated on **panel C**, which were normal but with slightly elevated pCO$_2$ in the arterial vessel of the umbilical cord.

to manage patterns, such as persistent unexplained tachycardia (Fig. 10.15) or loss of variability (Fig. 10.16), but without decelerations, are also patterns where $FSpO_2$ monitoring can be extremely helpful when persistently normal oxygen saturation values are found.

A nonreassuring $FSpO_2$ is defined as one in which the saturation falls below 30% for a significant time in the presence of a nonreassuring FHR pattern. The exact duration the saturation must remain below 30% for the fetus to be at risk for metabolic acidosis has not been definitively defined. Studies have suggested ranges of from 2 to 10 minutes. Obviously this duration also depends on the severity of the hypoxia. This does not really come into play clinically, because the most severe ranges of hypoxia usually produce prolonged decelerations and usually require intervention based on the FHR alone. In the U.S. randomized trial, a definition for nonreassurance was arbitrarily chosen as an $FSpO_2$ that stayed below 30% for the entire duration between two contractions (Fig. 10.17). Using this defini-

tion, no unexplained cases of severe metabolic acidosis were found in over 500 babies monitored with both FHR and $FSpO_2$.

RISKS AND BENEFIT

Like many diagnostic or monitoring modalities, the majority of early studies have been devoted to evaluating the accuracy of the device as well as exploring how best to use it in clinical practice. Subsequent to this, the device was implemented into clinical practice, especially in Europe, without a great deal of systematic study to define its real clinical value. Currently the available studies evaluating the benefit of this device in monitoring the fetus in labor are limited. There has been one large multicenter randomized controlled trial conducted before the introduction and approval of this device in the United States. This study, published in November 2000, was conducted in nine cen-

(text continues on page 164)

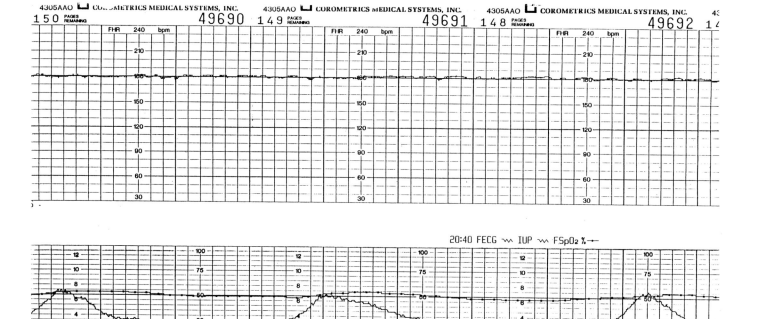

FIGURE 10.15. This patient is a gravida 1 para 0 at term admitted in active labor. She progressed normally with occasional variable decelerations that were not persistent. Later in labor, an unexplained fetal tachycardia developed up to 180 beats per minute with decreased variability but no decelerations. This is another situation where fetal pulse oximetry ultimately can provide reassurance because such patterns are not likely to be associated with fetal hypoxia. Several hours later this patient delivered a baby with Apgar scores of 9 at 1 minute and 9 at 5 minutes and normal umbilical blood gases (7.27 arterial, 7.36 venous).

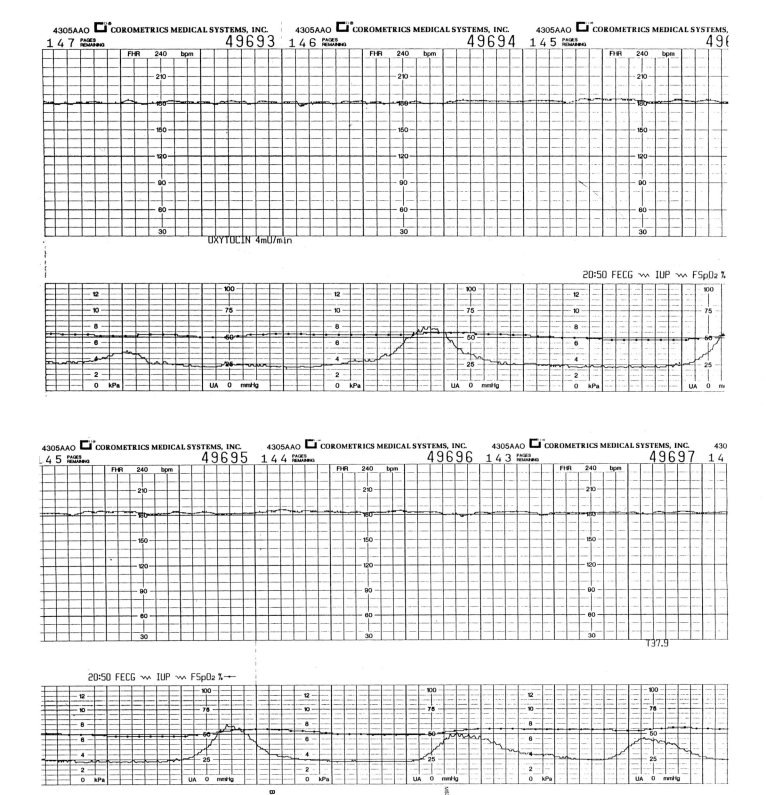

FIGURE 10.15. *(continued)*

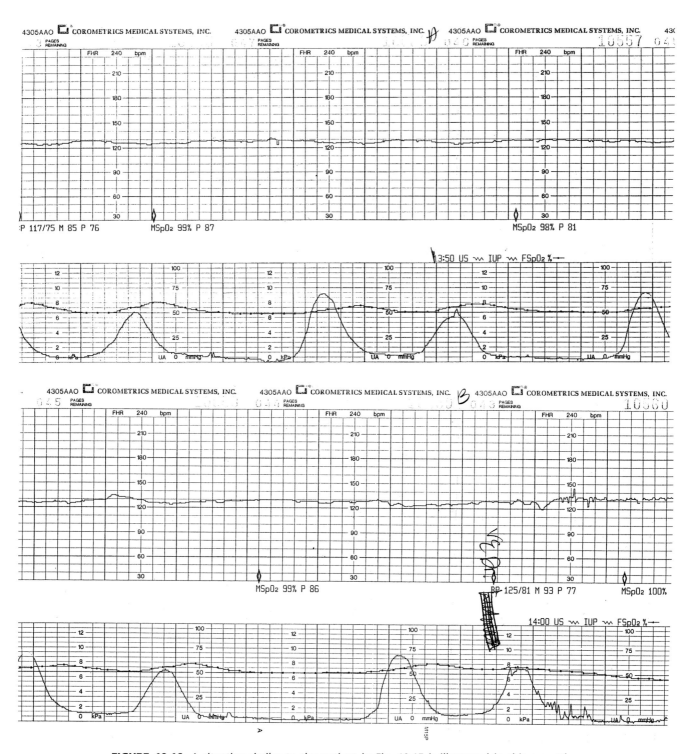

FIGURE 10.16. A situation similar to the patient in Fig. 10.15 is illustrated in this case. The patient presents with a fetal heart rate tracing with a normal heart rate of 130 beats per minute and no deceleration but with significantly decreased variability and absence of accelerations. Explanations for cases like this might include fetal anomalies, depressant drugs, sepsis, etc. In the absence of decelerations, it is unlikely that this is due to hypoxia. Fetal pulse oximetry can be used in such cases to rule out hypoxia as in this case where indeed oxygen saturations were normal with values between 50% and 60%. This patient subsequently delivered with normal Apgar scores and no explanation for the decreased variability that persisted throughout labor was found.

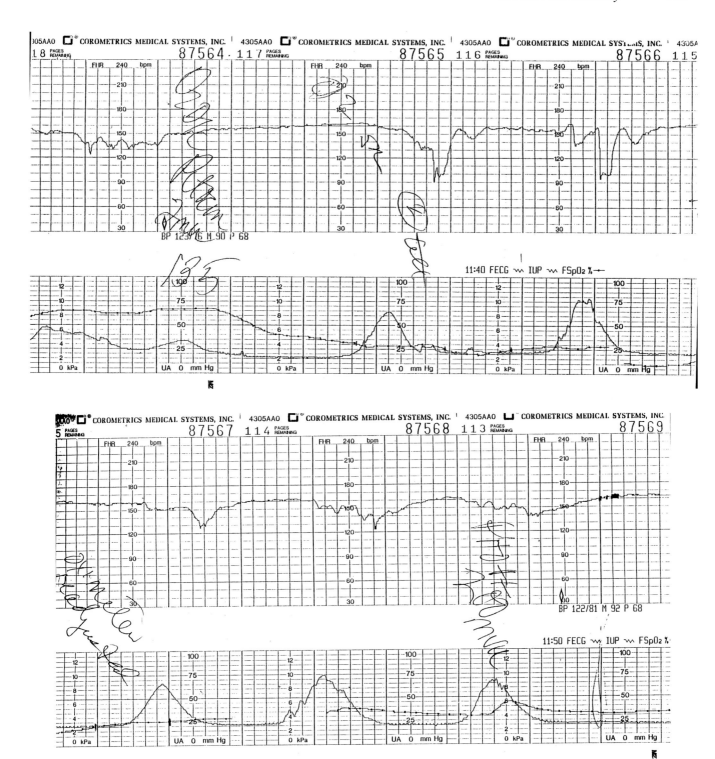

FIGURE 10.17. In the setting of the nonreassuring fetal heart rate (FHR) tracing as seen in this case, pulse oximetry must remain above 30% to provide reassurance. This patient is having persistent late decelerations with tachycardia and decreased variability. Initially the oxygen saturation at 60% to 70% is reassuring. However, in **panel 87565** the oxygen saturation drops down to 25% and persists below 30% for approximately 8 minutes. She underwent a primary cesarean section for a nonreassuring fetal status both from an FHR standpoint and oxygen saturation standpoint. At term a baby was delivered with Apgar scores of 9 at 1 minute and 9 at 5 minutes, arterial cord pH of 7.19 BE –5 and venous cord pH of 7.24 BE –4. *(Continued on next page)*

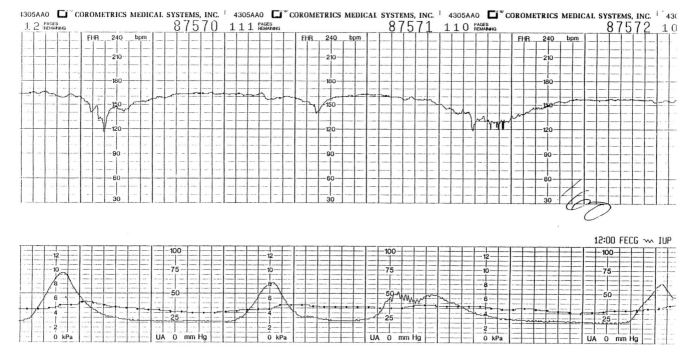

FIGURE 10.17. *(continued)*

ters, geographically distributed throughout the United States (12). The study included patients at 36 weeks or longer in active labor with a nonreassuring FHR pattern. Patients were randomized to be monitored by EFM alone versus EFM plus fetal pulse oximetry. Ultimately 1,010 patients were randomized, 508 to the study (oximetry and EFM) and 502 to the control (EFM alone) groups. There was a 50% reduction in the cesarean section rate for nonreassuring fetal status from 10% to 5%, but no reduction in the overall cesarean section rate because of a higher rate of cesarean section for dystocia in the study group. After detailed analysis, the authors concluded that this increase in cesarean section for dystocia was neither due to investigator bias nor the device. In addition, the study showed that both the specificity and sensitivity of $FSpO_2$ monitoring were improved using the decision to perform operative delivery for a nonreassuring fetal pattern compared to its correlation with neonatal depression, acidosis at birth, and need for resuscitation. This decrease in CS for NRFS and any delay in delivering babies with nonreassuring FHR patterns in the study group were accomplished without any apparent increase in adverse maternal or neonatal outcome. There were significantly more fetuses with severe metabolic acidosis (base excess >15) in the EFM alone group. The authors concluded that fetal pulse oximetry as a backup method for the fetus with a nonreassuring FHR pattern is a more accurate method for identifying the truly acidotic fetus in need of immediate delivery than EFM alone.

Safety

Outside of the United States and on study protocols in this country, over 30,000 patients were monitored with this device before its approval for use by the U.S. Food and Drug Administration in May 2000. The safety record of this device has been outstanding with no serious device-related complications despite this vast experience (personal communication, Debbie Reisenthal, Nellcor Perinatal, Pleasanton, California, February 2001). Numerous studies, including the multicenter trial previously discussed, have looked carefully for complications (12–14). The only common side effect is an indentation in the baby's face that disappears within hours of birth. No studies have shown an increase in maternal infectious complications, although most studies included patients who were monitored with other internal devices (scalp electrode, intrauterine pressure catheter). Dildy and Clark did report a statistically, but not clinically significant increase in maternal temperature in women whose labors were monitored with fetal pulse oximetry (14).

CURRENT UNRESOLVED PROBLEMS

There are several problems that remain unresolved before this device provides optimal value in intrapartum fetal evaluation. It is generally easy to insert, especially for individuals who have experience in inserting intrauterine pressure monitoring catheters, and the learning curve for introduction is short. The vast majority of fetuses will have the device successfully placed (>98%), and the only impediments include minimal cervical dilation (<2 cm), high station (< −2), complete dilation with low station, and rarely very thick vernix. The principal problem currently is maintaining a continuous signal. With fetal movement and descent during labor, the continuous recording of the device is frequently lost and relatively frequent adjustments of the catheter to reestablish contact are often necessary, particularly in the second stage of labor. While the exact frequency of these adjustments is unknown, the authors estimate it at about two to three times per hour. It is important to point out, however, that the device is designed not to display inaccurate values, as when either the electrical contact is inadequate or the fetal pulse amplitude is insufficient, no signal will be displayed. There are also other situations where the reliability of the device is currently unknown. These would include, but are not limited to, fetal sepsis, fetal anemia, and, of course, situations where fetal damage may be due to causes other than fetal hypoxia.

UTILITY OF FETAL PULSE OXIMETRY MONITORING

There is now substantial evidence that fetal pulse oximetry monitoring is a safe and accurate device for the evaluation of oxygenation in the term fetus in labor with a nonreassuring FHR pattern. Although the published studies are encouraging and give us assurance that the device can accurately do what it is purported to do, it remains to be seen whether the device will overcome the limitations of electronic FHR monitoring in actual practice.

Based on this lack of extensive clinical experience but on the reassurance the current studies provide, we can make the following recommendations on its use. FHR monitoring is reliable when reassuring and can be used externally in patients in early labor and in those with intact membranes. In addition, there is vast experience with electronic FHR monitoring and we know its benefits and limitations. FHR patterns not only often tell us when there is hypoxia, but they often tell us the mechanism of the hypoxia, and by their progression may help us prognosticate whether more serious problems will occur later in labor. Thus the pulse oximetry device should not replace FHR monitoring, nor should it be used when the FHR is reassuring, but rather it will complement the FHR monitor when a confusing or nonreassuring FHR is present.

Because fetal oximetry monitoring appears to be most valuable when the FHR pattern is nonreassuring, some specific recommendations may assist the clinician in deciding when to use this technology. FHR patterns where pulse oximetry monitoring may be most useful are listed in Table 10.1. Basically these are the same patterns used by those who use scalp pH or assessment of accelerations of the FHR

TABLE 10.1. FETAL HEART RATE PATTERNS WARRANTING THE USE OF FETAL PULSE OXIMETRY MONITORING

Persistent late decelerations
Variable decelerations with any of the following
  Those that become severe in depth and duration (e.g., <70 BPM × >60 sec)
  Slow return to baseline
  Associated tachycardia
  Associated loss of variability
Unexplained loss of variability for <30 minutes
Unexplained tachycardia
Baseline bradycardia
Tachycardia with loss of variability
Unexplained loss of accelerations <60 minutes
Apparent sinusoidal pattern
The confusing FHR pattern

to confirm a nonreassuring FHR pattern. As with scalp pH, with a clearly ominous pattern, one should not take the time to insert the pulse oximeter because any additional time spent could delay the need for urgent intervention.

Fetal pulse oximetry has many potential benefits. Pulse oximetry can clarify the confusing FHR pattern; has the potential to help the clinician with the decision of whether and how urgent there is a need for operative vaginal or cesarean delivery; and provides a more clear-cut end point, thus potentially eliminating disagreements over interpretation of the FHR pattern. Because many times, we overreact to patterns in labor often not associated with hypoxia, it also has the potential to help us learn which situations require interventions we also overuse and may unnecessarily increase patient anxiety, such as oxygen administration, hydration, and repositioning. Finally, by providing more clear end points, the device has the potential, as it did in anesthesia, to decrease lawsuits alleging neurologic damage and other complications were caused by hypoxia, when in reality significant hypoxia did not occur.

Only utilization in practice and future studies will determine how well this device will perform in actual practice. How should the device be used; will it decrease cesarean section rates, will it result in fewer lawsuits, will it be used widely, and someday will it be used universally? Only time will tell. Further confirmatory randomized and observational trials are needed. The device will open new doors to our understanding of normal and pathologic fetal oxygenation in labor, of FHR patterns in labor, and which therapies work and which do not. Finally the opportunity for new scientific studies are boundless.

REFERENCES

1. Seelbach-Gobel B, Heupel M, Kuhnert M, et al.: The prediction of fetal acidosis by means of intrapartum pulse oximetry. *Am J Obstet Gynecol* 80:73–81, 1991. Correction printed *Am J Obstet Gynecol* 180:1048, 1999.

2. Johnson N: Development and potential of fetal pulse oximetry. *Contemp Rev Obstet Gynecol* 3:193–200, 1991.

3. Nijland R, Jongsma HW, Nijhuis JG, et al.: Arterial oxygen saturation in relation to metabolic acidosis in fetal lambs. *Am J Obstet Gynecol* 172: 810–819, 1994.

4. Richardson B, Carmichael L, Homan J, et al.: Cerebral oxidative metabolism in fetal sheep with prolonged, graded hypoxemia. Presented at the 36th Meeting of the Society for Gynecologic Investigation, San Diego, California, March 1989.

5. Dildy GA, van den Berg PP, Katz M, et al.: Intrapartum fetal pulse oximetry: fetal oxygen saturation trends during labor and relation to delivery outcome. *Am J Obstet Gynecol* 171:679–684, 1994.

6. Goffinet F, Langer B, Carbonne B, et al., and the French Study Group on Fetal Pulse Oximetry: Multicenter study on the clinical value of fetal pulse oximetry. I. Methodologic evaluation. *Am J Obstet Gynecol* 177:1238–1246, 1997.

7. Kuhnert M, Seelback-Gobel B, Butterwegge M: Predictive agreement between the fetal arterial oxygen saturation and fetal scalp pH: results of the German multicenter study. *Am J Obstet Gynecol* 178:330–335, 1998.

8. Carbonne B, Langer B, Goffinet F, et al.: Multicenter study on the clinical value of fetal pulse oximetry. II. Compared predictive values of pulse oximetry and fetal blood analysis. *Am J Obstet Gynecol* 177:593–598, 1997.

9. Dildy G, Thorp J, Yeast J, et al.: The relationship between oxygen saturation and pH in umbilical blood: implications for intrapartum fetal oxygen saturation monitoring. *Am J Obstet Gynecol* 175:682–687, 1996.

10. Carbonne B, Audibert F, Segard L, et al.: Fetal pulse oximetry: correlation between changes in oxygen saturation and neonatal outcome. *Eur J Obstet Gynecol Reprod Biol* 57:73–77, 1994.

11. Lee R, Moore M, Brewster W, et al.: Late decelerations and severe variables are predictive of fetal hypoxia. *Am J Obstet Gynecol* 185:S130, 2001.

12. Garite TJ, Dildy GA, McNamara H, et al.: A multicenter controlled trial of fetal pulse oximetry in the intrapartum management of nonreassuring fetal heart rate patterns. *Am J Obstet Gynecol* 183:1049–1058, 2000.

13. Johnson N, Johnson VA, McNamara H, et al.: Fetal pulse oximetry: a new method of monitoring the fetus. *Aust NZ J Obstet Gynecol* 34:428–432, 1994.

14. Dildy GA, Loucks CA, Clark SL: Intrapartum fetal pulse oximetry puerperal morbidity. Paper presented at the Society for Perinatal Obstetricians 16th annual Meeting, Kamuela, HI, January 1996.

DIAGNOSIS AND MANAGEMENT OF NONREASSURING FETAL HEART RATE PATTERNS IN PREMATURE GESTATION

The potential for the beneficial effects of fetal heart rate (FHR) monitoring in the patient delivering prematurely is perhaps greater than in any other risk group. The continuation of dramatic improvements in the neonatal survival rates at progressively earlier gestational ages increases the necessity for evaluating fetal well-being in early pregnancies and for intervention in fetal indications. Delivering prematurely is, of course, an abnormal event, and as opposed to normal labor and delivery in the term pregnancy, the various pathologic causes of premature delivery are often scenarios in which the likelihood of fetal hypoxia is increased. The premature fetus is more likely not only to be exposed to hypoxia, but also to develop, and die from, the most common and serious complications of prematurity if born depressed and/or acidotic. FHR patterns in the premature fetus, both normal tracings and those indicative of distress, differ from those at term. It therefore seems appropriate to emphasize the evaluation and management of fetal hypoxia separately in the premature fetus.

EFFECTS OF HYPOXIA IN THE PREMATURE FETUS

It is clear that neonatal care is the major contributor to the ongoing improvements in survival and decreasing permanent morbidities in premature babies. A growing body of evidence indicates that the condition in which the premature newborn is delivered has an important impact on both its likelihood to survive and its odds of developing serious complications of prematurity.

Respiratory Distress Syndrome

In the early 1970s, when electronic FHR monitoring was initiated, Hobel et al. (1) and Martin et al. (2) showed that fetal distress had an impact on the outcome of the premature newborn. Both investigations demonstrated that premature babies with low Apgar scores, abnormal FHR patterns, or both, in labor had higher chances of developing respiratory distress syndrome (RDS), the most common serious complication of premature neonates, and had higher chances of dying of this complication. In the series of Martin and coworkers, abnormal FHR patterns were more predictive of RDS development than were low Apgar scores. Subsequent research has confirmed these findings. Physiologically this makes sense, as those enzyme systems responsible for the production of surfactant, which keeps the term baby's lungs open at birth, are very sensitive to acidosis in the preterm baby. Donald and coworkers (3) have shown that even those babies with amniotic fluid lecithin-to-sphingomyelin ratios that are indicative of fetal lung maturity may develop RDS if fetal distress and/or acidosis precede delivery.

Intraventricular Hemorrhage

With improved outcomes in even smaller babies, and as the treatment of RDS has become more successful, intraventricular hemorrhage (IVH) has assumed greater importance in the morbidity of the very premature newborn. Initially, intracranial compression forces were thought to be causative, but as data have accumulated, it has become apparent that route of delivery, per se, has little to do with IVH (4–6). The most important risk factor for IVH is the degree of prematurity, with newborns in the range of 500 to 1,000 g being at highest risk. Ventilator therapy probably ranks next in importance, due to the combination of RDS and patent ductus arteriosus in this very low birthweight group (7,8). Fetal distress in labor ranks next. Babies with no RDS and normal Apgar scores at birth are unlikely to develop the more severe degrees of IVH (grades 3 and 4), regardless of birthweight (8). Because fetal distress and RDS are integrally related, it becomes apparent that the labor process is of critical importance in determining whether the very low birthweight fetus will develop and possibly die of these two serious complications (IVH and RDS).

Necrotizing Enterocolitis

Necrotizing enterocolitis (NEC) is another important and potentially lethal complication in the premature infant. Although the cause is unknown, risk factors include infection, early feeding, umbilical arterial lines, exchange transfusion, and polycythemia (9). NEC is most likely to occur in premature infants with a history of perinatal asphyxia. The proposed mechanism is diversion of gastrointestinal blood flow to more critical organs with asphyctic conditions, resulting in ischemic injury to the bowel (9,10). In a review of FHR tracings of babies who developed NEC, Braly et al. (11) found that only 1 of 16 babies had a normal tracing, and 11 had severe FHR changes.

Death and Long-Term Injury

As one would expect, babies with fetal distress and the above complications are more likely to die in the neonatal period (1–15). Furthermore, the abnormal FHR patterns in labor that are indicative of potential compromise have also been found to correlate with immediate and long-term neurologic sequelae. Westgren and colleagues found abnormal FHR patterns to be highly predictive of fetal acidosis and that in acidotic babies with abnormal FHR patterns, neurologic problems in the neonatal period were more frequent than those in controls (12,13). They also found a relationship between abnormal FHR, acidosis, and death from asphyxia in the first 2 years of life.

In general, the earlier in pregnancy that delivery occurs, the more profound the correlation between abnormal FHR patterns, neonatal depression and acidosis, and immediate and long-term complications. Most studies find these relationships to be most persistent and most profound in babies of less than 33 weeks' gestation with birth weights of less than 1,500 g (12,13,15). For complications such as severe IVH, earlier gestations, such as those of less than 28 weeks and birth weights of less than 1,000 g, are more important.

RELATIONSHIP BETWEEN CAUSE OF PREMATURE BIRTH AND FETAL COMPROMISE

Many of the causes of prematurity are also situations that increase the probability that the fetus will be subjected to antepartum and/or intrapartum hypoxia, thus the premature baby not only is more likely to suffer complications if it becomes asphyxiated, but is also more likely to be subjected to asphyxia. The implications for management relate to the reasons for this increased exposure as it pertains to the various causes.

Abruptio Placentae

Abruption is an uncommon complication, occurring in only about 0.5% of term infants and in 5% to 10% of premature deliveries (16–18). Abruptio placentae increases hypoxic insults through two mechanisms. The separation of the placenta from the maternal blood supply, depending on degree, decreases placental surface area and thus oxygen exchange. In addition, there is often a marked increase in the frequency and, occasionally, duration of contractions, which prolongs the interval during which oxygen delivery to the intervillous space is interrupted. Because placental insufficiency is the mechanism of the fetal hypoxia, late decelerations will be the characteristic FHR pattern, and prolonged decelerations may occur in severe cases. One particular benefit of fetal monitoring is that patients sometimes present with preterm labor with minimal or no bleeding, and the contraction pattern and/or late decelerations are the earliest and only indication that abruptio placentae is the etiology of the premature labor (Fig. 11.1).

Preeclampsia

Preeclampsia is not an unusual cause of premature delivery resulting from associated premature labor, abruption, or induction of labor at an early gestational age because of the severity of the disease. Often, the onset of preeclampsia at very early gestational ages is associated with intrauterine growth retardation (IUGR) and chronic placental insufficiency. In such cases, FHR patterns may exhibit late decelerations if there is insufficient placental perfusion (Fig. 11.2) and/or variable decelerations if there is growth retardation and oligohydramnios leading to cord compression (Fig. 11.3). Clinical decisions regarding delivery of a very premature infant in a setting of nonreassuring FHR are complex and involve the integration of both maternal and fetal issues and prognoses.

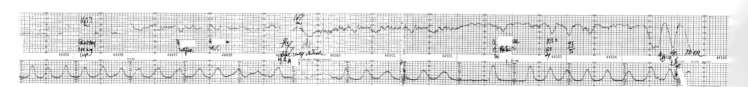

FIGURE 11.1. This patient presented in active labor with a maternal fever, no bleeding, and a gestational age of 32 weeks. The rise in baseline might be secondary to the maternal fever, but the onset of frequent ominous decelerations led to emergency cesarean section. A large retroplacental hematoma was present at surgery.

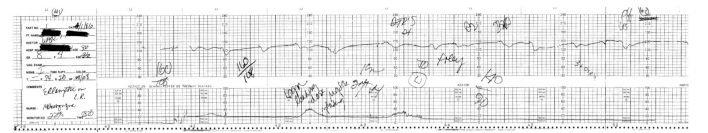

FIGURE 11.2. This patient presented with severe preeclampsia, and while receiving a loading dose of magnesium dulfate, she experienced an eclamptic seizure. Persistent late decelerations continued, and a cesarean section was performed following maternal stabilization. A severely growth-restricted infant with Apgar scores of 3 and 6 at 1 and 5 minutes, respectively, was delivered with evidence of moderate respiratory acidosis. Newborn course was benign.

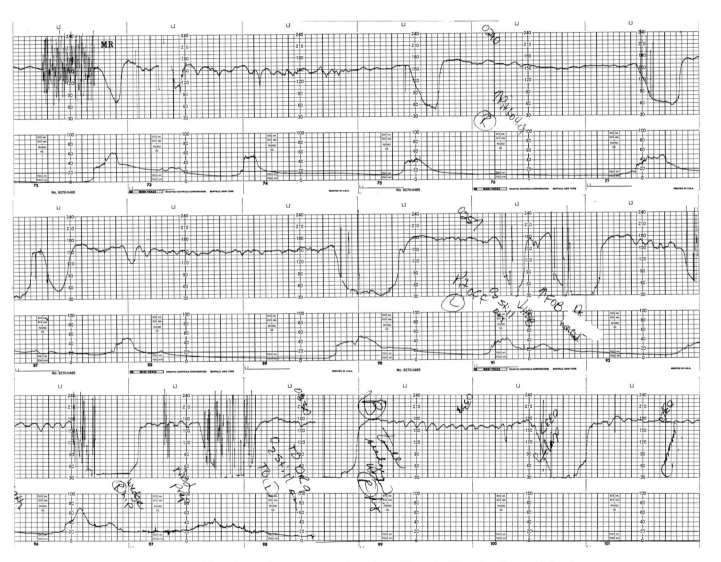

FIGURE 11.3. This patient with severe preeclampsia at 27 weeks illustrates the rapid development of progressively severe variable decelerations associated with developing fetal tachycardia. These patterns are similar to those seen with oligohydramnios secondary to premature rupture of membranes, but in this case the oligohydramnios was present with intact membranes. Cesarean section yielded an 860-g baby with Apgar scores of 1 and 4 and marked respiratory acidosis.

Preterm Premature Rupture of Membranes

Preterm premature rupture of membranes (PPROM) is the most common single circumstance leading to premature delivery and accounts for approximately 35% of preterm deliveries. Patients with PPROM in preterm labor have a sevenfold greater risk of fetal compromise requiring cesarean section than patients with preterm labor with intact membranes (19). The vast majority of such patients have variable or recurrent prolonged decelerative patterns consistent with umbilical cord compression secondary to oligohydramnios (Figs. 11.4 and 11.5). Prospective use of amnioinfusion has been demonstrated to decrease the frequency and severity of such decelerations and allow for vaginal delivery in such patients (20).

Intrauterine Growth Retardation

IUGR may result in preterm delivery either because the problem that caused the growth retardation also leads to preterm labor, as in preeclampsia or thyrotoxicosis, or because the physician detecting the IUGR decides to intervene prematurely. In such cases, fetal intolerance to labor is more likely due to the associated placental insufficiency resulting in late decelerations or to the associated oligohydramnios leading to umbilical cord compression patterns (Fig. 11.6). Fetuses with IUGR are even more susceptible to damage from asphyxia than their premature counterparts of similar gestational ages.

Infections

PROM or premature labor is commonly associated with clinical or occult chorioamnionitis. FHR patterns are affected by factors such as maternal fever or fetal sepsis. A variety of FHR changes may be seen. If there is maternal fever, the fetal temperature will increase and fetal tachycardia will develop. This tachycardia may be associated with a loss of variability from the rising FHR. The increased oxygen demands with the higher heart and

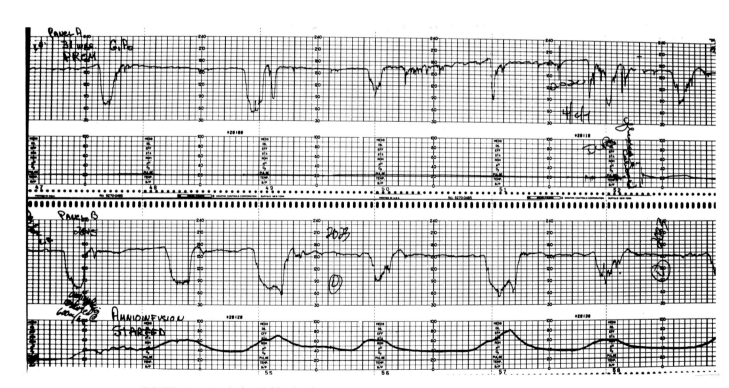

FIGURE 11.4. Typical variable decelerations seen in early labor (4 cm dilation) in a patient with premature rupture of membranes and oligohydramnios at 31 weeks. An attempt at amnioinfusion (seen on the **lower panel**) failed to relieve the cord compression, and the patient required cesarean section for a worsening pattern.

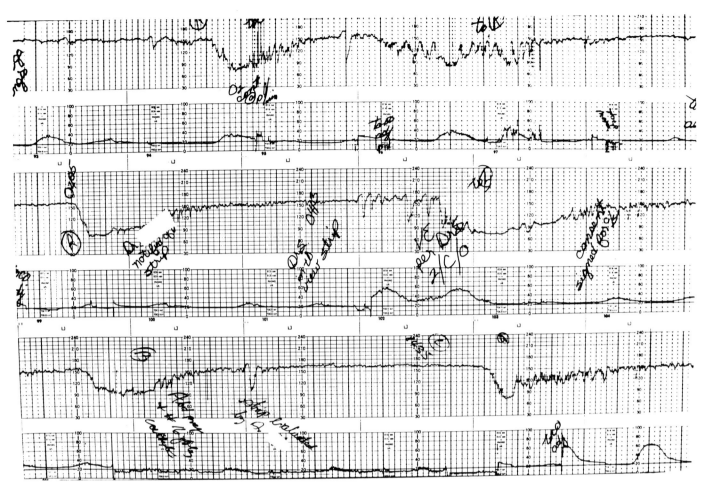

FIGURE 11.5. This patient was being treated expectantly in the hospital with premature rupture of membranes (PROM) at 34 weeks. She noticed mild contractions and was immediately monitored. Note the prolonged and variable decelerations that are occurring even though the patient is in early labor (irregular contractions, 2 cm dilated). With the presence of oligohydramnios secondary to PROM, the early development of such patterns is common.

metabolic rates may result in late decelerations. In septic fetuses there may be tachycardia, loss of variability, and loss of accelerations (reactivity) (Fig. 11.7). Often, this cannot be distinguished from changes secondary to maternal fever, and the use of the FHR to identify fetal infection is a problem.

A substantial proportion of premature infants are exposed to amniotic fluid infection and an associated proinflammatory response and cytokine production. Neonatal mortality is increased by prematurity, amniotic fluid infection, and associated maternal and fetal inflammatory responses. Morbidities such as respiratory distress syndrome, bronchopulmonary dysplasia, periventricular leukomalacia, and cerebral palsy are increased in the setting of amniotic fluid infection over and above those attributable to prematurity alone (21–25). Consequently, close attention needs to be directed to those at greatest risk to be complicated by amniotic fluid infection. There is no evidence to

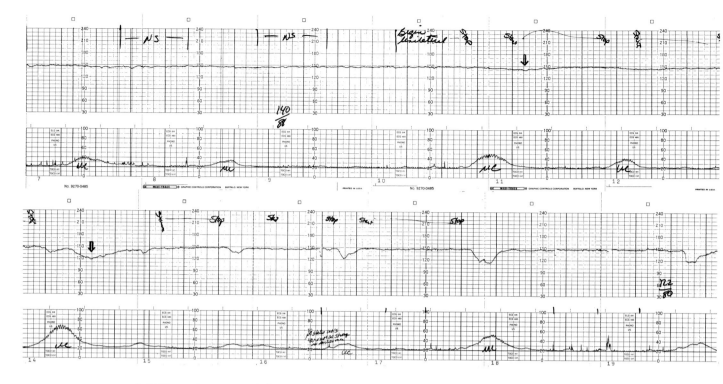

FIGURE 11.6. A 27-week fetus with suspected intrauterine growth retardation underwent a nonstress test, which was nonreactive. A contraction stress test was performed by nipple stimulation. Two late decelerations are seen with the stronger contractions (**arrows**) presumably secondary to the uteroplacental insufficiency, and multiple variable decelerations secondary to the oligohydramnios are also present.

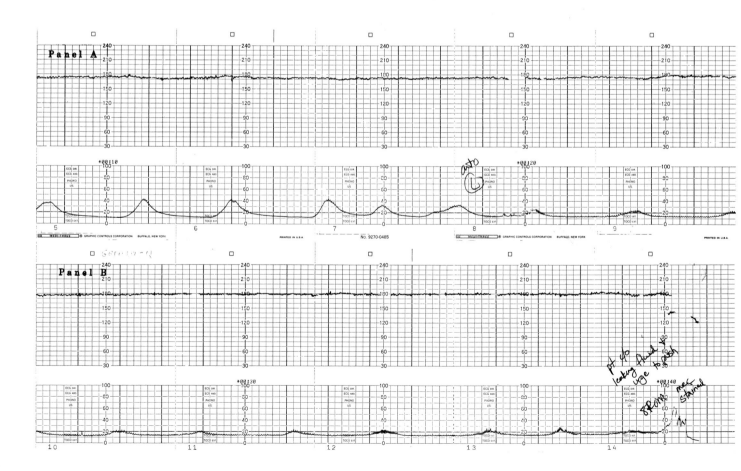

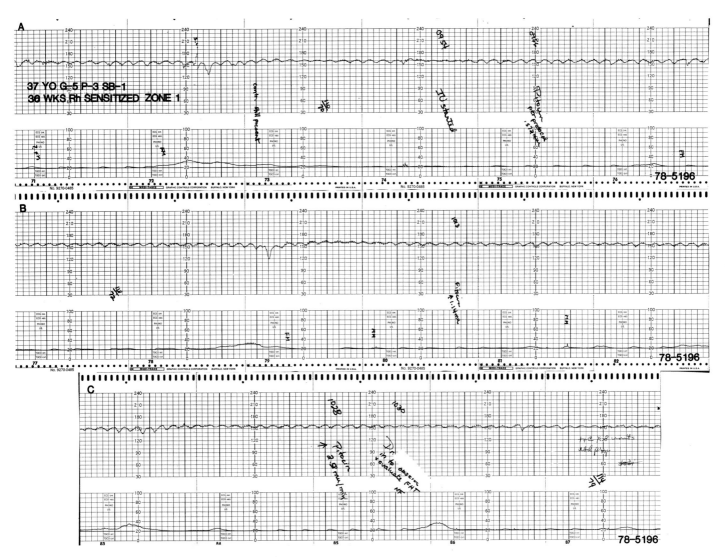

FIGURE 11.8. This Rh-sensitized patient at 36 weeks had an amniocentesis 2 weeks previously with a normal (Liley Zone I) delta OD450. On routine nonstress testing, this classic sinusoidal pattern was found. Note the absence of reactivity and the probable late deceleration on **panel B.** Immediate delivery resulted in a severely anemic, nonhydropic baby with a central hematocrit of 18%.

suggest that intrapartum intervention can alter these outcomes.

Fetal Isoimmunization

Fetal isoimmunization and subsequent hydrops may be identified in the preterm pregnancy. In an anemic fetus,

tachycardia, late decelerations, and sinusoidal patterns may occur (Fig. 11.8).

Malpresentations

Premature fetuses are more likely than those at term to present in labor with breech or other malpresentations. Simi-

FIGURE 11.7. External monitoring of this patient, being evaluated at 29 weeks for possible premature labor, revealed tachycardia (170 beats per minute) and no accelerations, although no decelerations were seen. The end of **panel B** notes where spontaneous rupture of membranes occurred. Labor progressed, and in view of a breech presentation, cesarean section was performed. The patient was delivered of a depressed baby (Apgar scores 1 and 3) with normal umbilical cord pH values. Clinically, the baby was septic, and blood culture specimens revealed *Listeria monocytogenes.* The combination of depressed Apgar scores and normal cord blood gas values is characteristic of the septic baby.

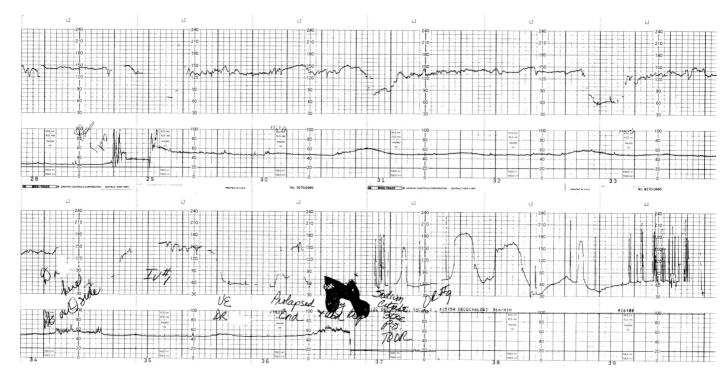

FIGURE 11.9. A patient with a breech presentation and premature rupture of membranes at 31 weeks was being managed expectantly: On noting some mild contractions, she was brought to the labor area for monitoring. The variable decelerations seen on the **upper panel** suggest significant umbilical cord compression. On the **lower panel** these have progressed rapidly, and pelvic examination revealed a cord prolapse. Elevation of the buttock, followed by immediate cesarean section, produced a 1,340-g baby with Apgar scores of 4 and 7 and a mild respiratory acidosis.

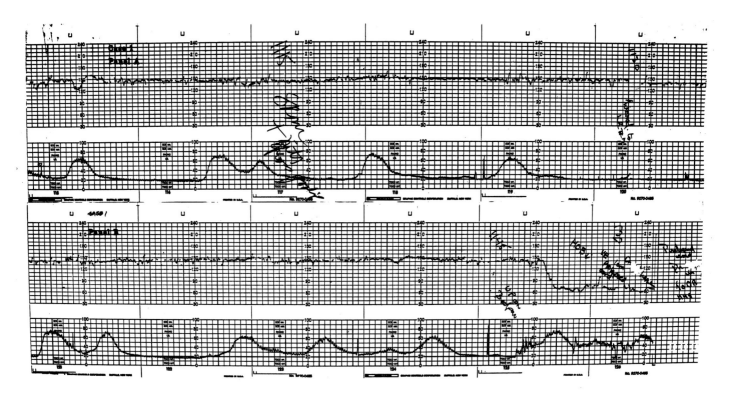

FIGURE 11.10. This patient is in active labor with a vertex presentation. Following a sudden gush of fluid from the vagina there was a deceleration of the fetal heart rate. Immediate pelvic examination revealed a small loop of umbilical cord between the cervix and fetal head. Immediate cesarean section ensued with delivery of a healthy newborn.

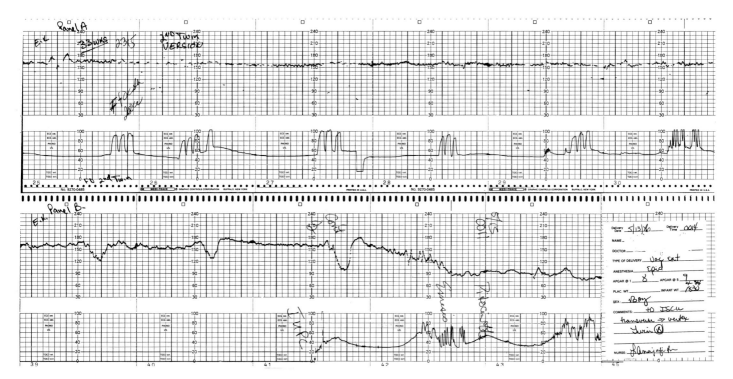

FIGURE 11.11. At 33 weeks, a patient with a twin gestation presenting vertex (twin A) and breech (twin B) was admitted in advanced premature labor. Following delivery of twin A, an external cephalic version of twin B was performed. As the vertex descended into the pelvis, an amniotomy was done and an internal electrode placed **(panel B)**. A prolonged deceleration developed with the vertex at +1 station, and a vacuum extraction yielded a 1830-g baby boy with Apgar scores of 8 and 9 with the cord adjacent to the baby's head.

larly, fetuses allowed to proceed to labor and delivery with nonvertex presentations are more likely than those with vertex presentations to have cord compression and cord prolapse (Figs. 11.9 and 11.10).

Multiple Gestation

Multiple gestations deliver prematurely at a higher rate than any other risk group. Twins are more likely to exhibit fetal distress for a number of reasons. More malpresentations, abruptions, cord prolapses, IUGR, preeclampsia, and PROM are exhibited in this group than in singleton gestations, and as explained previously, each of these risks has associated increases in fetal compromise (Fig. 11.11). In addition, monochorionic multifetal gestations with discordance of fetal growth, regardless of the cause of the discordance, exhibit more fetal compromise patterns. Therefore, the effects are additive. Twins are more likely to deliver prematurely and are more likely to have these associated complications.

DIFFERENCES IN FETAL HEART RATE PATTERNS IN PRETERM PREGNANCIES

In addition to being more susceptible to the effects of hypoxia and more likely to be subjected to these insults, preterm fetuses manifest FHR patterns in response to hypoxic insults that differ significantly from those of fetuses at term.

Antepartum Fetal Heart Rate Patterns

The normal preterm FHR and FHR patterns in the antepartum period differ somewhat from those of later gestations. The average FHR will be higher (see Fig. 2.6), up to 160 beats per minute (BPM) may be normal in the preterm fetus, whereas the normal-term FHR will rarely range above 150 to 155 BPM. Accelerations are generally of lower amplitude and less frequency in the preterm fetus (Fig. 11.12A); however, even at 24 to 26 weeks and beyond, the majority of FHRs meet the criteria for reactivity (>15 BPM of amplitude lasting at least 15 seconds) (Fig. 11.12B) (26,27). Similarly, FHR variability is somewhat less in the

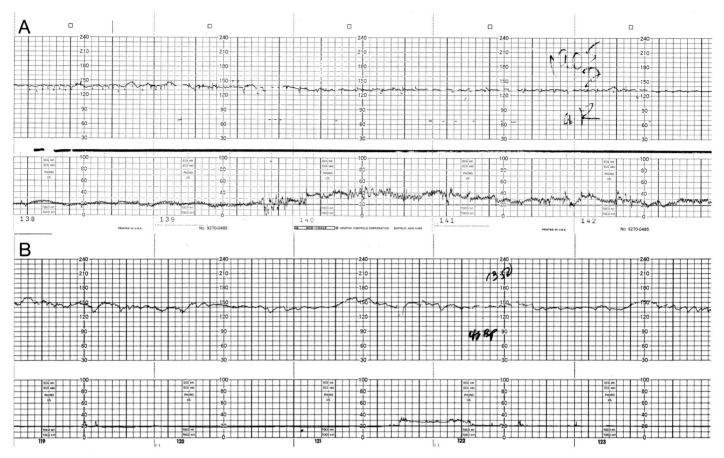

FIGURE 11.12. These external tracings of two different fetuses, both at 27 weeks, show the great variation in the amplitude and duration of accelerations that can be seen in healthy babies at this early gestational age. In the first part of **panel A,** three small accelerations of about 5 beats per minute (BPM) appear. Seen in **panel B** are numerous accelerations of 10 to 20 BPM above the baseline and lasting up to 1½ minutes.

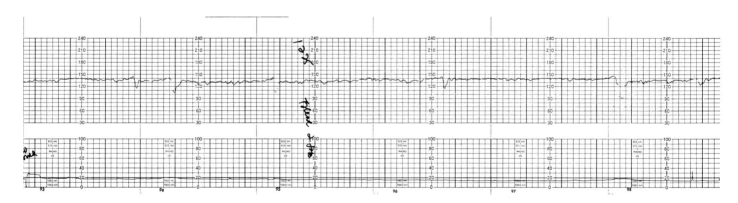

FIGURE 11.13. Frequent small decelerations, characteristic of the very premature fetal heart rate, are seen in this external tracing at 25 weeks.

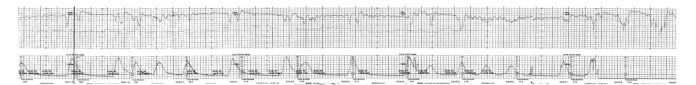

FIGURE 11.14. This tracing is that of a patient at 30 weeks' gestation with premature rupture of membranes for at least 2 days. She had no prenatal care, and maternal temperature was 101°F on admission. Note the significant baseline tachycardia and rapidly progressing and worsening decelerations. Emergency cesarean section resulted in delivery of a depressed 1,200-g premature infant with Apgar scores of 1 and 2 at 1 and 5 minutes, respectively. Cord gases revealed moderate to severe mixed metabolic and respiratory acidosis. The infant died secondary to overwhelming sepsis.

very premature fetus, although this has not been quantified. Sorokin et al. (28) have reported that variable decelerations commonly occur in fetuses at 20 to 30 weeks, even in the absence of contractions. These decelerations are, however, generally minimal in depth and duration, and deeper and longer decelerations appear to have a significance similar to that in term pregnancies (Fig. 11.13).

Intrapartum Fetal Heart Rate Patterns

The intrapartum differences in the normal FHR, in both baseline and periodic changes, are the same as those described previously for the antepartum period. However, there are marked differences in the appearance and progression of abnormal patterns.

During labor of a preterm fetus, variable decelerations are more common, occurring in 70% to 75% of such patients, compared with about 30% to 50% at term. (11,12). These decelerations may progress rapidly from reassuring to nonreassuring patterns in early gestations (11,13,29) and are more likely to be associated with loss of FHR variability (12,14). The combination of variable decelerations and loss of variability is strongly associated with low Apgar scores and fetal acidosis at birth in the preterm fetus (Fig. 11.14) (11,13,29–31).

Decreased or absent variability occurs more commonly in the premature fetus, and the progression of normal to absent variability is rapid (12,14). Most important, loss of variability in the early gestation is much more predictive of acidosis and depressed Apgar scores than at term (11,13,29–31). Whereas at term only approximately 20% of babies with abnormal or nonreassuring patterns will be depressed, in gestations of less than 33 weeks, approximately 70% to 80% of babies with nonreassuring FHR patterns will be depressed and/or acidotic.

Tachycardia is also more common in the premature neonate. Westgren et al. (13) found an FHR of greater than 160 BPM in 78% of babies under 33 weeks' gestation, as opposed to 20% of those beyond 33 weeks. Although maternal fever and tachycardia-inducing drugs are possible explanations in these earlier pregnancies, they do not adequately account for such a variation. Thus the development of tachycardia and loss of variability, and their correlation with low Apgar scores and acidosis, suggest that the early fetus develops residual hypoxia and acidosis more rapidly than at term, and that these FHR changes are indicative of changes in the metabolic state.

Late decelerations do not appear to be more or less common in premature pregnancies in labor per se (12,29); nonetheless, conditions that are more likely to provoke late decelerations—IUGR, abruptio placentae, and preeclampsia—are more frequent in premature deliveries. Prolonged decelerations appear to occur with frequencies similar to those in term pregnancies.

An additional factor needs to be considered. Because of threatened preterm delivery or pathologic conditions that are associated with preterm labor, drugs are often administered to the mother that have significant effects on the FHR. Beta-sympathomimetics such as ritodrine or terbutaline commonly increase the FHR to tachycardic levels (Fig. 11.15). This increase in FHR may itself diminish variability. The effects of other tocolytics such as magnesium sulfate, Indocin, and calcium channel blockers on FHR variability are minimal (Figs. 11.16 and 11.17A,B) (32).

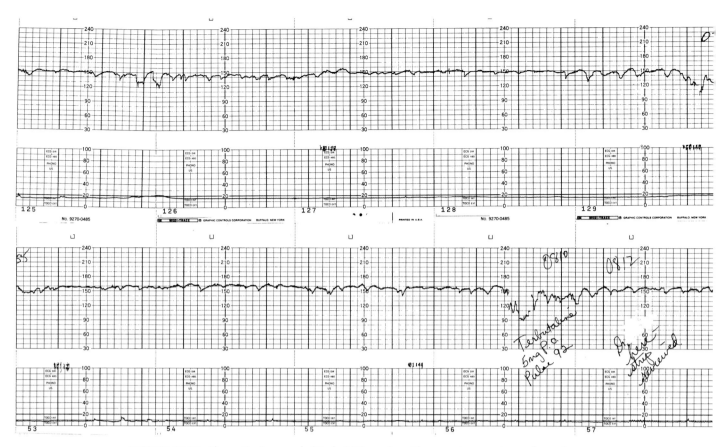

FIGURE 11.15. The patient was admitted at 28 weeks with premature rupture of membranes and without evidence of infection or labor. The baseline fetal heart rate (FHR) on the **upper panel** is 140 to 150 beats per minute (BPM). The patient was subsequently treated prophylactically with oral terbutaline. Five hours later (**lower panel**) the FHR rose somewhat to 155 to 160 BPM, presumably due to the passage of the beta-sympathomimetic into the fetal circulation.

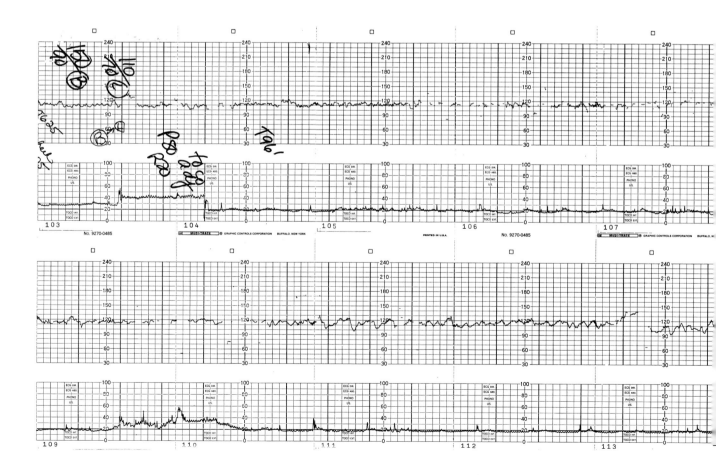

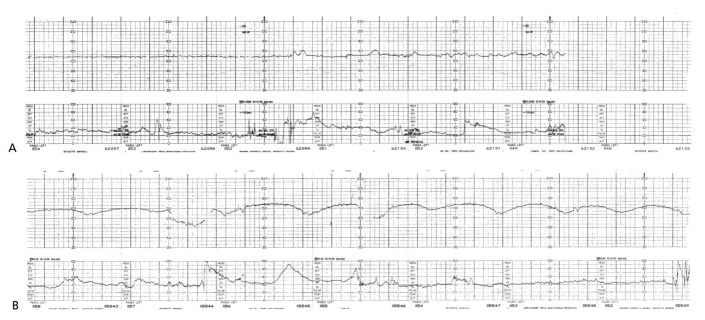

FIGURE 11.17. A,B: A patient in premature labor was admitted to the hospital for tocolysis. **Panel A** 54-49 demonstrates a fetus with a reassuring fetal heart rate (FHR) tracing. Despite tocolysis, the patient progresses in labor, and 3 hours later the FHR tracing has become nonreassuring with late decelerations and a loss of long-term variability (**panel B**). This patient went on to deliver a viable female infant with Apgar scores of 5 and 7 at 1 minute and 5 minutes, respectively.

APGAR SCORES IN THE PRETERM NEWBORN

When the Apgar score was introduced as a tool for immediate neonatal assessment, it was described in the term fetus. Despite the initial absence of data for the utility of this method in premature infants, it has become applied to describing the condition of all newborns, regardless of birth weight or gestational age. Studies have shown that the premature newborn is more likely to have a depressed Apgar score even in the absence of acidosis (15,33). In the series of Goldenberg et al. (33), only 50% of babies at 28 weeks with a 1-minute Apgar score less than 7 had an umbilical arterial pH of less than 7.25. In the series of Bowes et al. (16), consisting of premature newborns with birthweights of less than 1,500 g, 58% with Apgar scores of less than 4 and 69% with scores of less than 7 at 1 minute had normal umbilical artery pH values. This is in contrast to the very good correlation between neonatal depression and low cord pH values in the term newborn. It appears that prematurity alone is an explanation of depression at birth, and the Apgar score alone may not be a reliable indicator of metabolic abnormality in the premature baby.

SUMMARY

There appear to be substantial differences in normal FHR patterns and changes in these patterns in the preterm fetus. Tachycardia, loss of variability, and variable decelerations are more common. Compared to the term fetus, the progression of reassuring patterns to nonreassuring occurs more frequently and more rapidly. Once nonreassuring patterns develop in the preterm fetus, the correlation with neonatal depression, acidosis, neonatal complications, death, and long-term sequelae are stronger than at term. Hence, there is a much greater potential in the prematurely delivering baby for improving outcome with electronic

FIGURE 11.16. A patient in premature labor was successfully tocolyzed with intravenous MgSO₄. The fetal heart rate (FHR), before infusing the MgSO₄, was 140 beats per minute (BPM). Six hours later, the FHR baseline was showing mild bradycardia at 110 BPM. Note the accelerations on the **lower panel,** making this an overall reassuring tracing. The patient's temperature, as seen on the **upper panel,** was 35.6°C. The fetal bradycardia in this case was due to maternal (and thus fetal) hypothermia secondary to the MgSO₄.

FHR monitoring and an aggressive and rapid approach to intervention. Bowes et al. (15) attempted such an approach in pregnancies delivering at less than 33 weeks, and their results suggested a significant improvement in outcome. The only prospective randomized trial is by Luthy and colleagues (34), who could not demonstrate any difference in outcome when comparing electronic FHR monitoring to auscultation. These authors, however, required documentation of fetal acidosis by scalp pH before intervening. A relatively high incidence of more severe degrees of intraventricular hemorrhage was seen in this study, and since acidosis is known to correlate with IVH, it may be that waiting for acidosis to develop in the premature fetus before intervening for fetal distress may be waiting too long. Based on the available information, it is apparent that fetal compromise develops rapidly in the preterm fetus, and that this distress correlates with adverse outcome. Thus, an aggressive and rapid response is warranted in the patient delivering prematurely.

REFERENCES

1. Hobel CJ, Hyvarinen MA, Oh W: Abnormal fetal heart rate patterns and fetal acid base balance in low birth weight infants in relation to respiratory distress syndrome. *Obstet Gynecol* 39:83, 1972.
2. Martin CB Jr, Siassi B, Hon EH: Fetal heart rate patterns and neonatal death in low birthweight infants. *Obstet Gynecol* 44:503, 1974.
3. Donald IR, Freeman RK, Goebelsmann U, et al.: Clinical experience with amniotic fluid lecithin/sphingomyelin ratio. *Am J Obstet Gynecol* 115:547, 1973.
4. Rayburn WF, Donn SM, Kolin MG, et al.: Obstetric care and intraventricular hemorrhage in the low birth weight infant. *Obstet Gynecol* 61:408, 1983.
5. Papile LA, Burstein J, Burstein R, et al.: Incidence and evolution of subependymal and intraventricular hemorrhage: a study of infants with birth weights less than 1500 grams. *J Pediatr* 92:529, 1978.
6. Welch RA, Bottoms SF: Reconsideration of head compression and intraventricular hemorrhage in the vertex very-low-birth-weight fetus. *Obstet Gynecol* 68:29, 1986.
7. Volpe JJ: Neonatal intraventricular hemorrhage. *N Engl J Med* 304:886, 1981.
8. McGuinness GA, Smith WL: Head ultrasound screening in premature neonates weighing more than 1500 grams at birth. *Am J Dis Child* 138:817, 1984.
9. Towbin A, Turner GL: Obstetric factors in fetal-neonatal visceral injury. *Obstet Gynecol* 52:113, 1978.
10. Alward CT, Hook JB, Helmrath TA, et al.: Effects of asphyxia on cardiac output and organ blood flow in the newborn piglet. *Pediatr Res* 12:824, 1978.
11. Braly P, Garite TJ, German J: Fetal heart rate patterns in infants in whom necrotizing enterocolitis develops: a preliminary report. *Arch Surg* 115:1050, 1980.
12. Westgren M, Holmquist P, Svenningsen NW, et al.: Intrapartum fetal monitoring in preterm deliveries: prospective study. *Obstet Gynecol* 60:99, 1982.
13. Westgren M, Holmquist P, Ingemarsson I, et al.: Intrapartum fetal acidosis in preterm infants: Fetal monitoring and long term morbidity. *Obstet Gynecol* 63:355, 1984.
14. Westgren LMR, Malcus P, Svenningsen NW: Intrauterine asphyxia and long term outcome in preterm fetuses. *Obstet Gynecol* 67:512, 1986.
15. Bowes WA Jr, Halgrimson M, Simmons MA: Results of the intensive perinatal management of very-low-birth-weight infants (501 to 1,500 grams). *J Reprod Med* 23:245, 1979.
16. Tejani NA, Verma UL: Effect of tocolysis on incidence of low birth weight. *Obstet Gynecol* 61:556, 1983.
17. Zlatnik F: The applicability of labor inhibition to the problem of prematurity. *Am J Obstet Gynecol* 113:704, 1972.
18. Scholl JS: Abruptio placentae: clinical management in nonacute cases. *Am J Obstet Gynecol* 156:40, 1987.
19. Moberg LJ, Garite TJ, Freeman RK: Fetal heart rate patterns and fetal distress in patients with preterm premature rupture of membranes. *Obstet Gynecol* 64:60, 1984.
20. Nageotte MP, Bertucci L, Towers CV, et al.: Prophylactic amnioinfusion in pregnancies complicated by oligohydramnios or thick meconium: a prospective study. *Obstet Gynecol* 77:677, 1991.
21. Hitti J, Krohn MA, Patton DL, et al.: Amniotic fluid tumor necrosis factor-alpha and risk of respiratory distress syndrome among preterm infants. *Am J Obstet Gynecol* 177:50–56, 1997.
22. Yoon BH, Romero R, Kim KS, et al.: A systemic fetal inflammatory response and the development of bronchopulmonary dysplasia. *Am J Obstet Gynecol* 181:773–779, 1999.
23. Yoon BH, Romero R, Kim CJ, et al.: High expression of tumor necrosis factor-alpha and interleukin-6 in periventircular leukomalcia. *Am J Obstet Gynecol* 177:1406–1411, 1997.
24. Yoon BH, Romero R, Park KH, et al.: Amniotic fluid inflammatory cytokines (intertleukin-6, interleukin-1 beta and tumor necrosis factor-alpha), neonatal brain white matter lesions, and cerebral palsy. *Am J Obstet Gynecol* 177:19–26, 1997.
25. Grether JK, Nelson KB: Maternal infection and cerebral palsy in infants of normal birth weight. *JAMA* 278:207–211, 1997.
26. Lavin JP, Miovodnik M, Barden TP: Relationship of nonstress test reactivity and gestational age. *Obstet Gynecol* 63:338, 1984.
27. Devoe LD: Antepartum fetal heart rate testing in preterm pregnancy. *Obstet Gynecol* 60:431, 1982.
28. Sorokin Y, Dierker LJ, Pillay SK, et al.: The association between fetal heart rate patterns and fetal movements in pregnancies between 20 and 30 weeks gestation. *Am J Obstet Gynecol* 143:243, 1982.
29. Zanini B, Paul RH, Huey JR: Intrapartum fetal heart rate: correlation with scalp pH in the preterm fetus. *Am J Obstet Gynecol* 136:43, 1980.
30. Cibils LA: Clinical significance of fetal heart rate patterns during labor. *Am J Obstet Gynecol* 132:791, 1978.
31. Douvas SG, Meeks GR, Graves G, et al.: Intrapartum fetal heart rate monitoring as a predictor of fetal distress and immediate condition in low-birth-weight (<1800 grams) infants. *Am J Obstet Gynecol* 148:300, 1984.
32. Parsons MT, Owens CA, Spellacy WN: Thermic effects of tocolytic agents: decreased temperature with magnesium sulfate. *Obstet Gynecol* 69:88, 1987.
33. Goldenberg RL, Huddleston JF, Nelson KG: Apgar scores and umbilical arterial pH in preterm newborn infants. *Am J Obstet Gynecol* 149:651, 1984.
34. Luthy DA, Shy KK, Van Belle G, et al.: A randomized trial of electronic fetal monitoring in premature labor. *Obstet Gynecol* 69:687, 1987.

12

ANTEPARTUM FETAL MONITORING

Because more than two thirds of fetal deaths occur before the onset of labor (1), it would be natural to extend the principles of intrapartum fetal heart rate (FHR) monitoring to the antepartum period in an effort to prevent these fetal deaths. A substantial number of antepartum deaths occur in women who have risk factors for uteroplacental insufficiency (UPI) (2). Other causes include hydrops fetalis, intrauterine infections, cord accidents, congenital anomalies, and a number of unknowns. An ideal test for assessing the antepartum fetus would allow intervention before fetal death or asphyctic damage. Before the availability of such tests, the only method for attacking this problem was to prematurely deliver such fetuses based on empirical risk data, as in the method proposed by Priscilla White for managing diabetics (3). The problem with such an approach is twofold: The majority of such prematurely delivered fetuses were not in jeopardy, and the morbidity and mortality from premature intervention often exceed those of the original risk factor. It would be preferable to treat the disease process and allow the fetus to go to term; however, we have made few advances in treating UPI.

Several biochemical tests have been proposed to evaluate the antepartum fetus. Historically, these include maternal estriol, human placental lactogen, diamine oxidase, and heat stable alkaline phosphatase. Since these biochemical tests are no longer used, they will not be discussed here. Currently available methods for antepartum fetal assessment include:

1. Fetal movement counting
2. Assessment of uterine growth
3. Antepartum fetal heart rate (AFHR) testing
4. Biophysical profile (BPP) testing
5. Doppler velocimetry

PHYSIOLOGY AND PATHOPHYSIOLOGY

UPI implies inadequate delivery of nutritive and/or respiratory substances to appropriate fetal tissues. The term UPI may be applied specifically to inadequate exchange within the placenta due to decreased blood flow, decreased surface area, or increased membrane thickness. The term may also be applied more generally to problems of inadequate maternal delivery of nutrients or oxygen to the placenta, as in starvation or cyanotic cardiac disease, or to problems of inadequate fetal uptake (e.g., fetal anemia). Kubli et al. suggested that UPI be divided into nutritive and respiratory components: nutritive deficiency leading to intrauterine growth retardation (IUGR) and respiratory insufficiency leading to asphyctic damage and subsequent fetal death (4). Parer suggested that fetal nutritive function generally precedes fetal respiratory compromise (except in diabetics) (5). Figure 12.1 is a theoretical scheme of the stages through which a fetus with declining placental function might pass. The rapidity with which this occurs may vary, being gradual in such cases as chronic hypertension or happening very suddenly as in abruption. Other conditions, perhaps including diabetes, might bypass the stage of nutritive insufficiency completely.

RISK IDENTIFICATION

To apply this knowledge to patient treatment, one must first identify the patients at risk who need evaluation. This risk identification must include data from the patient's history, physical examination, ongoing patient assessment (including uterine growth and blood pressure), and laboratory data. Those conditions that place the patient at risk for UPI are listed in Table 12.1. In addition, some obstetric/fetal conditions apparently unrelated to maternal disease may also be associated with UPI. The most common reasons for AFHR testing are postdate pregnancy, hypertension, diabetes, clinical IUGR, and the history of a stillbirth. However, distribution or indications vary depending upon the reported testing protocol (Table 12.2) (6–8). Similarly, the rate of abnormal test result varies depending on the primary testing modality used (Table 12.3).

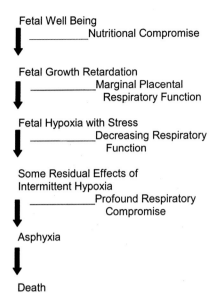

FIGURE 12.1. Theoretical scheme of fetal deterioration with progressive uteroplacental insufficiency.

TABLE 12.1. CONDITIONS PLACING THE FETUS AT RISK FOR UPI

Preeclampsia
Chronic hypertension
Collagen vascular disease
Diabetes mellitus
Renal disease
Fetal or maternal anemia
Blood group sensitization
Hyperthyroidism
Thrombophilia
Cyanotic heart disease
Postdate pregnancy
Fetal growth restriction

UPI, uteroplacental insufficiency.

TABLE 12.2. INDICATIONS FOR ANTEPARTUM TESTING BY PRIMARY SURVEILLANCE TEST

Indication	CST (%)	MBPP (%)	BPP (%)
Postdate	39	44	12
Hypertension	31	8	18
Diabetes			
Gestational	5	6	7
Insulin dependent	10	—	2
Intrauterine growth restriction	9	24	21
Previous stillbirth	4	2	4
Other	5	6	38

(Totals are >100% because some patients had more than one testing indication.)

BPP, biophysical profile; CST, contraction stress test; MBPP, modified biophysical profile.
From Freeman R, Anderson G, Dorchester W: A prospective multiinstitutional study monitoring. I. Risk of perinatal mortality according to antepartum fetal heart rate test results. *Am J Obstet Gynecol* 143:771, 1982; Manning F, Morrison I, Lange I, et al: Fetal assessment based on fetal biophysical profile scoring: experience in 12,620 referred high-risk pregnancies. *Am J Obstet Gynecol* 151:343, 1985; Nageotte M, Towers C, Asrat T, et al: Perinatal outcome with the modified biophysical profile. *Am J Obstet Gynecol* 170:1672, 1994, with permission.

TABLE 12.3. DISTRIBUTION OF TEST RESULTS BY PRIMARY SURVEILLANCE TEST

Result	CST (%)	MBPP (%)	BPP (%)
Negative	67	92	97
Equivocal	23	8	2
Positive	10	3[a]	1

[a]The positive test results for patients receiving MBPP were all in patients receiving back-up testing for an equivocal MBPP.
BPP, biophysical profile; CST, contraction stress test; MBPP, modified biophysical profile.
From Freeman R, Anderson G, Dorchester W: A prospective multiinstitutional study monitoring. I. Risk of perinatal mortality according to antepartum fetal heart rate test results. *Am J Obstet Gynecol* 143:771, 1982; Manning F, Morrison I, Lange I, et al: Fetal assessment based on fetal biophysical profile scoring: experience in 12,620 referred high-risk pregnancies. *Am J Obstet Gynecol* 151:343, 1985; Nageotte M, Towers C, Asrat T, et al: Perinatal outcome with the modified biophysical profile. *Am J Obstet Gynecol* 170:1672, 1994, with permission.

FETAL MOVEMENT COUNTING

Long before electronic monitoring devices were available, clinicians recognized that maternal perception of a decrease in fetal movements may be a sign of impending fetal death. In a prospectively randomized antepartum fetal surveillance study, Neldam had over 1,000 patients followed by a fetal movement counting protocol (9). In those women randomized to the protocol of daily monitoring of fetal movement there were no antepartum fetal deaths, whereas for over 1,000 patients followed with no fetal movement counting protocol there were eight fetal deaths. This method of fetal surveillance costs nothing, and when done in a systematic fashion, especially in low-risk populations, may contribute significantly to the detection of otherwise unsuspected fetal jeopardy.

Sadovsky has used fetal movement monitoring in developing a systematized approach to the assessment of fetal well-being (10). If there are more than three movements in 30 minutes, the fetus is considered to be in good condition. Less than three movements in 30 minutes is either indicative of a fetal sleep state or reason for concern and further counting should continue. We instruct our patients to count for another 30 minutes, and if there are still less than three movements in the second counting period, we ask the patient to come to the hospital for a nonstress test (NST). If the NST is nonreactive, subsequent management is according to antepartum FHR testing protocols. If the NST is reactive (which is usually the case), the patient is reassured and asked to continue her daily counting schedule. At the time of the NST, the patient is usually taught how to count movement, because the reason for her perceived decreased count is often her nonrecognition of movement that is there. When simultaneous real-time ultrasound scanning has been done with patients asked to note the perceived movements, more movements are observed by ultrasound than are perceived by the patient (11). Most patients will feel three movements in just a few minutes, so very little time is actually required for the patient. A fetal movement count that drops below three in 12 hours or that ceases for 12 hours is termed the "movement alarm signal" by Sadovsky, which correlates with impending fetal death (12–14). Moore and Piacquadio performed a pilot study in which all patients were instructed to monitor the elapsed time it took every day from 28 weeks to register ten fetal movements (15). A nonstress test was performed if 2 hours elapsed without ten movements. They report a fourfold reduction in fetal mortality associated with complaints of decreased fetal movement using this simple protocol.

ASSESSMENT OF UTERINE GROWTH

During the third trimester, assessment of uterine growth should be done on all patients at the time of their routine prenatal visits. As a general rule, the fundal height in centimeters as measured with a tape measure will equal the weeks of gestation. There are several things that may negate this relationship, including maternal obesity, multiple gestation, polyhydramnios, abnormal fetal lie, oligohydramnios, low fetal station, and fetal growth retardation. Except for maternal obesity and myomas, the other causes are all things about which the clinician should be interested. Specifically, abnormalities in the amniotic fluid volume may lead to the

diagnosis of a fetal malformation or intrauterine growth retardation. Thus, abnormalities in the gross uterine size or abnormal growth rates of the fundal height should lead to further investigation, specifically sonography and/or FHR testing. Unfortunately, the accuracy of clinical assessment leaves something to be desired. The diagnosis of IUGR by clinical estimates is a poor predictor of a subsequent growth retarded neonate. Generally speaking, whenever the uterine size is significantly larger than gestational age, the patient should be advised to have a sonogram. Likewise, if the uterine size is significantly below gestational age or if there is a lack of uterine growth or a decreased growth rate, the patient should be evaluated by sonography. If the findings suggest uteroplacental insufficiency, some form of fetal surveillance should be performed.

WHEN TO BEGIN TESTING

Indications for testing and the gestational age for beginning testing are listed in Table 12.4. Many factors go into the decision as to when to begin testing (16–22). Single factors with minimal to moderate increased risk for antepartum death nearly all warrant surveillance starting at about 32 weeks (e.g., chronic hypertension, gestational diabetes, previous stillbirth) (19,21). The highest maternal risk factors are chronic hypertension with preeclampsia and the more severe classes of diabetes mellitus (D, F, and R). In diabetics with hypertension, proteinuria, IUGR, or proliferative retinopathy, the risk of fetal deterioration before 34 weeks is high and fetal testing should begin as early as 26 weeks (20). In the patient without diabetes or hypertension, when the clinical diagnosis of IUGR is confirmed by ultrasound, fetal testing should begin as early as it is reasonable to expect a chance of neonatal viability (about 26 weeks). As a general rule, AFHR testing should not begin until esti-

TABLE 12.4. INDICATIONS AND GESTATIONAL AGE FOR AFHR TESTING

Indication	Gestational Age to Start Testing (wk)
Diabetes	
Class A (uncomplicated)	40
Class A (complicated)	32
Class B, C, D	32
Class F, R	26–30
Preeclampsia	At diagnosis >25–26
Chronic hypertension	32
Severe Rh disease	At diagnosis >26
Previous stillbirth	Gestational age of previous stillbirth
IUGR at diagnosis	>25–26
Post date pregnancy	41–42
Cyanotic heart disease	32
Hyperthyroidism	32
Oligohydramnios	At diagnosis >25–26

AFHR, antepartum fetal heart rate; IUGR, intrauterine growth retardation; Rh, rhesus isoimmunization.
From references 16–22.

mated fetal maturity is sufficient to expect a reasonable chance of survival should intervention (delivery) be necessary. This is especially difficult with twin gestations, because intervention for a compromised twin may adversely affect an apparently normal twin before maturity. Testing for patients exceeding their due date is a common indication. In most cases, testing in some form should begin between 41 and 42 weeks' gestation (22).

WHERE TO BEGIN TESTING

Experience is the key to obtaining quality tests in the shortest time. It is most desirable for nurses or technicians to specialize in antepartum testing. When testing is done in a hospital setting, an area separate from the labor and delivery suite is preferable to resist the temptation to have labor and delivery nurses cross-cover the antepartum testing area and not be able to devote enough attention to the patient being tested. Alternatively, provision of testing either in labor and delivery or in an office setting should be done in a quiet and stress-free environment.

The patient is placed in the semi-Fowler's position to avoid supine hypotension syndrome. Baseline blood pressure is recorded and repeated throughout the test, again to be sure that supine hypotension does not occur, as this may be a cause of decreased uteroplacental perfusion and false-positive test results. Baseline contractions and FHR are recorded for approximately 20 minutes. The baseline heart rate and reactivity are noted, as is the background uterine activity. Following this evaluation, if results are not reassuring, continued monitoring of FHR may be necessary. Alternatively, initiation of a contraction stress test or use of real-time ultrasound to measure amniotic fluid volume and assess various fetal parameters should ensue.

WHICH TEST TO USE?

In the previous editions of this text, we have presented the contraction stress test (CST) as the "gold standard" of antepartum fetal surveillance. Using the CST as the primary means of fetal surveillance for most indications results in a very impressive and remarkably low incidence of unexpected fetal death within 7 days of a negative test result (23). However, significant problems accompany the use of contraction stress testing as primary fetal surveillance. These include the increase in time, cost, and inconvenience of the CST compared with other forms of fetal testing. In addition, the high frequency of equivocal test results and lack of consensus over test interpretation makes the CST an often impractical if not inappropriate choice of testing for many caregivers. As a result, the CST has essentially been replaced by either the NST, the biophysical profile (BPP), or the modified biophysical profile (MBPP) for primary

FHR monitoring. In our centers, we now use the MBPP test as the primary means of antepartum fetal testing with the exception being the continued use of the CST for insulin-requiring diabetics. Other forms of fetal assessment include the use of ultrasound and Doppler of various fetal vessels or the maternal uterine arteries. What follows is a description of the various testing options available with particular emphasis on the evolution and reported application of the CST, NST, BPP, and the MBPP. Doppler application for fetal surveillance is briefly presented as well but is not extensively reviewed. There continues to be argument and controversy regarding the relative value and efficacy of these various types of fetal assessment despite their well-established place in the clinical practice of obstetrics (24).

CONTRACTION STRESS TEST

It can be surmised that, given a condition of borderline fetal oxygenation, a test that further stresses the fetus in terms of oxygen deprivation might produce some biophysical sign of such compromise, and that these data could be of prognostic importance. Early tests that attempted to accomplish this utilized the maternal exercise stress test and breathing gas mixtures with decreased oxygen concentrations (25). Animal data suggest that uterine contractions producing an intraamniotic pressure in excess of approximately 30 mm Hg create an intramyometrial pressure that exceeds mean intraarterial pressure, thereby temporarily halting uterine blood flow (26). A well-oxygenated fetus tolerates this limited period of intervillous stasis well; however, a hypoxic fetus will manifest late decelerations. It was therefore suggested that by inducing such contractions in the antepartum period, one might be able to detect the compromised fetus before death (and possible damage) occurred. In 1966, Hammacher studied 207 pregnancies in the antepartum period and found that late decelerations correlated with lower Apgar scores at subsequent delivery and that 17 of 23 that resulted in stillbirth had manifested such late decelerations with spontaneous contractions in the antepartum period (27). Subsequently, Pose and Escarcena (28), Kubli et al. (4), and Spurrett (29) found late decelerations in the antepartum period to correlate with stillbirth, IUGR, and low Apgar scores. Sanchez-Ramos et al. found no fetal deaths within a week of testing when no late decelerations were seen (30).

The first systematic trial of stress testing in this country was performed by Ray et al. in 1972 (31). They performed a prospective blinded trial on 66 patients and defined criteria for adequate testing, frequency of testing, and results, all of which are in common use in this country today. Of the 66 patients, 15 had positive test results, and of these, three had fetal deaths and six had low Apgar scores. Furthermore, there were no deaths within a week of a negative test result. Ray et al. called the test the oxytocin challenge test (OCT).

Because the test can use either spontaneously occurring contractions or contractions induced by breast stimulation, it has become known more properly as the contraction stress test or CST.

How to Perform the Contraction Stress Test

External monitors for contraction and FHR measurement are placed on the patient. With the patient in semi-Fowler's position or left lateral tilt to minimize supine hypotension, an initial monitoring period lasting from 20 to 30 minutes is obtained to assess the FHR baseline, to identify the presence or absence of periodic changes and to determine if there is evidence of spontaneous uterine activity. If there are three adequate spontaneously occurring contractions within a 10-minute period and the FHR recording is of sufficient quality, the test is concluded (Fig. 12.2). If the contractions are absent or of insufficient frequency, they must be stimulated. Historically, oxytocin infusion intravenously has been used to elicit contractions of the uterus. This is accomplished by beginning oxytocin through an infusion pump at a rate of 1.0 mU/minute. The infusion rate is initially doubled every 15 minutes until the appearance of contractions. Smaller incre-

ments for oxytocin increase are then used until three contractions lasting 40 to 60 seconds occur in 10 minutes. Patience and experience are valuable in obtaining an adequate CST and avoiding overstimulation of uterine activity (Fig. 12.3).

A widely used alternative to intravenous oxytocin infusion is that of breast stimulation. Oxytocin is released from the posterior pituitary following breast stimulation, and this technique has been used for both initiation of labor as well as for initiation of the CST (32–36). When used for fetal testing, breast stimulation has similar efficacy to oxytocin infusion with a shorter testing time with less expense, discomfort, and inconvenience. Breast stimulation has been associated with uterine hyperstimulation and fails to achieve adequate uterine activity in approximately 20% of tests (37–40). The test is best performed with the patient initially rolling or tugging on one nipple through her clothing until a contraction occurs. If no contraction results following 2 to 3 minutes, the patient is asked to perfom bilateral stimulation following a 5-minute rest period. This cycle of stimulation is then repeated until adequate uterine activity is documented. Figure 12.4 is an example of a reactive negative CST done with nipple stimulation. Following the appearance of adequate uterine activity, oxytocin infusion or breast stimulation is stopped and the patient continued

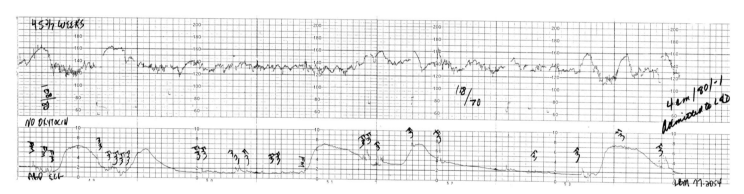

FIGURE 12.2. Spontaneous negative contraction stress test (no oxytocin needed). The patient is actually found to be in labor.

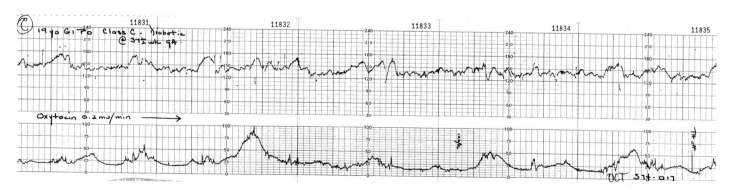

FIGURE 12.3. Negative contraction stress test result. Three contractions are obtained in 10 minutes, lasting more than 60 seconds each, with adequate quality fetal heart rate recording.

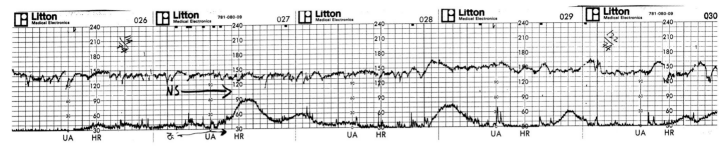

FIGURE 12.4. Reactive negative contraction stress test using breast stimulation.

to be monitored until activity significantly diminishes or disappears (41).

If late decelerations are present with every spontaneous contraction, yet the contraction frequency is less than three in 10 minutes, initiation of further uterine activity is not indicated and the CST result is positive.

Interpretation of the Contraction Stress Test

Negative

No late decelerations appearing anywhere on the strip, adequate contraction frequency (three in 10 minutes), and adequate FHR recording must be obtained (Figs. 12.2 to 12.4) for the interpretation to be negative.

Positive

In a positive CST result, late decelerations are present with the majority (greater than one half) of contractions during the period of maximum contraction stress without excessive uterine activity (see Hyperstimulation). If persistent late decelerations are present before the contraction frequency is

adequate, this is a positive test result and may be concluded. Figure 12.5 shows a reactive positive CST result, Fig. 12.6 a minimally reactive positive CST result, and Fig. 12.7 a nonreactive positive CST result.

Equivocal Test Results

Suspicious. A test result is considered suspicious if late decelerations are present with less than half of the contractions. It is sometimes necessary to keep a test going awhile longer to determine whether the late deceleration is persistent or only sporadic (Fig. 12.8).

Hyperstimulation. Decelerations after contractions lasting more than 90 seconds, or with contraction frequency greater than every 2 minutes, constitute hyperstimulation (Figs. 12.9 and 12.10). When such prolonged frequent contractions occur without late decelerations, it is not hyperstimulation (Fig. 12.11). Hyperstimulation may occur with either spontaneous or oxytocin-induced contractions.

Unsatisfactory. When adequate contraction frequency cannot be induced or when the FHR recording is not of sufficient quality to be sure about the presence of late decelerations, the test result is considered unsatisfactory (Fig. 12.12).

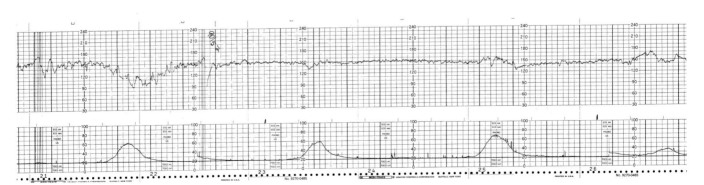

FIGURE 12.5. Reactive positive contraction stress test using breast stimulation.

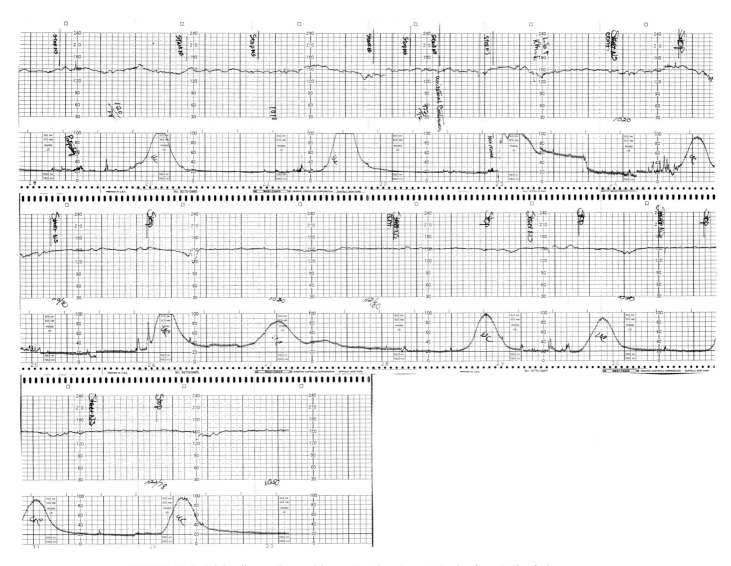

FIGURE 12.6. Minimally reactive positive contraction stress test using breast stimulation.

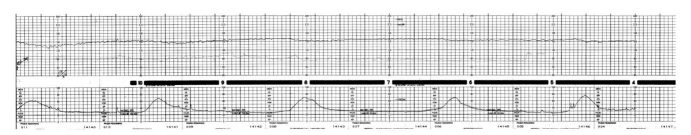

FIGURE 12.7. This is a nonreactive positive contraction stress test elicited with unilateral breast stimulation. The decelerations are subtle and frequently not appreciated. Note the complete absence of accelerations, which should always lead to a close evaluation of the heart rate.

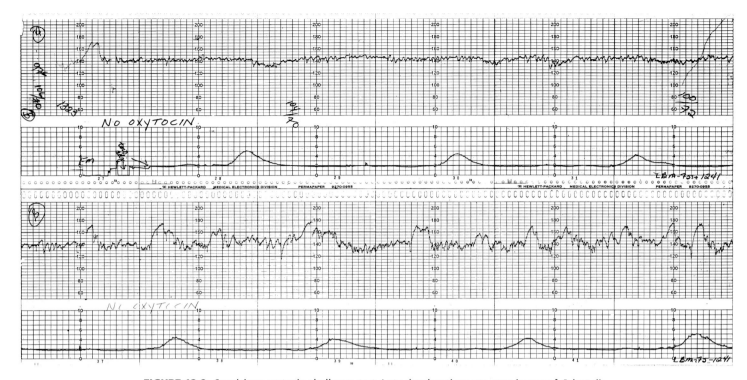

FIGURE 12.8. Suspicious oxytocin challenge test. Late decelerations are seen in **panel A** but disappear in **panel B**. As is often the case, the late decelerations are seen during a period of absent reactivity (no accelerations) but resolve when the fetus becomes reactive. The explanation for this is unclear.

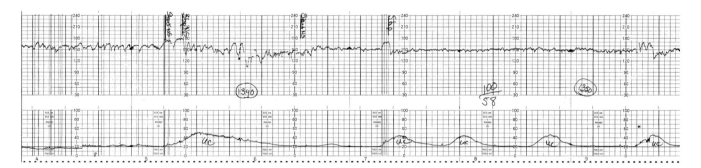

FIGURE 12.9. This tracing is read as equivocal due to hyperstimulation. Note the deceleration associated with a prolonged uterine contraction.

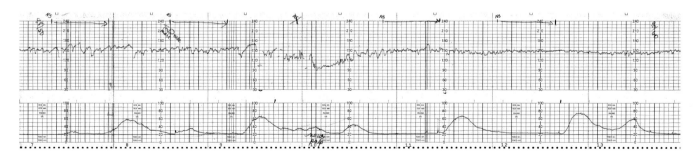

FIGURE 12.10. This tracing is read as equivocal due to hyperstimulation. Note the deceleration associated with frequent contractions.

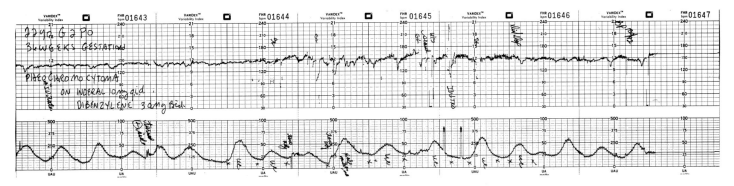

FIGURE 12.11. Very frequent uterine contractions are noted in this patient who was known to have a pheochromocytoma. The norepinephrine from the pheochromocytoma is thought to be responsible for this. Because no significant decelerations are noted, this tracing is read as a reactive negative spontaneous contraction stress test.

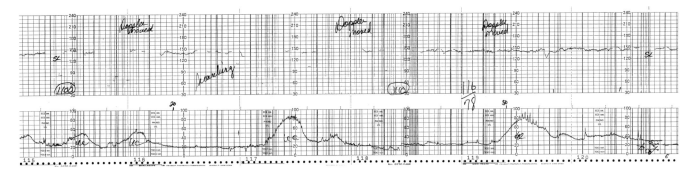

FIGURE 12.12. The quality of this recording is not sufficient for interpretation. It is therefore read as unsatisfactory.

Other Patterns

When variable decelerations are seen, they are suggestive of oligohydramnios or cord entrapment (Fig 12.13). Such test results are highly suspicious and usually suggest the need for a sonogram to look for oligohydramnios. The test should be repeated the next day when significant variable decelerations are present. Variables associated with loss of variability and blunting of decelerations have been observed by Freeman and James (42) and by Baskett and Sandy (43) and are found to be very ominous (Fig. 12.14).

The sinusoidal pattern consists of sine wave undulations of the FHR, with a cyclicity of approximately three to five per minute (Fig. 12.15). It is characterized by an absence of short-term variability with uniform long-term variability. The pattern is always nonreactive and should be present for more than a few minutes to be significant. Sinusoidal patterns fluctuate above and below the baseline and are uniform (44). Late decelerations are commonly seen in association with sinusoidal patterns. They have been reported to be associated with severe fetal anemia, as in Rh isoimmunization (45) or fetal-maternal hemorrhage (Fig. 12.16) (46). These patterns may also be seen with hypoxic fetal dis-

tress in the absence of fetal anemia. Generally, the sinusoidal pattern is ominous and has been associated with a high incidence of perinatal mortality. However, other tracings with increased long-term variability may be easily confused with sinusoidal patterns and might cause inappropriate intervention (Fig. 12.17). Although the literature is somewhat confusing on the significance of sinusoidal patterns, when the criteria described by Modanlou and Freeman (44) are used, we find the pattern to be uniformly ominous.

A very rare test result is a nonreactive negative CST. Theoretically, this should not occur if the appearance of late deceleration is an earlier finding than the loss of acceleration (47). A mistake commonly made in this situation is to miss very subtle late decelerations when the fetus may be severely hypoxic (Fig. 12.18). It is therefore important to be sure that no subtle late decelerations are present when reading a test as nonreactive negative. Grundy et al. (48) have shown that only 2 in 1,000 negative CST results are completely nonreactive. Fetuses with nonreactive negative CST results were often found in mothers taking central nervous system (CNS) depressant drugs and in fetuses with CNS abnormalities. When excluding those with CNS abnormal-

(text continues on page 192)

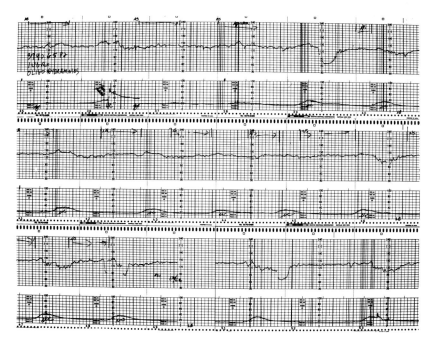

FIGURE 12.13. The variable decelerations noted on this contraction stress test are believed to be due to umbilical cord compression in this patient with known oligohydramnios.

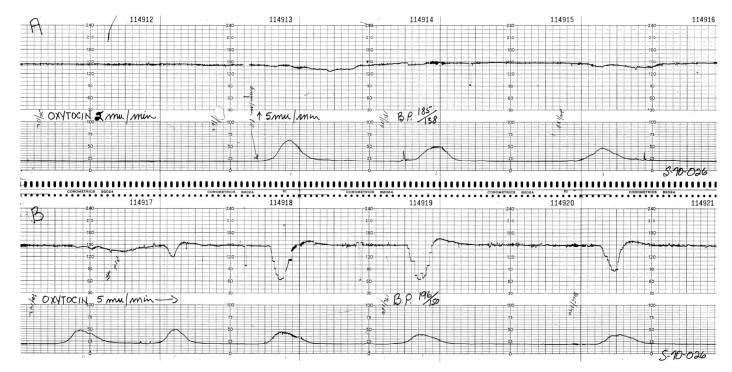

FIGURE 12.14. These variable decelerations are particularly ominous. They are deep, blunted, and associated with a prolonged terminal increase in fetal heart rate (overshoot) and with a smooth nonreactive baseline. Such patterns have been associated with a high rate of fetal death and neonatal depression.

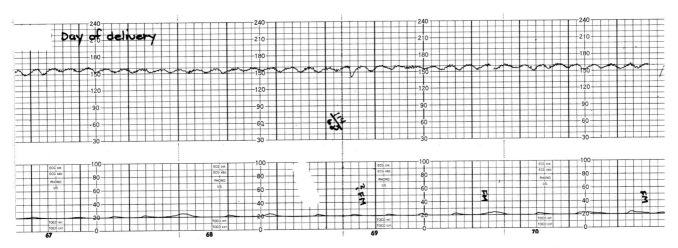

FIGURE 12.15. Sinusoidal pattern. This is an antepartum sinusoidal heart rate pattern. The sine wave, and long-term variability, may be seen to fluctuate above and below the baseline, is constant, and may be seen with late decelerations. This often represents severe fetal anemia or hypoxia.

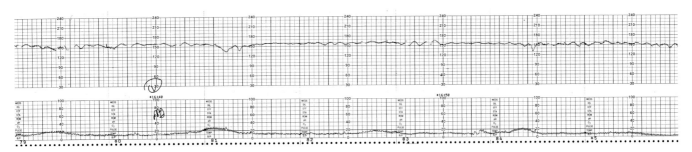

FIGURE 12.16. Sinusoidal pattern. This pattern is associated with a maternal history of Rh sensitization at 32 weeks' gestation.

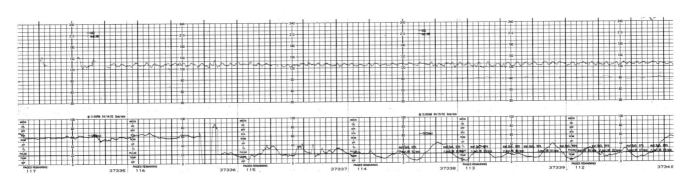

FIGURE 12.17. This is a pseudosinusoidal pattern. There is an increased cyclicity and presence of short-term variability. The fetal heart rate was reactive before and after this episode.

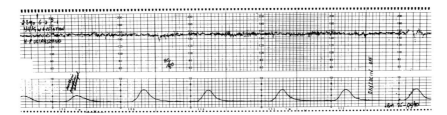

FIGURE 12.18. Nonreactive positive contraction stress test (CST) taken from a first-generation fetal monitor with significant baseline artifact. Note that there are very subtle late decelerations that are difficult to see. We have seen several similar recordings read as nonreactive negative CSTs followed by fetal death.

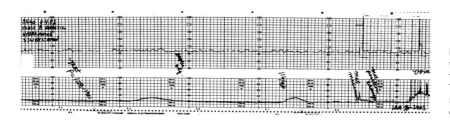

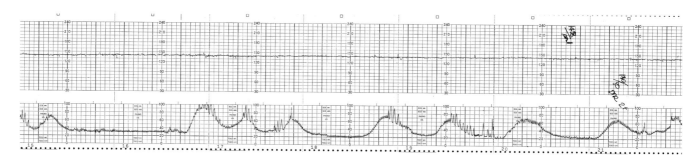

FIGURE 12.19. Tracing taken from a fetus with anencephaly. Note the absence of reactivity and the absence of late decelerations. This nonreactive negative reading is commonly found in fetuses with anomalies of the central nervous system.

FIGURE 12.20. Tracing taken from an eclamptic patient who received a dose of phenobarbital for her seizure activity. Note the absence of reactivity and the absence of late decelerations. This nonreactive negative reading is commonly found in patients taking central nervous system-depressant drugs.

ities, the immediate perinatal outcome in these rare situations did not differ from that of neonates with reactive negative tests. The long-term outcome would be guarded, however, since the lack of reactivity may indicate some preexisting CNS abnormality that was not immediately apparent in the neonate. When one encounters a fetus with a nonreactive negative CST result, it is reasonable to take a drug history and evaluate the fetus for CNS abnormalities with ultrasound and a biophysical profile (Figs. 12.19 and 12.20).

Management

One significant advantage of the CST is that the test is repeated weekly if there are negative test results unless there is some change in the clinical situation (Table 12.5). Equivocal test results require repeat testing the next day. Positive test results are acted on only in the context of the entire clinical condition. This includes gestational age, fetal maturity, maternal condition, and the results of other tests of fetal status. The limitations of nonreassuring tests must be considered and individualized to the specific clinical situa-

tion. Repeatedly equivocal CST results often require switching to another form of fetal assessment and should not alone be an indication for delivery. Further, an abnormal CST result may be due to a reversible maternal condition. We have seen abnormal test results in patients with various conditions that have reverted to reassuring tracings after treatment of the maternal condition (Table 12.6).

These maternal conditions would also place the mother at increased risk if operative intervention were undertaken on behalf of the fetus before their correction.

Contraindications

The only part of contraction stress testing that carries any potential risk is the stimulation of uterine contractions. Patients with previous classical cesarean sections or other uterine surgery that has left a scar through the thickness of the fundal portion of the uterus would generally not be candidates for stress testing. We have used fetal stress testing with oxytocin or nipple stimulation in those patients with previous cesarean sections of the low transverse type and have not observed any problems related to the scars.

TABLE 12.5. COMMON INDICATIONS FOR SHORTENING THE INTERVAL BETWEEN TESTING

Deterioration in diabetic control
Worsening hypertension
Need to introduce antihypertensives
Decreased fetal movement

TABLE 12.6. REVERSIBLE CAUSES OF ABNORMAL TESTING

Diabetic ketoacidosis
Sickle cell crisis
Asthma attack
Dehydration
Maternal anemia

TABLE 12.7. CONTRAINDICATIONS TO THE CST (WITH OXYTOCIN OR NIPPLE STIMULATION)

Premature rupture of membranes
Previous classical cesarean section
Placenta previa
Incompetent cervix
History of premature labor in this pregnancy
Multiple gestation

CST, contraction stress test.

Patients with documented placenta previa would also not be tested with the CST for obvious reasons. There is no indication that stress testing causes premature labor (49), but we have generally avoided the CST in patients at high risk for prematurity. This would include preterm patients with multiple gestations, premature rupture of membranes, bleeding, cervical cerclage in place, or previous treatment for preterm labor in this pregnancy (Table 12.7). There are unusual situations in which one might stress the patient even in the presence of such contraindications. This would occur when all other indices suggest antepartum fetal distress and the only alternative to the CST is intervention.

NONSTRESS TESTING

The examination of characteristics of the baseline FHR unrelated to contractions and its application to the antepartum period came as a result of observations by Hammacher (27) in 1966 and by Kubli et al. (4) in 1969. They observed that healthy fetuses displayed normal oscillations and fluctuations of the baseline FHR, and when these were absent there was an increased chance of depressed neonates and perinatal mortality. Trierweiler et al. pointed out that accelerations of the FHR during antepartum stress testing seemed to correlate with fetal well-being (50). Subsequently, several investigators have looked at accelerations of the FHR and other parameters of the nonstressed antepartum FHR as a means of evaluating the fetus at risk (45, 50–60). These other parameters include baseline heart rate, apparent heart rate variability, and the presence or absence of spontaneously occurring decelerations.

Accelerations of the FHR occur in association with fetal movement (Fig. 12.21) or uterine contractions (Fig. 12.22), or in response to external stimuli (Fig. 12.23). Rabinowitz et al. have shown that accelerations are virtually always associated with fetal movement on simultaneous ultrasound imaging, but movement also frequently occurs without heart rate acceleration (11). Clinically, therefore, it is not necessary to document fetal movement to satisfy the criteria for fetal reactivity. Accelerations of the FHR seem to be an objective reflection of FHR variability, which is not monitored well externally. Fetal sleeplike states and CNS depressant drugs reduce both variability and reactivity (61). Accelerations may also be caused by partial compression of the umbilical cord resulting in venous occlusion and fetal hypotension without interference in umbilical arterial flow. Therefore, FHR accelerations appear to be a reflection of CNS alertness and activity, and their absence seems to

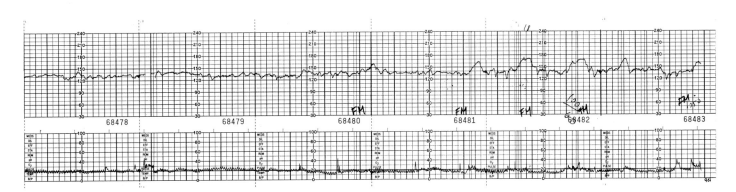

FIGURE 12.21. Reactive nonstress test showing accelerations associated with fetal movement, marked by the notation "FM."

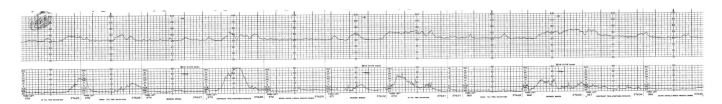

FIGURE 12.22. These accelerations appear to occur in association with uterine contractions.

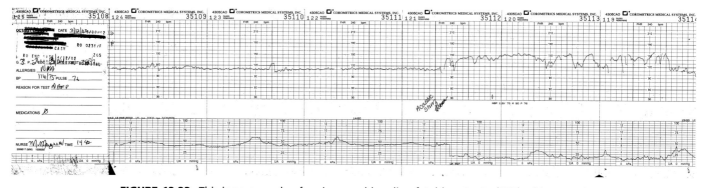

FIGURE 12.23. This is an example of an increased baseline fetal heart rate (FHR) with arousal from sleep. The fetus had been nonreactive for 30 minutes with an FHR baseline in the 110s when the sound stimulation (noted in **panel 121**) was administered. Note the acceleration induced by the sound stimulation.

depict CNS depression caused by hypoxia, drugs, fetal sleep, or congenital anomalies.

In 1977, Read and Miller first studied the fetal response to sound as a test for fetal well-being (62). In 1984, Sarafini et al. reported on the correlation between the lack of accelerations in response to sound and subsequent fetal distress in labor (63). They reported that the sound stimulation test also decreased the time necessary for an NST. Smith and associates have evaluated the use of sound stimulation with an artificial larynx as a means of eliciting reactivity and shortening the time for an NST (64). The same group showed that there was also a good correlation between response to sound with acceleration and fetal pH during labor (65). The use of sound stimulation decreases the time for an NST, and the accelerations produced are as reassuring as spontaneously occurring accelerations.

The endpoint of the NST is the presence or absence of FHR accelerations within a specific time. A great variety of criteria have been set by different authors for what constitutes a reactive NST. Most clinicians use two accelerations of 15 beats per minute (BPM) for 15 seconds in a 20-minute period as satisfying the criteria for reactivity. Brown and Patrick pointed out in 1981 that the length of time a fetus is nonreactive is highly correlated with fetal compromise, and when the fetus remains nonreactive for more than 80 minutes, it is virtually always found to have evidence of significant compromise and remains nonreactive (66). Leveno and associates confirmed this finding (67). One of the problems with using FHR accelerations as an endpoint for fetal well-being is the extension of this to pregnancies of less than 32 weeks' gestation. A healthy fetus under 32 weeks may not have reactivity or accelerations that meet the magnitude requirement of 15 BPM peak and an acceleration duration of 15 seconds. Because nonreactivity may be due to prematurity and not fetal jeopardy, one must consider this fact in the interpretation of NST results before 32 weeks' gestation. The more remote from term that testing occurs, the more likely that nonreactivity will be due to fetal

prematurity (68, 69). We generally use 28 to 30 weeks as the gestational age at which we expect reactivity to be present or strongly suspect fetal CNS dysfunction. Devoe et al. have used the percentage of acceleration time as well as sequential analysis of tests in a given patient to increase the accuracy of NST surveillance (70, 71).

Performing the Nonstress Test

In the United States, the most common method of antepartum testing is the nonstress test. The patient is placed in the semi-Fowler's position (72), blood pressure is recorded, and the external monitors are applied. The tocodynamometer is included for recording of spontaneous contractions and fetal movement. Fetal movement is recorded on the lower channel in one of two ways.

Either the patient informs the nurse, who charts the fetal movement (FM) on the tracing (Fig. 12.21), or an event marker (supplied with many monitors) is given to the patient to push each time the fetus moves (Fig. 12.24). This is recorded on the lower channel, usually with an arrow or vertical line (Fig. 12.25). A 20-minute period is recorded. According to the criteria of Evertson et al., if there are two or more accelerations in 20 minutes, the test result is interpreted as reactive and is concluded (Fig. 12.26) (60). Accelerations are defined as an increase of at least 15 BPM above the baseline lasting at least 15 seconds. If there are insufficient accelerations, fetal sound stimulation will often elicit an acceleration response. Manual manipulation of the uterus and fetus may elicit accelerations of the FHR, but Druzin et al. showed no effect in a controlled study (73). Should the lack of accelerations (less than two) in a 20-minute period persist, the test is interpreted as nonreactive and a back-up test or continued monitoring should be performed (Figs. 12.27 and 12.28).

There has not been universal agreement on the number of accelerations required to consider a test result reactive. Evertson et al. looked at this question specifically (60).

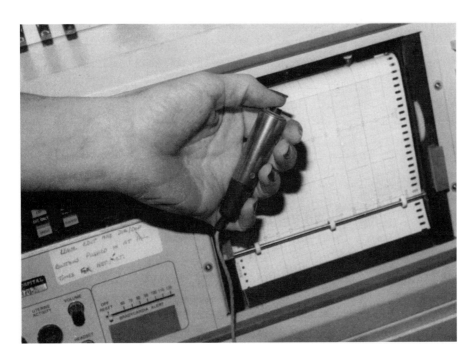

FIGURE 12.24. Event marker for recording fetal movement. When the patient presses the button, an arrow is printed on the lower channel of the fetal monitor record (see Fig. 12.25).

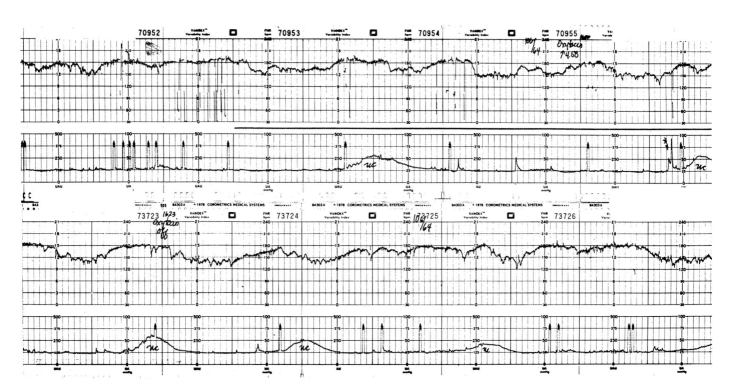

FIGURE 12.25. Note the vertical arrows produced by the fetal monitor when the patient pushed the event marker at the time of perceived fetal movement.

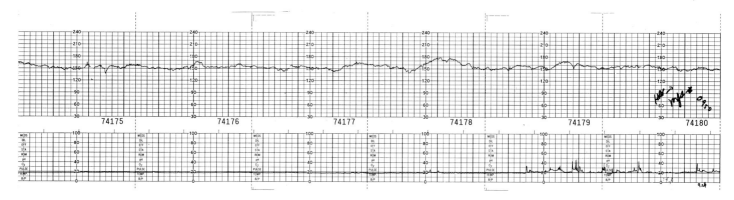

FIGURE 12.26. Reactive nonstress test characterized by fetal heart rate accelerations of 15 beats per minute or greater lasting 15 seconds or more from onset to offset.

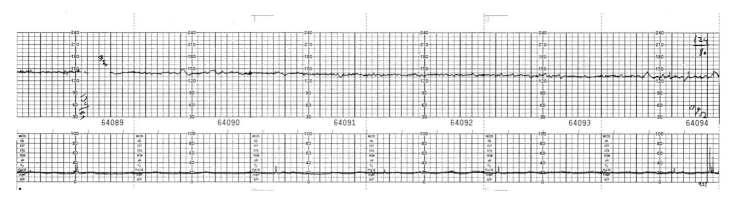

FIGURE 12.27. This nonreactive nonstress test does not show adequate fetal heart rate acceleration to meet the criteria for reactivity. It must be further evaluated.

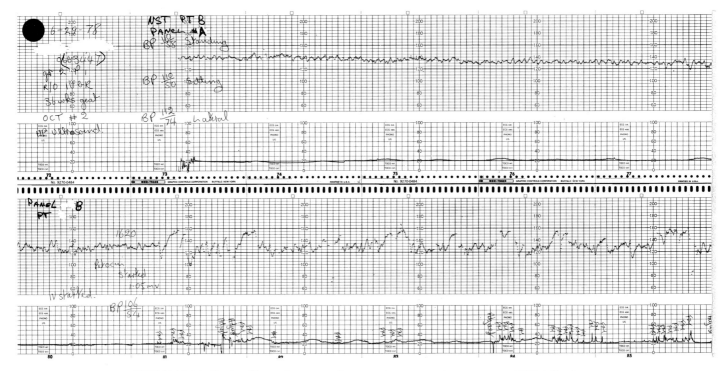

FIGURE 12.28. Tracing illustrating a reactive negative contraction stress test (CST) following a nonreactive CST. This is a reassuring test, and repeat testing is indicated in 1 week.

They found that in NSTs followed by CSTs, there were no positive CST results when two or more accelerations were seen in 20 minutes. These are the only objective data available, and this seems the most appropriate way of choosing this endpoint. However, in our extensive experience with CSTs, we have seen many positive CST results with more than two accelerations in the prestress recording period. When interpreting a CST, we recommend including the presence or absence of fetal movement and heart rate accelerations.

BIOPHYSICAL PROFILE TESTING

The BPP has become a common means of providing antepartum fetal assessment. The BPP score is based on a composite of four dynamic fetal variables (fetal breathing, movement, tone, and the nonstress test) and one long-term variable (amniotic fluid volume) (Table 12.8). When first reported in 1980 by Manning et al., the BPP score showed a very high correlation with fetal well-being when normal (i.e., scores of 8 or 10) as well as with fetal compromise when abnormal (i.e., scores of 4 or less) (74). Further, there is a highly significant inverse relationship between the BPP score and pH in the fetal blood obtained either with antepartum cordocentesis (75) or at elective cesarean section in nonlaboring patients (76), with a normal BPP score always associated with the absence of fetal acidemia. Although commonly used as originally described, the BPP has undergone two modifications by Manning's group. The definition of oligohydramnios was changed from the largest pocket of amniotic fluid being no greater than 1 cm to a pocket no greater than 2 cm (77). A further modification was reported in 1987 with the NST being performed only when one or more of the dynamic ultrasound variables was abnormal (78). Other definitions of oligohydramnios using a composite amniotic fluid index of 5 cm or less have also been reported with the BPP.

When used as the primary fetal surveillance test, the BPP has a very low false-negative rate reported between 0.7 and 2.3 per 1,000 tested patients (80). In specifically evaluating the various components of the BPP, Vintzileos et al. reported that the strongest correlation with perinatal mortality was the absence of fetal tone (81). However, in cases of severe oligohydramnios (e.g., IUGR or preterm premature rupture of membranes), tone may be hard to evaluate. The use of the BPP in a setting of a nonreactive NST was found to be helpful. With a reactive NST, the addition of other BPP parameters did not improve predictability of fetal status. These findings supported the current common approach of using the BPP as a back-up test for patients with nonreactive or equivocal nonstress testing.

MODIFIED BIOPHYSICAL PROFILE

As experience had been gained with antepartum fetal testing, it has become evident that the tests with the best predicative value have both an acute marker (acceleration of FHR, fetal movement, fetal tone, fetal breathing) and a chronic marker reflecting uteroplacental reserve (amniotic fluid volume, FHR response to uterine contractions). Although, easy to perform, the NST has a relatively high false-negative rate of 3.2 per 1,000 (23). With accelerations of the FHR, fetal tone and movement are present. The addition of a semiquantitative amniotic fluid assessment to the NST provides a chronic marker to an acute marker. Using twice-weekly "modified BPP" testing, Clark et al. suggested that such an approach was comparable in results to the weekly CST (82). In a large, prospective study we report that the modified BPP had similarly low false-negative results to the CST, and using the BPP as back-up for equivocal tests was associated with fewer interventions than with the CST as back-up (8,79).

Performing the Modified Biophysical Profile Test

The modified BPP can be performed by antepartum testing nurses trained in the ultrasound measurement of amniotic fluid volume and the dynamic fetal assessments of tone, movement, and breathing. A standard NST is combined

TABLE 12.8. BIOPHYSICAL PROFILE SCORING

Biophysical Variable	Normal (Score = 2)	Abnormal (Score = 0)
1. Fetal breathing movements	≥1 episode of ≥30 sec in 30 min	Absence or <30 sec in 30 min
2. Gross body movements	≥3 discrete body/limb movements in 30 min	≤2 discrete body/limb movements in 30 min
3. Fetal tone	≥1 active extension/flexion of limb, trunk, or hand	Slow or absent fetal extension/flexion
4. Reactive fetal heart rate	≥2 accelerations of ≥15 BPM for ≥15 sec in 20 min	>2 accelerations
5. Qualitative amniotic fluid volume	≥1 pocket of fluid >1 cm in 2 perpendicular planes	No pocket >1 cm in 2 perpendicular planes

Our protocol uses a 5.0 cm AFT cutoff for normal score.
BPM, beats per minute.
From Manning FA, Platt LW, Sipos L: Antepartum fetal evaluation: development of a biophysical profile. *Am J Obstet Gynecol* 136:787, 1980, with permission.

with an amniotic fluid index (AFI) (83). The test result is considered negative if the NST is reactive without decelerations and the AFI is greater than 5.0 cm. If the NST is nonreactive, has decelerations, or if the AFI is 5.0 cm or less, a BPP is performed for back-up test. If the BPP score is 8 or 10, the MBPP is repeated in 3 to 4 days. If the BPP score is 6 or less, clinical management may include delivery, continuous monitoring, or repeat testing in 1 day. As with all forms of fetal testing, decisions regarding clinical management must be individualized with consideration given to maternal status, gestational age, and fetal maturity.

Negative test results are repeated every 3 to 4 days. If the AFI is greater than 5.0 cm, a repeat assessment of amniotic fluid is not indicated for 1 week (84). We use the modified BPP in all indications for antepartum fetal surveillance with the exception of patients with insulin-dependent diabetes mellitus. In such patients, we perform weekly modified BPP with a mid-week CST because AFI is not a reliable chronic marker in the insulin-dependent diabetic.

PRIMARY FETAL SURVEILLANCE

Historically, the CST, NST, BPP, and modified BPP have been reported as means of primary fetal surveillance testing. Although efforts have been made to establish the "best" test based upon various outcome parameters, there have been no adequate prospective randomized studies comparing the various testing modalities (85). Each method of antepartum testing has unique advantages and disadvantages. Although requiring only once a week testing and associated with a false-negative rate of 0.4 per 1,000, the CST is more difficult and costly to perform and has a relatively high rate of false-positive and equivocal results (23). The NST, although easy to perform and interpret, has a false-positive rate approaching 50% and a high false-negative rate of 3.2 per 1,000 (23). The complete biophysical profile is more time-consuming than the NST and includes necessary technology and experience in ultrasound measurements of various parameters. It may also be significantly more expensive, depending on the specific costs applied to the BPP performance and interpretation. The most recent and largest report of cumulative false-negative rate was between 0.7 and 2.29 per 1,000 (80). The false-positive rate for the complete BPP is approximately 40% if the endpoint is fetal or neonatal compromise (86). The clinical significance of this is dependent on the gestational age and the specific perinatal endpoint examined. The modified BPP has a low false-negative rate of 0.8 per 1,000 and an intermediate false-positive rate of iatrogenic prematurity in 1.5% of women tested preterm (86). The final decision regarding choice of fetal surveillance test is most often determined by institutional preference and experience. What is clear is that all forms of fetal testing are valuable and need to be interpreted cautiously with full knowledge of the spe-cific test limitations as well as the physiology of the indication for testing. Testing frequency of the CST and the BPP is generally weekly, but it is recommended that the BPP be performed twice weekly for certain high-risk conditions (postdate pregnancy, insulin-dependent diabetes mellitus) (7). Unpredictable morbid events such as massive fetomaternal hemorrhage may explain some cases of fetal demise following negative test results (80,87).

PRETERM PREMATURE RUPTURE OF MEMBRANES

Antepartum assessment in a pregnancy complicated by preterm premature rupture of membranes (PPROM) is both challenging and important because of the high degree of associated perinatal morbidity and mortality (88–91). Major risks include infection, cord prolapse, stillbirth, fetal deformity, and compromise. Although the CST is contraindicated with PPROM, various investigators have reported on the use of amniotic fluid assessment, nonstress testing, and BPP for this clinical condition (92–96). There appears to be a correlation between a low AFI and the development of variable decelerations and nonreactivity (92). The initial AFI is possibly associated with duration of latency period, response to tocolytic therapy, and possibly with infection, although there is not consensus on all these relationships (92,93,96,97). Following an initial period of clinical assessment and continuous FHR monitoring, a daily 1-hour nonstress test is a reasonable protocol to follow in patients with PPROM.

Clinical Management with Nonstress Testing for Primary Surveillance

The NST is the most popular method for antepartum fetal surveillance because it is easy to perform, easy to interpret, has fewer equivocal results, and has excellent patient and physician acceptance. Traditionally it has been offered on a weekly basis, but some authors have suggested increasing the frequency to twice weekly (72), especially in postdate and diabetic pregnancies. When the NST result is nonreactive or has spontaneous decelerations, further testing is necessary. We recommend a full BPP as the back-up test.

Some data indicate that the loss of reactivity occurs later than the appearance of late decelerations in a chronically deteriorating fetus. Murata and colleagues showed that in the monkey fetus undergoing progressive intrauterine hypoxia ultimately leading to death, the first evidence of hypoxia on the FHR pattern was the appearance of late deceleration (36). Only after the development of significant fetal acidosis did the fetuses lose FHR acceleration. For this reason, it should be kept in mind that if a fetus is truly nonreactive it may be in very serious condition.

Clinical Management with the Biophysical Profile and Modified Biophysical Profile for Primary Surveillance

As clinicians have gained experience with real-time ultrasound and the equipment has been improved, there has been an increasing interest in using this method for primary fetal surveillance. Manning and associates have been the primary proponents of this approach and currently only use the NST as a backup about 3% of the time (78). Using this method twice weekly, Manning et al. report results that are comparable to those with the weekly CST and that identify more anomalous babies.

The most common finding triggering intervention is oligohydramnios, yet there is no universal agreement on what constitutes oligohydramnios. Manning et al. (74) originally said that a 1-cm vertical pocket was adequate, but Vintzileos et al. (81) advocated intervention with pockets measuring less than 2 cm. Perhaps a better approach is to use the four-quadrant measurement of 5 cm total or greater, as described by Rutherford et al. (83). Clearly, there is a very high perinatal morbidity among patients with significant oligohydramnios (74,75). Most studies have shown that primary NST surveillance has a higher antepartum fetal death rate than primary CST surveillance or primary BPP surveillance. Perhaps this is because, in the fetus with clinically significant oligohydramnios, the condition will not be detected unless there are contractions or the patient has an ultrasound study. Current recommendations for the frequency of testing with the BPP are not well established, varying from once weekly testing to twice weekly.

DOPPLER VELOCIMETRY

Because Doppler velocimetry is arguably still considered investigational for antepartum fetal assessment, it will not be extensively presented (98–101). However, Doppler velocimetry remains an attractive method with great potential in the assessment of the fetus. In normal pregnancy, the physiologic conditions of the placenta present an area of low vascular impedance, which allows continuous forward blood flow throughout the cardiac cycle. With increases in placental impedance, the mostly passive blood flow in diastole in the umbilical artery decreases to low, absent, or revered end-diastolic flow. It is suggested that the abnormal change in the pattern of umbilical artery blood flow reflects the presence of a structural placental lesion and that such abnormal Doppler test results require specific management protocols and intensive fetal surveillance (102,103). Umbilical artery Doppler is a placental test more than a fetal test. It is a poor indicator of fetal compromise or adaptation to the placental abnormality but does identify patients at risk for increased perinatal mortality.

Clinical studies employing Doppler velocimetry have revealed a strong correlation between high systolic to diastolic (S/D) ratios and IUGR (104–107). Similar associations between increased S/D ratio, absent or reversed diastolic flow, and adverse outcome have been reported in poorly controlled diabetes in pregnancy (108,109) and postdate pregnancies (110). Correlations between abnormal antepartum FHR tests and high S/D ratio have also been reported (111).

As with other forms of fetal surveillance, umbilical artery velocimetry appears to have clinical utility in the management of high-risk pregnancies. Meta-analyses of published, peer-reviewed, randomized controlled trials reveal a reduction in perinatal mortality in the Doppler group without apparent increase in the rate of inappropriate obstetric interventions (102,112). However, the question that remains unanswered should not be whether or not Doppler velocimetry should be used instead of other forms of fetal surveillance but rather does it have a role in concert with the other fetal tests? Further, Doppler may serve in helping to determine the timing of delivery particularly in a setting where all measures of fetal status are nonreassuring. As with all other forms of fetal testing, randomized controlled clinical trials are necessary to answer these specific questions.

REFERENCES

1. Predictors of fetal distress. In: *Antenatal diagnosis*. United States Department of HEW/NIH. NIH Publication no. 79-1973, 1979.
2. Garite TJ, Freeman RK, Hochleutner I, et al.: Oxytocin challenge test; achieving the desired goals. *Obstet Gynecol* 51:614, 1978.
3. White P: Pregnancy and diabetes, medical aspects. *Med Clin North Am* 49:1015, 1965.
4. Kubli FW, Kaeser O, Hinselmann M: Diagnostic management of chronic placental insufficiency. In: Pecile A, Finzi C, eds. *The feto-placental unit*. Exercepta Medica Foundation, Amsterdam, 1969:323.
5. Parer JT: Normal and impaired placental exchange. *Contemp Obstet Gyncecol* 7:117, 1976.
6. Freeman R, Anderson G, Dorchester W: A prospective multiinstitutional study monitoring. I. Risk of perinatal mortality according to antepartum fetal heart rate test results. *Am J Obstet Gynecol* 143:771, 1982.
7. Manning F, Morrison I, Lange I, et al.: Fetal assessment based on fetal biophysical profile scoring: experience in 12,620 referred high-risk pregnancies. *Am J Obstet Gynecol* 151: 343, 1985.
8. Nageotte M, Towers C, Asrat T, et al.: Perinatal outcome with the modified biophysical profile. *Am J Obstet Gynecol* 170: 1672, 1994.
9. Neldam S: Fetal movements as an indicator of fetal well-being. *Lancet* 2:1222, 1980.
10. Sadovsky E: When prompt delivery is indicated. *Contemp Obstet Gynecol* 16:109, 1980.
11. Rabinowitz R, Persitz E, Sadovsky E: The relation between fetal heart rate accelerations and fetal movements. *Obstet Gynecol* 61:16, 1983.

12. Sadovsky E, Polishuk W: Fetal movements in utero. *Obstet Gynecol* 50:49, 1977.

13. Sadovsky E, Yaffe H: Daily fetal movement recording and fetal prognosis. *Obstet Gynecol* 31:845, 1973.

14. Sadovsky E, Yaffe H, Polishuk W: Fetal movements monitoring in normal and pathological pregnancy. *Int J Gynecol Obstet* 12:75, 1974.

15. Moore T, Piacquadio K: A prospective evaluation of fetal movement screening to reduce the incidence of antepartum fetal death. *Am J Obstet Gynecol* 160:1075, 1989.

16. Freeman RK: The use of the oxytocin challenge test for antepartum clinical evaluation of uteroplacental respiratory function. *Am J Obstet Gynecol* 121:481, 1975.

17. Gabbe SG, Freeman RK, Mestman JH: Management and outcome of the class "A" diabetic. *Am J Obstet Gynecol* 127:465, 1977.

18. Gabbe SG, Mestman JH, Freeman RK, et al.: Management and outcome of diabetes mellitus, classes *Br Am J Obstet Gynecol* 129(7):723, 1977.

19. Pircon RN, Lagrew DC, Towers CV, et al.: Antepartum testing in the hypertensive patient: when to begin? *Am J Obstet Gynecol* 164:1563, 1991.

20. Lagrew DC, Pircon RA, Towers CV, et al.: Antepartum surveillance in the diabetic: when to start? *Am J Obstet Gynecol* 168:1820, 1993.

21. Weeks JW, Asrat T, Morgan MA, et al.: Antepartum surveillance for a history of stillbirth: when to begin? *Am J Obstet Gynecol* 172:486, 1995.

22. Porto M, Merril PA, Lovett SM, et al.: When should antepartum testing begin in post-term pregnancy? Presentation at Society of Perinatal Obstetricians Annual Conference, San Antonio, January 1986.

23. Freeman RK, Anderson G, Dorchester W: A prospective multi-institutional study of antepartum fetal heart rate monitoring. II. Contraction stress test versus non stress test for primary surveillance. *Am J Obstet Gynecol* 143:778, 1982.

24. Thacker SD, Berkelman RL: Assessing the diagnostic accuracy and efficacy of selected antepartum fetal surveillance techniques. *Obstet Gynecol* 41:121, 1986.

25. Hon EH, Wohlgemuth R: The electronic evaluation of fetal heart rate. IV. The effect of maternal exercise. *Am J Obstet Gynecol* 81:361, 1961.

26. Hendricks CH: Amniotic fluid pressure recordings. *Clin Obstet Gynecol* 9:535, 1966.

27. Hammacher K: Fruherkennung intrauterineo gefahrenzustande dutch electrophonocardiographie and focographie. In: Elert R, Hates KA, eds. *Prophylaxe Frunddkindicher Hirnschaden.* Thieme Verlag, Stuttgart, 1966:120.

28. Pose SV, Escarcena L: The influence of uterine contractions on the partial pressure of oxygen of the human fetus. In: *Effects of labour on the foetus and newborn.* Pergamon Press, Oxford, 1967:48.

29. Spurrett B: Stressed cardiotocography in late pregnancy. *J Obstet Gynaecol Br Commonw* 78:894, 1971.

30. Sanchez-Ramos J, Santisimo JL, Peman FC: La prueba del la oxitocina en el diagnostico del estado fetal anteparto. *Acta Ginecol (Madrid)* 22:697, 1971.

31. Ray M, Freeman RK, Pine S, et al.: Clinical experience with the oxytocin challenge test. *Am J Obstet Gynecol* 114:1, 1972.

32. Jhirad T, Vago T: Induction of labor by breast stimulation. *Obstet Gynecol* 41:347, 1978.

33. Oki E, Keegan K, Freeman R, Dorchester W: The breast stimulated contraction stress test. *J Reprod Med* 32:919, 1987.

34. MacMillan JB, Halr R: Contraction stress testing with mammary self-stimulation. *J Reprod Med* 29:219, 1984.

35. Capeless E, Mann LI: Use of breast stimulation for antepartum stress testing. *Obstet Gynecol* 64:641, 1984.

36. Copel JA, Otis CS, Steward E, et al.: Contraction stress testing with nipple stimulation. *J Reprod Med* 30:465, 1985.

37. Schellpeffer M, Hoyle D, Johnson JWC: Antepartum uterine hypercontractility secondary to nipple stimulation. *Obstet Gynecol* 65:588, 1985.

38. Viegas O, Arulkumaran S, Gibb D, et al.: Nipple stimulation in late pregnancy causing uterine hyperstimulation and profound fetal bradycardia. *Br J Obstet Gynaecol* 91:364, 1984.

39. Viegas O, Arulkumaran S, Gibb D, et al.: Nipple stimulation in late pregnancy causing uterine hyperstimulation and profound fetal bradycardia. *Br J Obstet Gynaecol* 91:364, 1984.

40. Huddleston JF, Sutlieff G, Robinson D: Contraction stress test by intermittent nipple stimulation. *Obstet Gynecol* 63:669, 1984.

41. American College of Obstetricians and Gynecologists (ACOG): Fetal heart rate patterns: Monitoring, interpretation and management. ACOG Technical Bulletin, No. 207, 1995.

42. Freeman RK, James J: Clinical experience with the oxytocin challenge test. II. An ominous atypical pattern. *Obstet Gynecol* 46:255, 1975.

43. Baskett TF, Sandy E: The oxytocin challenge test: an ominous pattern associated with severe fetal growth retardation. *Obstet Gynecol* 54:365, 1979.

44. Modanlou H, Freeman R: Sinusoidal fetal heart rate pattern: its definition and significance. *Am J Obstet Gynecol* 142:1033, 1982.

45. Rochard F, Schifrin BS, Goupil F, et al.: Nonstressed fetal heart rate monitoring in the antepartum period. *Am J Obstet Gynecol* 126:699, 1976.

46. Modanlou HD, Freeman RK, Ortiz O, et al.: Sinusoidal fetal heart rate pattern and severe fetal anemia. *Obstet Gynecol* 49:537, 1977.

47. Murata Y, Martin CB, Ikenoue T, et al.: Fetal heart rate accelerations and late decelerations during the course of intrauterine death in chronically catheterized rhesus monkeys. *Am J Obstet Gynecol* 144:218, 1982.

48. Grundy H, Freeman R, Lederman S, et al.: Nonreactive contraction stress test: clinical significance. *Obstet Gynecol* 64:337, 1984.

49. Braly PB, Freeman RK, Garite TJ, et al.: Premature labor and the oxytocin challenge test. *Am J Obstet Gynecol* 141:5, 1981.

50. Trierweiler M, Freeman R, James J: Baseline fetal heart rate characteristics as an indicator fetal status during the antepartum period. *Am J Obstet Gynecol* 125:618, 1976.

51. Freeman RK, Goelbelsmann U, Nochimson D, et al.: An evaluation of the significance of a positive oxytocin challenge test. *Obstet Gynecol* 47:8, 1976.

52. Farahani G, Vasudeva K, Petrie R, et al.: Oxytocin challenge test in a high risk pregnancy. *Obstet Gynecol* 47:159, 1976.

53. Weingold AB, DeJesus TPS, O'Keeffe J: Oxytocin challenge test. *Am J Obstet Gynecol* 123:466, 1975.

54. Braly PB, Freeman RK: The significance of fetal heart rate activity with a positive oxytocin challenge test. *Obstet Gynecol* 50:689, 1977.

55. Kubli F, Boos R, Ruttgers H, et al.: Antepartum fetal heart rate monitoring. In: Bear R, Campbell S, eds. *The current status of FHR monitoring and ultrasound in obstetrics.* Royal College of Obstetrics and Gynaecology, London, 1977:28.

56. Lee CY, DiLoreto PC, Logrand B: Fetal activity acceleration determination for the evaluation of fetal reserve. *Obstet Gynecol* 48:19, 1976.

57. Tushhuizen PBT, Stoot JEGM, Ubachs JMH: Clinical experience in nonstressed antepartum cardiotocography. *Am J Obstet Gynecol* 128:507, 1977.

58. Flynn AM, Kelly J: Evaluation of fetal well-being by antepartum fetal heart rate monitoring. *BMJ* 1:936, 1977.

59. Krebs HB, Petries RE: Clinical application of a scoring system for evaluation of antepartum fetal heart rate monitoring. *Am J Obstet Gynecol* 130:765, 1978.

60. Evertson LR, Gauthier RJ, Schifrin BS, et al.: Antepartum fetal heart rate testing. I. Evaluation of the non stress test. *Am J Obstet Gynecol* 133:29, 1979.

61. Keegan KA, Paul RH, Broussard PM, et al.: Antepartum fetal heart rate testing. III. The effect of phenobarbital on the nonstress test. *Am J Obstet Gynecol* 133:579, 1979.

62. Read JA, Miller FC: Fetal heart rate acceleration in response to acoustic stimulation as a measure of fetal well-being. *Am J Obstet Gynecol* 141:512, 1977.

63. Serafini P, Lindsay MBJ, Nagey D, et al.: Antepartum fetal heart rate response to sound stimulation: the acoustic stimulation test. *Am J Obstet Gynecol* 148:41, 1984.

64. Smith CV, Phelan JP, Paul RH, et al.: Fetal acoustic stimulation testing: a retrospective experience with the fetal acoustic stimulation test. *Am J Obstet Gynecol* 153:567, 1985.

65. Smith C, Hguyen H, Phelan J, et al.: Intrapartum assessment of fetal well-being: a comparison of fetal acoustic stimulation with acid base determinations. *Am J Obstet Gynecol* 155:726, 1986.

66. Brown R, Patrick J: The non stress test: how long is enough? *Am J Obstet Gynecol* 141:646, 1981.

67. Leveno K, Williams L, DePalma R, et al.: Perinatal outcome in the absence of antepartum fetal heart rate acceleration. *Obstet Gynecol* 61:347, 1983.

68. Devoe L: Antepartum fetal heart rate testing in preterm pregnancy. *Obstet Gynecol* 60:431, 1982.

69. Druzin M, Fox H, Kogut E, et al.: The relationship of the nonstress test to gestational age. *Am J Obstet Gynecol* 153:386, 1985.

70. Devoe LD, Castillo R, Saad S, et al.: Percent acceleration time; a new method of fetal assessment. *Obstet Gynecol* 67:191, 1986.

71. Devoe L, Castillo R, McKenzie J, et al.: Sequential nonstress testing with use of each fetus as its own control. *Am J Obstet Gynecol* 154:931, 1986.

72. Nathan EB, Haberman S, Burgess T, et al.: The relationship of maternal position to the results of brief nonstress tests: a randomized clinical trial. *Am J Obstet Gynecol* 182:1070, 2000.

73. Druzin ML, Gratacos J, Paul RH, et al.: Antepartum fetal heart rate testing. XII. The effect of manual manipulation of the fetus on the nonstress test. *Am J Obstet Gynecol* 151:61, 1985.

74. Manning FA, Platt LW, Sipos L: Antepartum fetal evaluation: development of a biophysical profile. *Am J Obstet Gynecol* 136:787, 1980.

75. Manning FA, Snijders R, Harman CR, et al.: Fetal biophysical profile scoring. VI. Correlations with antepartum umbilical venous pH. *Am J Obstet Gynecol* 169:755, 1993.

76. Vintzileos AM, Fleming AD, Scorza WE, et al.: Relationship between fetal biophysical activities and cord blood gas values. *Am J Obstet Gynecol* 165:707, 1991.

77. Manning FA: Fetal biophysical profile scoring. In: Manning FA, ed. *Fetal medicine: principles and practice*. Appleton and Lange, Norwalk, CT, 1995:241.

78. Manning F, Morrison M, Lange I, et al.: Fetal biophysical profile scoring: selective use of the nonstress test. *Am J Obstet Gynecol* 156:709, 1987.

79. Nageotte MP, Towers CV, Asrat T, et al.: The value of a negative antepartum test: contraction stress test and modified biophysical profile. *Obstet Gynecol* 84:231, 1994.

80. Dayal AK, Manning FA, Berck DJ, et al.: Fetal heath after normal biophysical profile score: An eighteen year experience. *Am J Obstet Gynecol* 181:1231, 1999.

81. Vintzileos A, Campbell W, Nochimson D, et al.: The use and misuse of biophysical profile. *Am J Obstet Gynecol* 156:527, 1987.

82. Clark S, Sabey P, Jolley K: Nonstress testing with acoustic stimulation and amniotic volume assessment: 5973 tests without unexpected fetal death. *Am J Obstet Gynecol* 160:694, 1989.

83. Rutherford S, Phelan J, Smith C, et al.: The four quadrant assessment of amniotic fluid volume: an adjunct to antepartum fetal heart rate testing. *Obstet Gynecol* 70:689, 1977.

84. Lagrew DC, Freeman RK, Pircon RA, et al.: How frequently should the amniotic fluid index be repeated? *Am J Obstet Gynecol* 167:1129, 1992.

85. Alfirevic Z, Neilson JP: Biophysical profile for fetal assessment in high risk pregnancies (Cochrane review). In: *The Cochrane library*, issue Z. Update Software, Oxford, 2002.

86. Miller DA, Rabello YA, Paul RH: The modified biophysical profile: antepartum testing in the 1990s. *Am J Obstet Gynecol* 174:812, 1996.

87. Samadi R, Greenspoon JS, Gviazda I, et al.: Massive fetomaternal hemorrhage and fetal death: are they predictable? *J Perinatol* 19(3):227, 1999.

88. Mead PB: Management of the patient with premature rupture of the membranes. *Clin Perinatol* 7:243, 1980.

89. Nimrod C, Varela-Gittings F, Machin G, et al.: The effect of very prolonged membrane rupture on fetal development. *Am J Obstet Gynecol* 148:540, 1984.

90. Blott M, Greenough A: Neonatal outcome after prolonged rupture of the membranes starting in the second trimester. *Arch Dis Child* 63:1146, 1988.

91. Naeye RL, Jackson DM, Lewis DF, et al.: Correlation of amniotic fluid index and nonstress test in a patients with preterm premature rupture of membranes. *Am J Obstet Gynecol* 165:1088, 1991.

92. Harding JA, Jackson DM, Lewis DF, et al.: Correlation of amniotic fluid index and nonstress test in patients with preterm premature rupture of membranes. *Am J Obstet Gynecol* 165:1088, 1991.

93. Ghidini A, Salafia C, Kirn V, et al.: Biophysical profile in predicting acute ascending infection in preterm premature rupture of membranes before 32 weeks. *Obstet Gynecol* 96:201, 2000.

94. Vintzileos AM, Campbell WA, Nochimson DJ, et al.: Fetal biophysical profile versus amniocentesis in predicting infection in preterm premature rupture of the membranes. *Obstet Gynecol* 68:488, 1986.

95. Romero R, Athayde N, Maymon E, et al.: Premature rupture of the membranes. In: Reece EA, Hobbins JC, eds. *Medicine of the fetus and mother*. Lippincott-Raven, Philadelphia, 1999:1581.

96. Vintzileos AM, Campbell WA, Nochimson DJ, et al.: The use of the nonstress test in patients with premature rupture of the membranes. *Obstet Gynecol* 155:149, 1986.

97. Gonik B, Bottoms SF, Cotton DB: Amniotic fluid volume as a risk factor in preterm premature rupture of the membranes. *Obstet Gynecol* 65:456, 1985.

98. Dornan JC, Harper H: Where are we with Doppler? *Br J Obstet Gynecol* 101:190, 1994.

99. Low JA: The current status of maternal and fetal blood flow velocimetry. *Am J Obstet Gynecol* 164:1049, 1991.

100. American College of Obstetricians and Gynecologists: Utility of antepartum Doppler for estimating fetal umbilical and uterine artery flow. American College of Obstetrician and Gynecologists, Washington, 1992, Committee Opinion no. 116.

101. American College of Obstetricians and Gynecologists: Antepartum fetal surveillance Washington: American College of Obstetricians and Gynecologists, Washington, Technical Bulletin no. 188.

102. Alfirevic Z, Neilson JP: Doppler ultrasonography in high-risk pregnancies: systematic review with meta-analysis. *Am J Obstet Gynecol* 172:1379, 1995.

103. Divon, MY: Umbilical artery Doppler velocimetry: clinical utility in high-risk pregnancies. *Am J Obstet Gynecol* 174:10, 1996.

104. Almstrom H, Axelsson, O, Cnattingius S, et al.: Comparison of umbilical artery velocimetry and cardiotocography for surveillance of small-for-gestational age fetuses. A multicenter randomised controlled trial. *Lancet* 340:936, 1992.

105. Campbell S, Pearce J, Hackett G: Qualitative assessment of uteroplacental blood flow: Early screening test for high risk pregnancies. *Obstet Gynecol* 68:649, 1986.

106. Pattison RC, Norman K, Odendal HJ: The role of Doppler velocimetry in the management of high risk pregnancies. *Br J Obstet Gynecol* 101:114, 1994.

107. Laurini R, Laurin L, Marsal K: Placental histology and fetal blood flow in intrauterine growth retardation. *Acta Obstet Gynecol Scand* 73:529, 1994.

108. Bracero L, Schulman H, Fleischer A, et al.: Umbilical artery velocity waveforms in diabetic pregnancy. *Obstet Gynecol* 68:654, 1986.

109. Trudinger B, Cook C, Jones W, et al.: A comparison of fetal heart rate monitoring and umbilical artery waveforms in the recognition of fetal compromise. *Br J Obstet Gynaecol* 93:171, 1986.

110. Guidetti DA, Divon MY, Cavalieri RL, et al.: Fetal umbilical artery flow velocimetry in postdate pregnancies. *Am J Obstet Gynecol* 157:1521, 1987.

111. Farmakides G, Schulman H, Ducey J, et al.: Prenatal testing using non-stress testing and Doppler velocimetry. *Obstet Gynecol* 71:184, 1988.

112. Giles W, Bisits A: Clinical use of Doppler in pregnancy: information for six randomized trials. *Fetal Diagn Ther* 8:247, 1993.

ANTEPARTUM MANAGEMENT OF THE HIGH-RISK PATIENT

The previous chapter was devoted to introducing antepartum fetal surveillance, including fetal heart rate (FHR) testing and biophysical profile (BPP), describing methodology, interpretation, and understanding the associated limitations and pitfalls. The appropriate application of these methods in various clinical situations is critically important.

First we must decide which patients require antepartum testing. Almost half of the antepartum deaths occurring beyond 26 weeks of gestation are in patients at risk for some form of uteroplacental insufficiency (UPI) (1,2). Patients at increased risk for UPI comprise approximately 10% to 20% of the prenatal population, and various means have been used to attempt to correctly identify these women (3). The other half of antenatal deaths, however, occur in patients who would generally be classified as low risk. Low-risk women make up the majority of the obstetric population. One choice is to limit antepartum fetal surveillance to the 10% to 20% of patients at risk for UPI and thereby attempt to prevent this one-half of fetal deaths. Another choice is to test all patients in an effort to attempt to avoid all fetal deaths. This latter choice is an extreme alternative, and there is no study that shows a benefit to the routine fetal testing (beyond fetal movement assessment) of all low-risk patients. The more reasonable and well-accepted approach for identifying the low-risk patient destined to have a fetal death is to carefully observe all patients for normal fetal growth and fetal movement. Many patients with unexpected fetal death will have a growth-restricted fetus. Thus the general approach is to routinely measure fundal height in all patients receiving prenatal care, and evaluate the fetus with ultrasound when the fundal height is significantly less than expected. In addition, although not necessarily recommended, many patients do have a routine ultrasound in the late second or early third trimester. When these examinations, for whatever reason, confirm intrauterine growth restriction (IUGR), antepartum testing becomes indicated. Routine fetal movement testing has been shown in large well-controlled studies to decrease the rate of antepartum fetal deaths in low-risk patients (4,5). Thus all patients should be counseled at some time in the early third

trimester to do some kind of daily assessment of fetal movement (Fig. 13.1). There is a great deal of variation in the exact method used for fetal movement counting, as outlined in the previous chapter. Regardless of the specific method chosen, when the patient calls with absent or substantially reduced fetal movement, and when this has been confirmed by having her concentrate for an hour or two in a quiet room, the patient must come in for an immediate nonstress test regardless of the time of day. Keep in mind, however, that whatever the indication, testing should be implemented until a gestational age is reached where the clinician, if faced with definitely ominous data, is ready to intervene. Thus in the 80% of otherwise low-risk patients, the main indications for testing are the development of suspected IUGR and decreased or absent fetal movement. In the remaining high-risk patients, the indications for antepartum FHR testing are summarized in Table 13.1.

TESTING PROTOCOL BY CLINICAL SITUATION

We shall attempt to describe an approach to antepartum testing in terms of categories of risk and specific diagnoses or risk factors that place the patient at increased risk for fetal death from UPI. We shall present our approach to antepartum testing and use this format to provide examples for illustration. It should be clear that there are many different approaches in terms of when to begin testing, when to intervene, different ancillary tests, etc. The approach presented here is based on extensive clinical experience with antepartum heart rate testing in high-risk patients and on data that have been published by the authors and many others (1,6,7).

Which Test to Use

Controversy exists as to which form of antepartum surveillance provides optimal results. Issues such as patient population, available facilities, cost, convenience, testing inter-

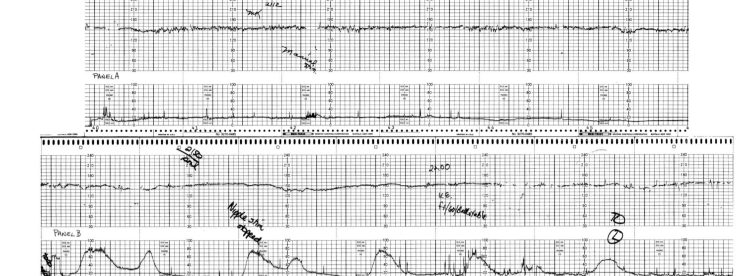

FIGURE 13.1. A primigravida woman at 39 weeks complained of no fetal movement for 1 day. Previously, there had been a decrease in movement frequency over 2 days. A nonstress test was performed **(panel A)** and was read as nonreactive with suspicious areas. This was immediately followed by a nipple stimulation contraction stress test (CST) **(panel B).** The CST result was interpreted as nonreactive and positive. Because the cervix was unfavorable, an immediate cesarean section was performed with delivery of a 3,180-g infant with Apgar scores of 4 at 1 minute and 7 at 5 minutes. Umbilical artery pH was 7.10 with a pCO$_2$ of 49 and a base deficit of 11. Fresh meconium was noted; there was no evidence of placental separation. The infant did well in the newborn period.

TABLE 13.1. INDICATIONS FOR ANTEPARTUM FETAL SURVEILLANCE

Postdate pregnancy
Diabetes
   Class A$_2$ through R
   Class A$_1$ with:
      Elevated fasting blood sugar,
      History of stillbirth, or
      Pregnancy complicated by hypertension or suspected
      IUGR
   Class A at term
Preeclampsia
Chronic hypertension
Decreased fetal movement
Previous stillbirth
Suspected IUGR
Discordant twins
Preterm premature rupture of membranes
Rh isoimmunization
Cyanotic cardiac disease
Hemoglobinopathy/severe anemia
Asthma
Hyperthyroidism
Chronic renal disease
Collagen vascular disease

IUGR, intrauterine growth retardation.

val, and the specific indication for testing must be considered when selecting the particular means of fetal assessment for your patient.

As described in the previous chapter, the most frequently used method for primary surveillance is the **modified biophysical profile**. The nonstress test (NST) is almost always performed at least twice weekly. The frequency of the amniotic fluid volume assessment may be once or twice weekly. In a review of a large series of amniotic volume testing, Lagrew and coworkers found that in patients with an amniotic fluid index (AFI) of 8 cm or greater, that a change to significant oligohydramnios (AFI < 5) rarely occurred in less than a week, except in patients with IUGR and who go beyond 41 weeks (8). Thus it is logical to test these latter two groups of patients and those with borderline AFI (5.0 to 7.9 cm) with twice-weekly NSTs and AFIs and the remainder with twice-weekly NSTs and once-weekly AFIs. One group of patients that we approach differently are those with diabetes for reasons described in the following section on that complication. In general, other tests of fetal well-being are then reserved for "back-up" testing in those patients with an abnormal NST or AFI result (Fig. 13.2). The one exception perhaps is with Doppler testing of umbilical artery flow. This modality may have additional utility in clarifying the diagnosis of IUGR, prognosticating which babies are destined to develop abnormal tests that will require early deliv-

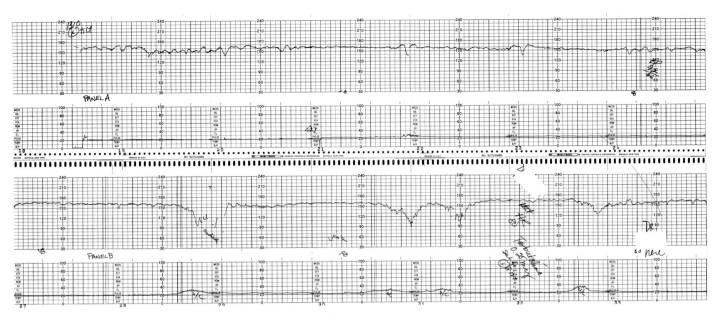

FIGURE 13.2. A 21-year-old gravida 1 para 0 at 34½ weeks was being observed for suspected intrauterine growth retardation with biweekly modified biophysical profiles (nonstress test and amniotic fluid index). Her initial nonstress test result **(panel A)** was reactive with occasional mild variable decelerations of unknown significance. Because her amniotic fluid index was 2.8 cm, she received a backup test, which was a contraction stress test (CST) **(panel B)**. The CST result was read as positive and did not meet reactivity standards. The patient underwent immediate delivery by cesarean section, delivering a 1,730-g newborn with Apgar scores of 8 at 1 minute and 9 at 5 minutes. Umbilical cord gases were normal. Nuchal cord was noted with no amniotic fluid at delivery. The infant subsequently did well in the nursery.

ery, and perhaps sort out the diagnosis of mid-trimester preeclampsia versus chronic hypertension. The exact clinical utility of Doppler to say the least is unclear and controversial, but in the extreme will help identify the highest risk patients for intensive antepartum testing.

Moderate Risk Groups

There is a group of conditions in which the risk for fetal death from UPI is only moderately increased above that of the low-risk population. Furthermore, in this group, fetal death tends to occur late in gestation. Thus in general, for these patients, we recommend beginning testing at approximately 34 weeks. These clinical situations include advance maternal age, maternal hyperthyroidism, and previous stillbirth. Women over the age of 35 years have previously been thought to represent a risk group for whom fetal surveillance is indicated. However, at least up to the age of 40 years, unless the pregnancy is complicated by diabetes, hypertension, or other problems, women do not have any increased risk for stillbirth or abnormal FHR tests secondary to UPI (9).

Women with a diagnosis of hyperthyroidism or a history of hyperthyroidism may be at risk for fetal compromise. The etiologic agent is a thyroid-stimulating immunoglobulin (TSIG) of the IgG class. Thus, this antibody can cross the

placenta and cause fetal hyperthyroidism and tachycardia. Women with a history of hyperthyroidism who are euthyroid following an ablative procedure (i.e., surgery or radioactive iodine) may still have the antibody present during a subsequent pregnancy, with potential fetal compromise. Even without the fetus being directly involved, poorly controlled hyperthyroidism may divert blood and oxygen from the fetus because of the increased metabolic demands of maternal tissues. For these reasons, we recommend testing in these women. Similarly, women with a history of an unexplained stillborn are begun on fetal surveillance at some point before the gestational age at which the loss occurred. Although this primarily provides maternal reassurance, we have found an increased incidence of abnormal test results in these patients, particularly in women with a history of previous stillbirth associated with a current diagnosis of hypertension or suspected IUGR (10).

Postdate Pregnancy

In most series, "postdate" pregnancy is the condition accounting for the majority of patients undergoing antepartum testing. Often this is because many patients have wrong dates. Postdate testing is relatively controversial, primarily from the standpoint of when to begin testing and when to deliver. Studies of contemporary practice suggest that the majority of practitioners will recommend delivery for patients at or beyond 41 weeks with a favorable cervix and for all patients after 42 weeks regardless of the condition of the cervix (11), which is our practice as well. Although the data suggest no substantial increase in asphyxia or stillbirth until after 42 weeks, a relationship exists between the incidence of abnormal antepartum testing results and advancing gestational age with positive test results increasing at and after 41 weeks (12) (Fig. 13.3). Thus we begin testing at 41 weeks. Postdate patients also have a high frequency of oligohydramnios. Oligohydramnios (AFI <5.0 cm) in a patient with a well-dated pregnancy beyond 41 weeks is virtually always an indication for delivery. The FHR during an NST or CST in patients with oligohydramnios will frequently demonstrate recurrent prolonged or variable decelerations, as the protection the fluid

offers the umbilical cord is diminished. Such patients pose an additional dilemma as cervical ripening agents often result in uterine hyperstimulation and prolonged cord compression. Often it is wise to precede the placement of the ripening agent with a negative CST result, which can indicate how well the fetus will tolerate uterine contractions. If there are decelerations associated with contractions in such patients, it is preferable not ripening at all or alternatively to choose an agent which is not likely to result in uncorrectable prolonged contractions (e.g., Foley catheter).

Currently, it appears that most clinicians use the modified biophysical profile for primary surveillance in the postdate pregnancy. As previously mentioned, we perform twice-weekly NSTs and AFIs in these patients. Because the only reason not to deliver these patients is an unfavorable cervix, which may increase the likelihood of failed induc-

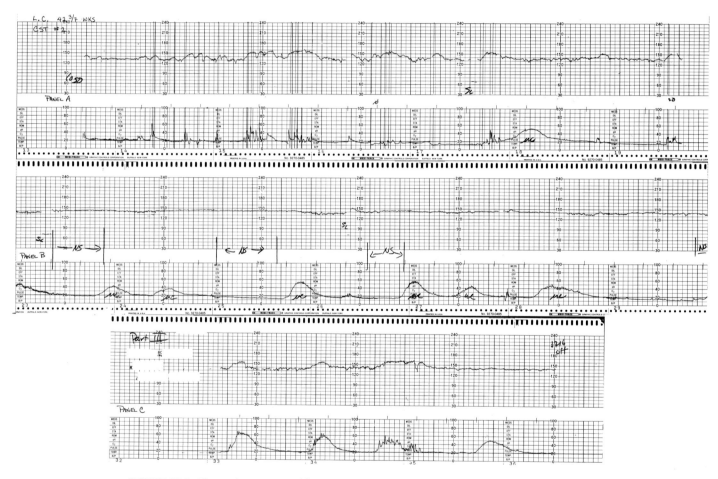

FIGURE 13.3. The patient was gravida 3 para 1 AB 1 at 42½ weeks by excellent dates and early ultrasound. A contraction stress test (CST) performed 7 days earlier had been reactive and negative. The initial portion of the CST **(panel A)** remains reactive. However, during the CST **(panel B)** there are late decelerations without reactivity. Because reactivity returned as the CST was continued **(panel C),** this test result was interpreted as reactive and positive. The patient was admitted and had artificial rupture of membranes and oxytocin augmentation. Other than passage of thick meconium requiring DeLee suctioning, labor and delivery were uneventful. Intermittent late decelerations were noted but were not persistent. The infant did well in the nursery. Some critics might call this a false-positive CST result; however, we believe that the discovery of late decelerations is potentially of critical importance in deciding whether or not to allow the pregnancy to continue.

tion and cesarean section, the threshold for delivery for abnormal tests is relatively low in this group of patients (13,14). Certainly, a positive CST result or low BPP (4 or less) is an indication for delivery (14–16). Most often however, these patients will be delivered for a low AFI and/or significant variable or prolonged decelerations. In these patients, these less ominous results may also be an indication for delivery since the only reason not to deliver the postdate patient is the risk of failed induction and cesarean section, and thus the risk benefit ratio requires less impetus to weigh in favor of delivery.

Preeclampsia

Preeclampsia is a disease for which it is particularly difficult to outline a routine for antepartum evaluation. This is because management is more often guided by maternal condition than by fetal condition. Conservative treatment of the maternal disease (i.e., bedrest) can improve fetal condition, and, conversely, deterioration of the maternal condition can result in worsening UPI. Gant et al. showed that UPI precedes the clinical manifestations of preeclampsia by 1 to 3 months (17,18). The fact that IUGR can be seen in patients many weeks before developing signs and symptoms of preeclampsia corroborates these data.

Antepartum testing in patients with preeclampsia should be conducted with the following basic rules in mind:

1. Fetal jeopardy may exist even in the patient whose blood pressure normalizes at bedrest.
2. The clinical condition may change rapidly. Should such changes occur, repeat evaluation of the fetus must be performed even when the most recent assessment was reassuring.
3. Fetal condition is but one variable in the equation of evaluation and management of these patients.
4. Occasionally, nonreassuring antepartum heart rate patterns improve when the maternal condition significantly changes for the better (e.g., control of severe hypertension).
5. Patients with severe preeclampsia require continuous monitoring of FHR even if the decision is made to delay delivery for extreme prematurity or to take the time to administer corticosteroids.

Antepartum fetal monitoring is begun when the disease is first recognized and viability is considered likely. In our institution, this is around 24 weeks of gestation (Fig. 13.4). As with other antepartum conditions, testing should occur every 3 to 4 days using the modified BPP, although amniotic fluid (AF) volume can be assessed every week if the previous value was normal (≥8 cm). If the preeclampsia is moderate to severe and the patient is not being delivered only in an effort to gain additional maturity, consideration should be given to daily NSTs because the situation is very dynamic and the patient is in the hospital. In severe cases where there is any delay in delivery, such as for stabilization or when corticosteroids are used to accelerate fetal pulmonary maturity, continuous FHR monitoring is indicated.

Chronic Hypertension

In terms of fetal jeopardy from UPI, chronic hypertension, especially when poorly controlled, is one of the most profound antepartum risk factors. Many cases of chronic hypertension are complicated with IUGR. In these cases, the risk is especially high, and fetal death may occur at any point. Consequently, we recommend initiation of antepartum surveillance beginning as early as 26 to 28 weeks in these patients, or sooner if there is suspicion of IUGR (19). As with other patients, testing can be conducted using the modified BPP with the NST done every 3 to 4 days and the AF volume assessed weekly unless there is IUGR or the previous value is less than 8 cm, where AF volume should be checked at least twice weekly. Often when beginning testing in early gestation the fetus may be nonreactive because of gestational age. It is reasonable to start with an NST regardless, because 50% of fetuses will meet criteria for reactivity by 24 to 26 weeks (20). One should also use the patient as her own baseline because those fetuses that were previously reactive will not become nonreactive because of immaturity. Patients with chronic hypertension and reassuring fetal surveillance, stable blood pressure, and no evidence of IUGR can be delivered at 38 weeks or later.

Many patients with chronic hypertension develop superimposed preeclampsia. These patients should then be treated as preeclamptics. Patients with chronic hypertension are also at risk for placental abruption; this can rarely be predicted, but vaginal bleeding or premature uterine activity requires immediate fetal evaluation with the potential of abruptio placentae in mind.

Patients with chronic hypertension may require changes or adjustments in their medications to control blood pressure during pregnancy. Commonly used antihypertensive medications are beta-blockers, which, among other things, may affect the amount of reactivity of the FHR, especially in high doses. This must be considered when attempting to interpret FHR information either antepartum or intrapartum in patients taking these medications. Another important point regarding hypertension control and FHR monitoring is that when patients with chronic hypertension develop severe deterioration of their blood pressure control, or in patients with severe preeclampsia, acute lowering of blood pressure may adversely affect uterine perfusion. Care should be taken to avoid rapid reduction to normal or below normal blood pressure because the fetus may become acutely hypoxic and will exhibit late decelerations with too vigorous antihypertensive therapy (see Figure 9.33). Continuous monitoring of FHR while treating severe hypertension is critically important to ensure adequate placental perfusion

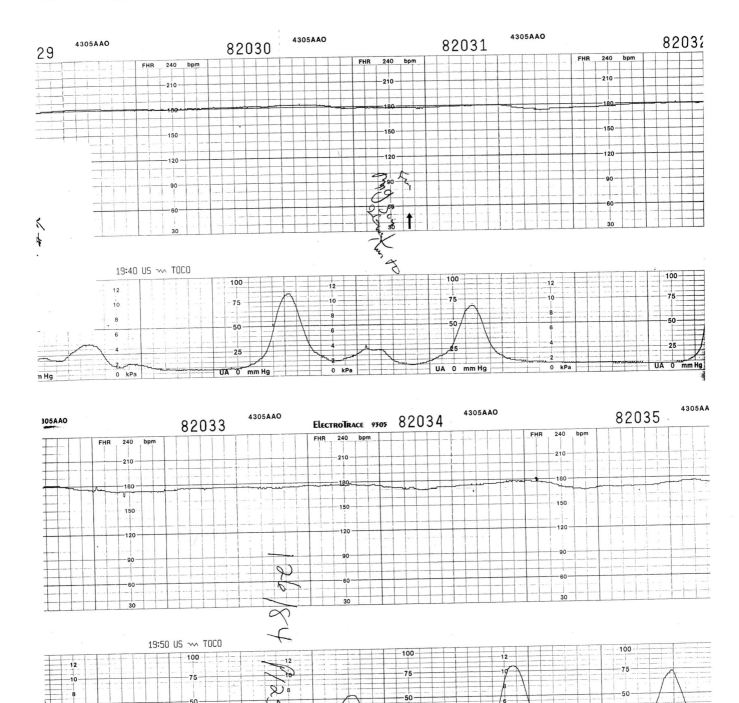

FIGURE 13.4. This is a 38-year-old gravida 4 para 3 at 29½ weeks admitted with mild blood pressure elevation, 1+ proteinuria, thrombocytopenia, and increased liver enzyme concentrations. She was seen 2 weeks previously without problems. The external fetal monitor revealed a flat baseline tachycardia and persistent late decelerations. After administration of magnesium sulfate, a primary cesarean section was done and a baby was delivered with Apgar scores of 0 at 1 minute, 3 at 5 minutes, and 5 at 10 minutes, weighing 1,330 g. Cord pH arterial was 6.90 with BE −22 and venous 7.01 with BE −17. The baby ultimately survived.

and identify possible fetal distress. Indeed, using FHR information is of great assistance in establishing an acceptable blood pressure endpoint for both fetus and mother.

Diabetes Mellitus

Pregnancy complicated by diabetes mellitus is an excellent example to demonstrate how the combination of antepartum testing and fetal pulmonary maturity studies has had a positive impact in improving perinatal outcome. In many centers, the perinatal mortality in pregnancies complicated by insulin-dependent diabetes has been reduced to that of non-diabetics when corrected for congenital abnormalities (21,22). Data suggest that uncomplicated class A diabetics have no increase in antenatal fetal mortality over the general population (23). This is true only for a class A diabetic who has a normal fasting blood sugar (without insulin therapy), is not preeclamptic, and has not had a previous stillbirth. Therefore, we do not use antepartum fetal testing in uncomplicated class A diabetics before 40 weeks' gestation. In the remainder of diabetics, there is some concern that the modified BPP may not be as effective a surveillance technique as in other pregnancy complications. This is based on both theoretical and experiential grounds. Presumably,

because of the diuretic effect of elevated glucose levels in the fetus, these patients often have elevated or high normal AF volumes. This is especially true in the more poorly controlled diabetic who is at the highest risk of stillbirth. Thus a high normal fluid volume may drop significantly but still remain in the normal range. Some centers with a high volume of diabetic patients have reported high unexpected fetal death rates with NSTs and AFV testing in diabetics (24). For this reason, in this group of patients only, we revert to using weekly CSTs and midweek NSTs for primary surveillance. For patients with diabetes complicating their pregnancies, both complicated class A (previous stillbirth, abnormal fasting blood sugar, or preeclampsia) and all insulin-dependent diabetics are managed with weekly CSTs and midweek NSTs. For the majority of these women, testing is begun at 34 weeks of gestation. For diabetic patients whose pregnancies are further complicated by hypertension, suspected IUGR, or renal disease, fetal surveillance is begun earlier (Fig. 13.5). These are started at 28 to 30 weeks (25). With continued tight diabetic control, good fetal growth, and reassuring fetal surveillance tests, we allow diabetic pregnancies to continue to 38 weeks' gestation and beyond, depending on diabetes control, patient compliance, testing, and cervical condition.

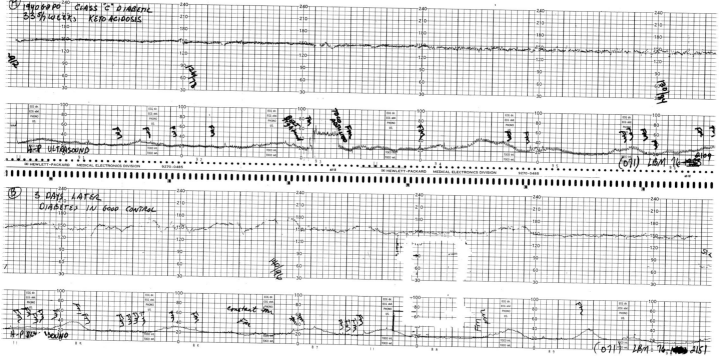

FIGURE 13.5. This case illustrates the effect of ketoacidosis on the fetus. **Panel A** is the fetal heart rate (FHR) tracing of a diabetic admitted in ketoacidosis at 33½ weeks. Note the nonreactive pattern. Three days later **(panel B)**, with the patient euglycemic and nonketotic, a normally reactive spontaneous contraction stress test result was seen. This illustrates the potential reversibility of FHR patterns when treatable conditions exist.

Third Trimester Bleeding

Patients with third trimester bleeding are a difficult problem in antepartum management, and care must be individualized. With an acute episode of bleeding, the fetal condition is a critical factor in any decision about immediate delivery. Once it has been established that bleeding is not excessive and there is no maternal coagulopathy, then fetal condition becomes the next concern. With, and subsequent to, any bleeding episode, continuous fetal monitoring is indicated. Occasionally, even with only minimal uterine activity, late decelerations can alert the physician to a significant abruption (Fig. 13.6). In premature gestations, especially those with contractions, even a small amount of bleeding is abnormal and should alert the clinician to the possibility of an underlying etiology. The characteristic picture of abruptio placentae on the fetal monitor are late decelerations and a tachysystolic uterine contraction pattern. One, both, or neither may be present and may or may not correlate with the apparent size of the abruption. With a major bleeding episode, a normal FHR tracing is an essential variable in the decision to attempt tocolysis or allow a trial of labor.

Once the acute episode is resolved and a reasonable time (usually at least 24 hours) of continuous fetal monitoring has provided reassurance, the patients can revert to intermittent antepartum testing. Our mainstay of testing for preterm gestations complicated by vaginal bleeding is the modified BPP. There is some debate as to whether patients with placenta previa have an increased risk of uteroplacental insufficiency as do those with non-previa bleeding. Markers of UPI, such as IUGR and stillbirth rates, do not appear increased in those with placenta previa. Thus, it may not be necessary to test these patients unless they have an acute bleeding episode. Because there is not universal agreement on this point, either approach (i.e., routine testing or not) appears reasonable. Generally, uterine bleeding before term contraindicates CST. Often these patients have sufficient uterine activity for a spontaneous CST. With a nonreactive NST, the BPP should be the primary backup test in these patients. Patients with significant third or late second trimester bleeding are observed until fetal pulmonary maturity is documented, usually at or beyond 36 to 37 weeks of gestation, and then delivery is effected.

Hemoglobinopathy/Severe Anemia/Cyanotic Cardiac and Pulmonary Disease

Patients with substantially decreased effective oxygen-carrying red blood cells or with other reasons for decreased oxygen delivery to the placenta (e.g., cyanotic maternal cardiac disease or pulmonary disease) can have a form of preplacental UPI. Such UPI may lead to growth restriction and/or hypoxic compromise. Patients with sickle cell disease, severe anemia (hematocrit less than 25%), or chronic

maternal hypoxemia should be observed during pregnancy, with fetal surveillance starting at 26 to 28 weeks. Sudden deterioration in maternal status, such as a sickle cell crisis or an acute asthmatic exacerbation, necessitates immediate FHR monitoring. Treatment of the maternal condition with oxygen therapy or transfusion may improve ominous FHR patterns (Fig. 13.7). If the clinical condition is stable and antepartum tests remain normal, these patients may be delivered after 36 to 38 weeks, with pulmonary maturity.

Suspected Intrauterine Growth Restriction

Even in patients without other risk factors, a lag in fundal growth or ultrasound findings may suggest IUGR. The ability to correctly diagnose IUGR depends on a high level of suspicion and accurate ultrasound measurements of different fetal parameters over time. Although the predictive value of any single parameter varies dramatically, the sensitivity of multiple ultrasound measurements in ruling out IUGR is very high. A normal ultrasound in a suspected case is very reassuring, as is the finding of normal interval growth. Umbilical artery Doppler may also be helpful in such cases (Fig. 13.8). Doppler may help both diagnostically, as IUGR from UPI will usually be associated with an index of increased resistance to flow in the umbilical artery, and as a prognostic test, as absent or reversed umbilical flow often portends the need for subsequent delivery based on a nonreassuring FHR or BPP, which often then deteriorates either immediately or in the next few days to weeks with such a Doppler finding.

The clinical management of suspected IUGR is very controversial. The primary issue centers around the timing of delivery. The issue is whether such patients should be delivered as soon as IUGR is severe and the baby has a likelihood of surviving in the nursery versus as soon as pulmonary maturity can be documented versus using antepartum testing and only delivering these babies early with nonreassuring surveillance. The basis of this issue is the unanswered question over whether the nutritional UPI with resultant IUGR alone causes the neurologic damage often seen in these babies or if intervening before hypoxic/asphyctic damage occurs is enough to avoid these injuries. If IUGR is suspected and delivery is not elected, some form of antepartum testing should be instituted. If testing is reassuring, expectant management with close follow-up of in utero growth should be continued until the decision for delivery is made.

Discordant Twins

Occurring in both monozygotic and dizygotic twin gestations, discordant growth is usually a form of growth restriction. The etiology may be typical UPI in one fetus either as

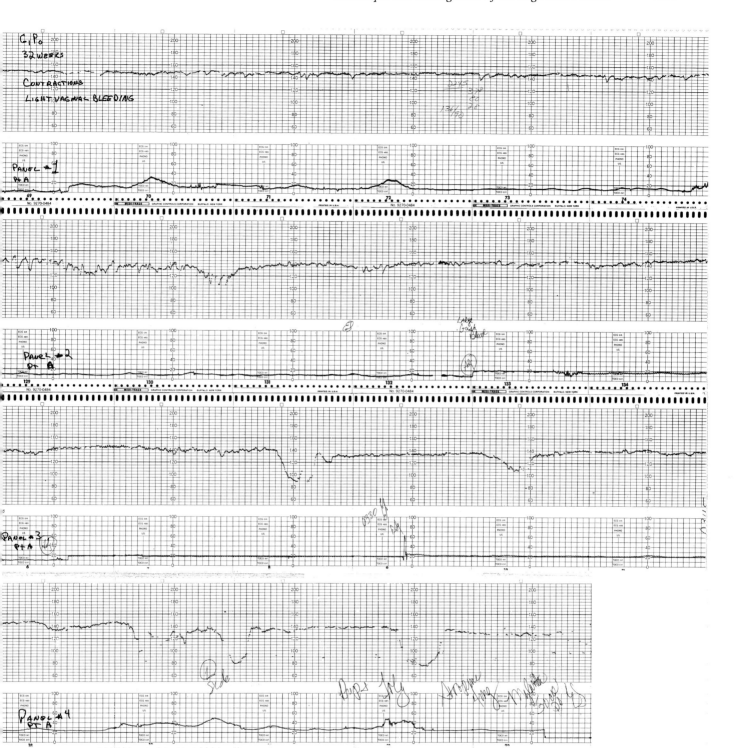

FIGURE 13.6. A gravida 1 was admitted at 32 weeks with mild uterine activity and light vaginal bleeding. The uterus was soft between contractions and nontender. Vital signs were normal. External monitoring revealed irregular uterine contractions that were difficult to record. At the **second panel**, the patient had a large gush of blood. Late decelerations are seen on the **second, third,** and **fourth panels.** Immediate cesarean section produced a 1,000-g female with Apgar scores of 1 at 1 minute and 6 at 5 minutes; the infant had moderate respiratory distress syndrome but subsequently did well. A 30% to 40% placental abruption was found. This case illustrates how fetal monitoring may be a sensitive indication of significant abruption.

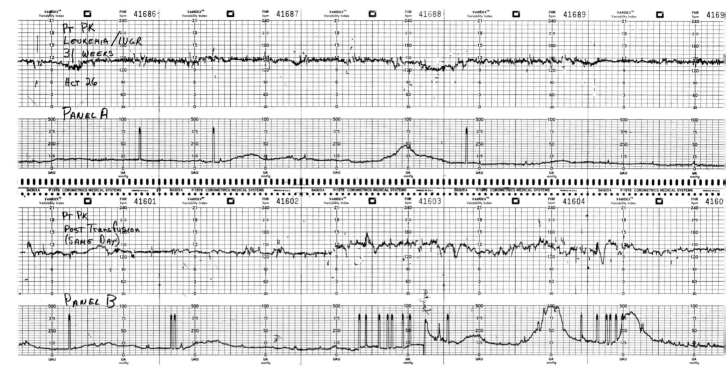

FIGURE 13.7. This 25-year-old gravida 1 para 0 presented with acute lymphocytic leukemia and suspected intrauterine growth retardation. At 16 weeks, the leukemia exacerbated and chemotherapy was reinstituted. Uterine growth was lagging from 20 weeks. The patient was anemic secondary to bone marrow suppression. The initial nonstress test (NST) performed at 31 weeks **(panel A)** was nonreactive and a contraction stress test (CST) was done with a positive result. After transfusion of 2 units of packed red blood cells, the test was repeated **(panel B)**. This is now a reactive NST result with a negative CST result. The patient did well until 37 weeks when the CST result was again positive, and she was delivered of a somewhat growth-restricted but otherwise normal female. Unfortunately the mother died 18 months later from pneumonia secondary to a recurrence of her leukemia.

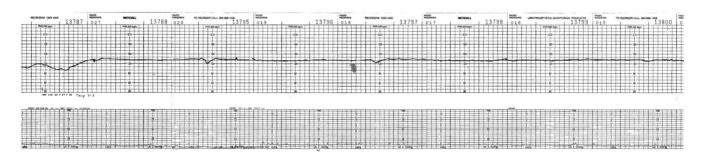

FIGURE 13.8. This patient was a 19-year-old gravida 1 para 0 at 26 weeks' gestation. She had a history of arthritis and laboratory abnormalities suggestive of possible systemic lupus erythematosis. An ultrasound done at the time of the initial consultation revealed a symmetrically growth-restricted fetus and an umbilical cord Doppler with reversal of end-diastolic flow. She was sent immediately to labor and delivery for fetal monitoring. The tracing was flat with spontaneous decelerations. The biophysical profile was 2 of 10 for fluid only. She underwent immediate cesarean section delivering a 526-g male with Apgar scores 6 at 1 minute and 6 at 5 minutes and cord gases of arterial 7.06 BE −12, venous 7.18, and BE −8. The baby ultimately survived and is developing normally at age 2.

a result of some maternal condition or from the other fetus being more successful in achieving adequate placental perfusion. Alternatively, in monozygotic twins, the discordance is often due to twin-to-twin transfusion, and there will be oligohydramnios in the smaller twin and polyhydramnios and even hydrops fetalis in the larger one. Ultrasound is the primary means of suspecting such a problem in utero. All twins should be scanned every 3 to 4 weeks after viability to rule out IUGR and discordance. When using the NST for fetal surveillance in twins, the only yield has been in patients whose twin pregnancy is complicated by discordancy. If ultrasound does not suggest a 20% to 25% or greater difference in estimated fetal weight between the twins, or IUGR in one or both, antepartum testing is not indicated. Just as with singleton pregnancies, fetal testing in multiple gestations should only be started at a gestational age when intervention might be entertained (Fig. 13.9). The finding of discordant growth in twins or triplets is not that rare, but intervention in the very premature gestation for an abnormal FHR of the small fetus can only be supported after careful assessment of the other sibling(s) in utero. At times, decisions about intervention are perhaps medically indicated but ethically a major dilemma, in that intervention will result in undue prematurity for the normally grown sibling fetus(es) without evidence of compromise.

One highly unusual condition is monoamniotic twins. These are monozygotic twins in one sac. The fetal mortality in such twins is approximately 50% and occurs primarily from cord entanglement but also can result from the other complications, such as twin-to-twin transfusion, seen in diamniotic monozygotic twins. Surveillance and timing of delivery in these patients is highly controversial as they are rare, less than 1% of all twins, and most reports of current management are based on very small series (26). Once viability is reached, these patients are usually hospitalized and monitored with daily NSTs, looking primarily for FHR findings suggestive of progressive umbilical cord entangle-

ment with resultant intermittent compression/interruption of cord blood flow. If evidence of significant variable decelerations or occasional prolonged decelerations exist, continuous fetal monitoring may be warranted. Delivery may be for either nonreassuring/worsening evidence of cord compression or when the fetus reaches 33 to 34 weeks as soon as fetal lung maturity can be ensured.

Decreased Fetal Movement

Not uncommonly, patients without other risk factors will complain of decreased or absent fetal movement. Clearly, all patients should be counseled to monitor fetal movement with some method beginning in the third trimester. Because 50% of stillbirths may come from the 85% of patients who are not at risk, fetal movement counting may be the only way to have an impact on this larger group. Although usually not a cause for true alarm, decreased fetal movement may be the only sign of impending fetal death in an otherwise normal pregnancy. In counseling patients with this concern, the first step should be to ask the patient to lie down on her side for 30 to 60 minutes and concentrate on counting movements. If she feels three or more movements in that time, she should be reassured. If the patient feels less than three movements in an hour and is beyond 26 weeks' gestation, the patient should be instructed to come in as soon as possible for an NST. An NST should not be postponed until the next day for a patient with this complaint. If the NST is reactive, no further testing is necessary if the patient has no other risk factors and the test does not need repeating. If decelerations are present and/or the tracing is nonreactive, further assessment is indicated immediately.

It is also important for high-risk patients to monitor fetal movement every day. Should a high-risk patient report decreased fetal movement, the same policy as described above is followed, regardless of when the last fetal surveillance was performed. It is of interest to note that the only type of prospective study employing some form of fetal sur-

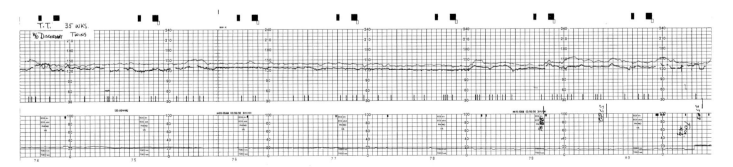

FIGURE 13.9. This patient had a twin gestation at 35 weeks with suspected discordancy. Biweekly nonstress tests were performed. Simultaneous monitoring of both fetuses is now possible using external Doppler. It is interesting to observe the degree of concordance of accelerations between the twins as well as similar changes in baseline.

veillance that has been shown to be of significant value in decreasing antepartum stillbirth is one comparing patients instructed in monitoring fetal movements daily with a group not noting daily movements (27).

Premature Rupture of Membranes

Approximately 10% to 15% of pregnancies are complicated by preterm premature rupture of the membranes (PROM), which accounts for 30% of premature deliveries (27). Although controversy exists over the optimal management for this complication in the term gestation (i.e., expectant management versus oxytocin induction, with or without allowed latency period), there is continued disagreement over the management of this complication in the preterm gestation. Most schemes of expectant management include the supplemental use of some means of fetal surveillance. Concern regarding infection, cord accidents, and abruption justifies the efforts to use frequent fetal monitoring in women with this complication. In pregnancies complicated by PROM that are being managed expectantly, we perform daily NST monitoring for 1 hour. The FHR baseline and the presence or absence of accelerations and decelerations are specifically noted. Variable decelerations, suggesting possible cord compression secondary to decreased amniotic fluid volume, are not uncommon and may indicate early labor or fetal distress (28). Furthermore, from studies using ultrasound there appears to be a relationship between the degree of oligohydramnios and the incidence of variable decelerations in patients with preterm PROM (29).

Vintzileos and coworkers (30), using a daily fetal biophysical profile in patients with PROM followed serially, found a relationship between progressively lower BPP scores and findings suggestive of infection in the fetus. However, these patients will also have a nonreactive NST. A randomized trial comparing daily NST with the daily BPP by Lewis et al. concluded that the NST was equivalent to the BPP in this situation and significantly less time-consuming and more cost-effective except in babies less than 28 weeks where nonreactivity was common due to early gestational age (31). Thus, the NST is an appropriate screen for cord compression and fetal infection. Because of these significant maternal and fetal risks in patients with preterm PROM, careful and frequent determination of fetal well-being is critically important when expectant management is elected. Our patients with PROM and a nonreactive NST result have a biophysical profile performed as their backup test.

MANAGEMENT OF PATIENTS WITH NONREASSURING TESTS

Nonreactive Nonstress Test

The NST should be viewed as a screening test when used as the primary means of antepartum testing. Nonreactive pat-

TABLE 13.2. ACOUSTIC STIMULATION TEST

Patient in left lateral recumbent position
External monitor of FHR and contractions
Establish baseline FHR for 5 to 10 min
Apply artificial larynx over fetal head and stimulate for 1 sec
Restimulate if no acceleration within 10 sec (repeat up to four times)
Continue to monitor for 15 min following acclerations

FHR, fetal heart rate.

terns may be caused by fetal hypoxia, previous CNS injury, anomalies, sleep states, or CNS-depressant drugs. In performing the NST, if there are not two or more 15 beats per minute (BPM) accelerations above the baseline FHR within the initial 20 to 30 minutes, stimulation of the fetus with uterine manipulation or sound (Table 13.2) is indicated. Another 20-minute period is then monitored, and if the fetus is still nonreactive, an alternative form of assessment (backup test) should be done immediately. In this setting we have historically used the CST if the NST is nonreactive. Alternatively a BPP may be done. If the fetus becomes reactive during the CST, it may be discontinued or completed but will be interpreted as any other reactive tracing (Fig. 13.10).

An NST that remains nonreactive and is followed by a negative CST result or an otherwise normal BPP may be repeated in 1 week. In these cases, there is an increased incidence of fetal anomalies. In addition, consideration should be given to the possible use of sedative drugs (e.g., phenobarbital, illicit depressant drugs, or antihypertensive medications such as beta-blockers) (32). A very careful review of the test for subtle late decelerations is critical, because the combination of true nonreactivity with a negative CST is unusual and should heighten one's clinical suspicion (Fig. 13.11).

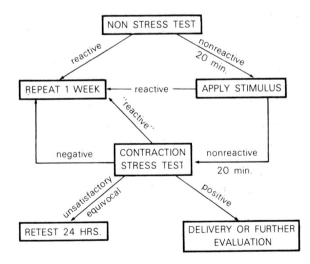

FIGURE 13.10. Outline for conducting the nonstress test. (From Evertson LR, Gauthier RJ, Schifrin BS, et al.: Antepartum fetal heart rate testing. I. Evolution of the nonstress test. *Am J Obstet Gynecol* 133:31, 1979, with permission.)

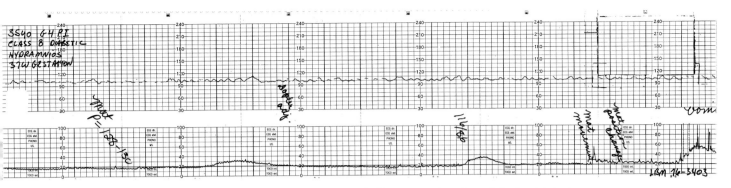

FIGURE 13.11. Nonreactive negative oxytocin challenge test done in a diabetic with hydramnios. There is a baseline bradycardia of 100 beats per minute. No late decelerations are seen, but no accelerations are seen. This unusual pattern occurred in a patient who later delivered a baby with multiple congenital anomalies including congenital heart disease, meningomyelocele, and hydrocephaly.

AMNIOTIC FLUID VOLUME

In doing the modified BPP, often the NST result will be reactive but the AFI abnormal. AFIs in the borderline range (5 to 8 cm) are not an indication for delivery, but the AFI should be repeated at least twice weekly in these patients. An AFI 5 cm or less is abnormal and requires careful consideration of fetal condition. The first important issue to realize is that the AFI may be considerably dynamic. As many as 30% to 40% of AFIs in the 3- to 5-cm range will be greater than 5 cm in 24 hours (8). Thus, except in the postdate pregnancy where virtually any abnormality warrants delivery, consideration should be given to repeating the test in 24 hours before deciding on delivery. An AFI 3 cm or less in the term patient is usually an indication for delivery. In the 33- to 36-week gestational ages, consideration of amniocentesis and delivery if maturity is found is reasonable. Before 33 weeks, testing frequency may be increased or a CST considered if such a finding occurs and delivery reserved for patients who have additional nonreassuring FHR patterns, a nonreassuring BPP, or other additional indications (Fig. 13.12).

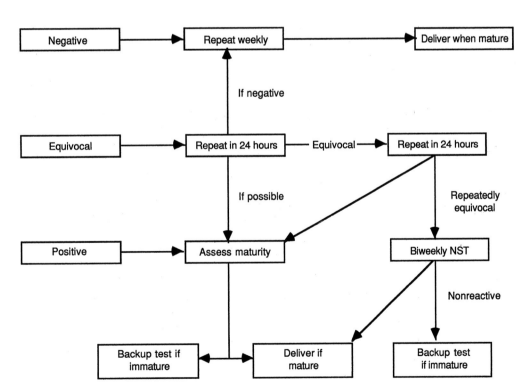

FIGURE 13.12. Contraction stress test management protocol.

Equivocal Tests

In doing an NST, or with a spontaneous CST or an OCT, any late deceleration, significant variable deceleration (deceleration dropping more than 15 BPM lasting more than 15 seconds), and/or prolonged decelerations are often seen, even when the fetus is reactive, and require further evaluation of repeat testing. When this occurs with an NST, a CST or BPP may be performed and if reassuring, the test repeated the next day. With the CST, approximately 20% to 30% of test results are equivocal. An equivocal CST only suggests that the test cannot be used to be sure that the fetus can be safely left alone for 1 week. There are basically two types of equivocal CSTs: the equivocal hyperstimulation and the equivocal suspicious. The equivocal hyperstimulation is seen in a CST that has a late deceleration associated with a prolonged contraction or contractions more frequent than every 2 minutes. The equivocal suspicious test has late decelerations with less than half of the uterine contractions that are not prolonged or of high frequency. With an equivocal test result, we require that the test be repeated the next day or acted upon sooner. Equivocal tests are rarely indications for delivery, although the repeatedly equivocal test in the postterm patient, or significantly complicated pregnancy (e.g. diabetes) may warrant delivery on a cost-effective basis alone.

Positive Contraction Stress Test Results

As previously stated, positive CST results have a high correlation with fetal and neonatal morbidity and even with

fetal mortality if not acted on. However, there is a high rate of false-positive test results. In a premature gestation this is an important consideration when making decisions about delivery. A term or preterm mature fetus with a positive CST result should be delivered (Fig. 13.12). Although fetal pulmonary maturity does not ensure that the newborn will not have other complications of prematurity, lung maturity is generally the limiting factor in normal survival of the premature neonate. Furthermore, if hypoxic UPI is allowed to persist and a depressed newborn is delivered, many complications of prematurity are more likely, including respiratory distress syndrome, even with a mature lecithin-to-sphingomyelin ratio (33). Therefore, a reactive positive CST result is generally an indication for an amniocentesis in preterm gestation (32 to 36 weeks). In a well-dated pregnancy at or beyond 37 weeks, however, delivery is indicated following a positive CST result without need for documentation of fetal pulmonary maturity (Fig. 13.13). With an immature fetus, a reactive positive CST requires further evidence of fetal jeopardy before intervention is justified. Daily testing with NST and/or BPP is appropriate in these immature fetuses with a reactive positive CST result (Fig. 13.14).

For the fetus with a persistently nonreactive positive CST result, the likelihood of a false-positive result is very low, unless the absence of reactivity is due to immaturity. Therefore, at or beyond 28 to 30 weeks, a nonreactive positive test result, where the nonreactivity continues for at least 90 minutes justifies delivery. In the more premature fetus we have successfully used BPP testing and usually

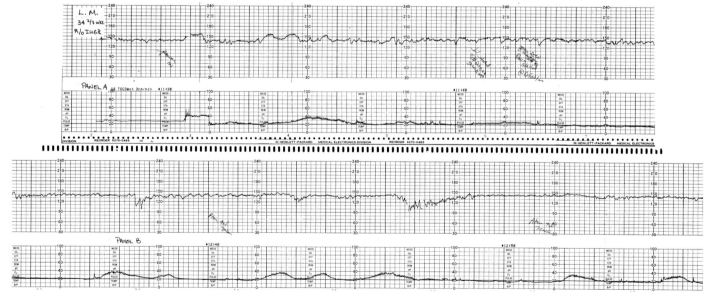

FIGURE 13.13. The history of this gravida 3 para 0 included a stillborn at 34 weeks. The etiology of the stillbirth was unknown. This pregnancy was further complicated by possible intrauterine growth retardation. During the initial portion of the contraction stress test **(panel A)**, the fetus was reactive. However, persistent late decelerations appeared with contractions **(panel B)**. Because of this positive test result, an amniocentesis was performed revealing meconium-stained amniotic fluid with a lecithin:sphingomyelin ratio of 2.6. Delivery was accomplished by cesarean section because of persistent late decelerations in labor. The infant did well following delivery.

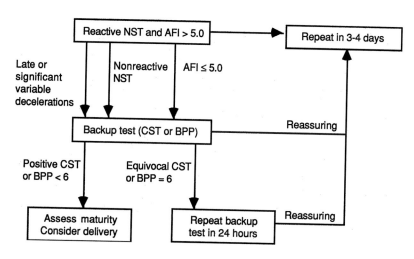

FIGURE 13.14. Modified biophysical profile: non-stress test with amniotic fluid index.

repeat these daily. Daily BPP testing in these situations has allowed us to gain time to attempt acceleration of pulmonary maturity with corticosteroids or delay delivery for several days to weeks (34).

ABNORMAL BIOPHYSICAL PROFILE

When using the BPP, either as primary surveillance or as backup to the nonreactive or equivocal CST result, the response should be, as with the CST, based on the entire clinical situation. A BPP of 8 or 10 is normal and requires repeating in 3 to 4 days with an NST, or sooner if there were decelerations or oligohydramnios. A BPP of 6 is equivocal and usually requires repeating the next day. If part of the reduction in BPP score is due to decreased AF volume, the management will be as outlined in the previous section on AF volume. A BPP of 4 may be treated similarly to the reactive positive CST, with delivery warranted for term fetuses and those with mature lung profiles, and if delivery is not undertaken, either continuous monitoring or repeat BPP in 6 hours. Finally a BPP of 0 to 2 is almost always an

indication for delivery in the viable fetus. The only exception may be the very premature gestation (e.g., ≤27 weeks), where the decision for delivery should never be undertaken unless all tests indicate an absolute need, and thus the addition of the nonreactive positive CST result and the BPP of 0 to 2 would be enough to warrant delivery at this time in gestation (35) (Table 13.3).

Choosing the Route of Delivery

Once the decision has been made to intervene on behalf of the fetus, the route of delivery must be considered. The presence or absence of reactivity is definitely a factor in a patient's ability to tolerate labor following a positive CST result (36,37). Virtually all patients with persistently nonreactive positive CST results have persistent late decelerations in labor. On the other hand, when accelerations are present, 50% of patients will tolerate labor without persistent late decelerations.

In performing the induction, the patient should be placed on her left side to maximize uterine perfusion. Oxygen should be administered by mask or nasal canula. Mem-

TABLE 13.3. BIOPHYSICAL PROFILE SCORING, MANAGEMENT PROTOCOL

Score	Interpretation Management
10	Normal infant, low risk. Repeat testing at weekly intervals for chronic asphyxia. Repeat twice weekly in diabetics and patients ≥42 weeks gestation.
8	Normal infant, low risk. Repeat testing at weekly intervals for chronic asphyxia. Repeat testing twice weekly in diabetics and patients ≥42 weeks. Oligohydramnios an indication for delivery.
6	Suspect chronic asphyxia. Repeat testing in 24 hours. Deliver if oligohydramnios present.
4	Suspect chronic asphyxia. If ≥36 weeks and favorable, then deliver. If <36 weeks and L/S=2.0, repeat test in 6 hours. If repeat score ≤4, deliver.
0–2	Strong suspicion of chronic asphyxia. Extended testing time to 120 minutes. If chronic asphyxia persistent score ≤4, deliver regardless of gestational age.

L/S, amniotic fluid lecithin: spingomyelin.
From Manning FA, Baskett TF, Morrison I, et al.: Fetal biophysical profile scoring: A prospective study in 1,184 high-risk patients. *Am J Obstet Gynecol* 140:289,1981.

branes should be artificially ruptured from the start of the induction, FHR monitored by scalp electrode, and the contractions monitored with an internal pressure transducer. Oxytocin is administered with special care to avoid uterine hyperstimulation. Should late decelerations persist despite all these measures, the patient should be delivered by cesarean section. The patient with an unfavorable cervix and/or nonvertex presentation can be delivered by cesarean section without a trial of labor. Additionally, patients with positive CST results with no accelerations present should be delivered by cesarean section without a trial of labor, as it is very unlikely that these fetuses will tolerate labor.

Finally, a note that is partly philosophy and partly good practice. Once the decision has been made to intervene, proceed without undue delay. This is not a delivery reasonably put off until the next day. While preparing for cesarean section with a delay for blood cross-match, mobilization of a surgical team, or whatever reason, the fetus should be continually monitored until the time of the abdominal preparation in the operating room. This is not a situation where a 30-minute rule for delivery after the decision is made exists. The fetus with a nonreassuring antepartum test result does not have the ongoing stress of labor. However, it is a situation that requires integration of all the variables available in making a decision regarding the urgency of delivery. For example, a patient who comes in with vaginal bleeding and a nonreactive baseline with late decelerations even with occasional contractions probably has an abruption and needs delivery urgently. Alternatively the 41-week fetus with the nonreactive test result that becomes reactive during an OCT that is positive and has an unfavorable cervix should probably be delivered by cesarean section that same day, but the urgency is much less. No cookbook statements can be made regarding how soon these patients should be delivered and judgment is key.

SUMMARY

Managing the antepartum patient is a difficult and challenging problem. Decisions regarding intervention have potentially grave consequences and should never be made on one parameter alone without knowledge of gestational age and maturity, or of maternal condition. The goal should be to deliver a healthy baby as near term as possible by the safest route for mother and fetus. Antepartum heart rate monitoring can contribute significantly toward this goal if understood well and used appropriately. Equivocal tests are rarely an indication for delivery, and unnecessary inductions may result in unnecessary cesarean sections, or worse yet, unnecessary premature delivery may have dire neonatal and long-term consequences. One other point to make is that no matter what means of surveillance is chosen, remember that negative tests are very reassuring with a very low likelihood of false negativity. However, positive test

results should be thoroughly evaluated to avoid unnecessary premature intervention. Therefore, we recommend the use of backup tests as assistance in making the decision whether to deliver, rather than relying on one test, particularly in very premature gestations (Figs. 13.11 to 13.13).

REFERENCES

1. Garite TJ, Freeman RK, Hochleutner I, et al.: Oxytocin challenge test: achieving the desired goals. *Obstet Gynecol* 15:614, 1978.
2. Nesbitt REL, Aubry RH: High risk obstetrics. II. Value of semi-objective grading system in evaluating the vulnerable group. *Am J Obstet Gynecol* 103:972, 1969.
3. Hobel CJ, Hyvarinen MA, Okada DM, et al.: Prenatal and intrapartum high risk screening. I. Prediction of the high risk neonate. *Am J Obstet Gynecol* 117:1, 1973.
4. Neldam S: Fetal movements as an indicator of fetal well-being. *Lancet* 1:1222, 1980.
5. Moore TR, Pacquadio K: A program evaluating fetal movement screening to reduce the incidence of antepartum fetal death. *Am J Obstet Gynecol* 160:1075, 1989.
6. Freeman RK: The use of the oxytocin challenge test for antepartum clinical evaluation of uteroplacental respiratory function. *Am J Obstet Gynecol* 121:481, 1975.
7. Freeman RK, Goelbelsmann U, Nochimson D, et al.: An evaluation of the significance of a positive oxytocin challenge test. *Obstet Gynecol* 47:8, 1976.
8. Lagrew DC, Pircon RA, Nageotte M, et al.: How frequently should the AFI be repeated? *Am J Obstet Gynecol* 167:1129, 1992.
9. Kirz DS, Dorchester W, Freeman RK: Advanced maternal age: the mature gravida. *Am J Obstet Gynecol* 152:7, 1985.
10. Freeman RK, Dorchester W, Anderson G, et al.: The significance of a previous stillbirth. *Am J Obstet Gynecol* 151:7, 1985.
11. Sue-A-Quan AK, Hannah ME, Cohn MM, et al.: How has clinical practice changed for post term pregnancy? *Am J Obstet Gynecol* 176:S124, 1997.
12. Porto M, Merrill PA, Lovett SM: When should antepartum fetal heart rate testing begin in post term pregnancy? Presented at the Society of Perinatal Obstetricians, San Antonio, Texas, February 1, 1986.
13. Freeman RK, Garite TJ, Modanlou H, et al.: Post date pregnancy: utilization of contraction stress testing for primary fetal surveillance. *Am J Obstet Gynecol* 140:128, 1981.
14. Eden R, Gergely R, Schifrin B: Comparison of antepartum testing schemes for the management of the postdate pregnancy. *Am J Obstet Gynecol* 144:683, 1982.
15. Phelan J, Platt L, Yeh S, et al.: The role of ultrasound assessment of amniotic fluid volume in the management of the post date pregnancy. *Am J Obstet Gynecol* 151:304, 1985.
16. Crowley P, O'Herlihy C, Boylan P: The value of ultrasound measurement of amniotic fluid in the management of prolonged pregnancies. *Br J Obstet Gynaecol* 91:444, 1984.
17. Gant NF, Daley GL, Chand S, et al.: A study of angiotensin II pressor response throughout primigravid pregnancy. *J Clin Invest* 52:2682, 1973.
18. Gant NF, Chand S, Worley RJ, et al.: A clinically useful test for predicting the development of acute hypertension in pregnancy. *Am J Obstet Gynecol* 120:1, 1974.
19. Pircon RA, Lagrew DC, Towers CV, et al.: Antepartum testing in the hypertensive patient: when to begin. *Am J Obstet Gynecol* 164:1563, 1991.

20. Druzin ML, Fox A, Kogut E, et al.: The relationship of the non-stress test to gestational age. *Am J Obstet Gynecol* 153:386, 1985.

21. Gabbe SG, Mestman JH, Freeman RK, et al.: Management and outcome of pregnancy in diabetes mellitus, classes B to R. *Am J Obstet Gynecol* 129:723, 1977.

22. Goldstein AI, Cronk DA, Garite TJ, et al.: Perinatal outcome in the diabetic pregnancy: a retrospective analysis. *J Reprod Med* 20:61, 1978.

23. Gabbe SG, Freeman RK, Mestman JH, et al.: Management and outcome of class A diabetes mellitus. *Am J Obstet Gynecol* 127:465, 1977.

24. Platt LD, Paul RH, Phelan J, et al.: Fifteen years of experience with antepartum testing. *Am J Obstet Gynecol* 156:1509, 1987.

25. Lagrew DC, Pircon RA, Towers CV, et al.: Antepartum fetal surveillance in diabetes: when to start. *Am J Obstet Gynecol* 168:1820, 1993.

26. Beasley E, Megerian G, Gerson A, et al.: Monoamniotic twins: case series and a proposal for antenatal management. *Obstet Gynecol* 93:130, 1999.

27. Kaltreider DF, Kohl F: Epidemiology of preterm delivery. *Clin Obstet Gynecol* 23:17, 1980.

28. Moberg LJ, Garite TJ, Freeman RK: Fetal heart rate patterns and fetal distress in patients with preterm premature rupture of membranes. *Obstet Gynecol* 64:60, 1984.

29. Vintzileos AM, Campbell WA, Nochimson DJ, et al.: Degree of oligohydramnios and pregnancy outcome in patients with premature rupture of membranes. *Obstet Gynecol* 66:165, 1985.

30. Vintzileos AM, Campbell WA, Nochimson DJ, et al.: The fetal biophysical profile in patients with premature rupture of the membranes - an early predictor of fetal infections. *Am J Obstet Gynecol* 152:510, 1985.

31. Lewis DF, Adair CD, Weeks JM, et al.: A randomized clinical trial of daily non-stress testing vs. biophysical profile in the management of preterm premature rupture of membranes. *Am J Obstet Gynecol* 181:1495, 1999.

32. Grundy H, Freeman RL, Lederman S, et al.: Nonreactive contraction stress test: clinical significance. *Obstet Gynecol* 64:337, 1984.

33. Cruz AC, Buhi WC, Birk SA, et al.: Respiratory distress syndrome with mature lecithin:sphingomyelin ratios: diabetes mellitus and low Apgar scores. *Am J Obstet Gynecol* 126:78, 1976.

34. Merrill PA, Porto M, Lovett SM, et al.: Evaluation of the non-reactive positive contraction stress test prior to 32 weeks gestation: the role of the biophysical profile. *Am J Perinatol* 12:229, 1995.

35. Manning F, Baskett T, Morrison I, et al.: Fetal biophysical profile scoring: a prospective study in 1,184 high risk patients. *Am J Obstet Gynecol* 140:289, 1981.

36. Braly PB, Freeman RK: The significance of fetal heart rate reactivity with a positive oxytocin challenge test. *Obstet Gynecol* S0:689, 1977.

37. Bisonette JM, Johnson K, Toomey C: The role of a trial of labor with a positive contraction stress test. *Am J Obstet Gynecol* 135:292, 1979.

FETAL HEART RATE PATTERNS ASSOCIATED WITH FETAL CENTRAL NERVOUS SYSTEM DYSFUNCTION

For some time it has been known that fetal heart rate (FHR) patterns preceding hypoxic fetal death in utero have characteristics that are not usually found in well-oxygenated fetuses or in fetuses with hypoxia that is not severe and/or prolonged (1–6). Martin et al. (7) have shown that with progressive fetal hypoxemia, late deceleration is first produced by a central nervous system (CNS) reflex that can be inhibited by autonomic blockade. When hypoxia advances to a point where significant fetal acidemia occurs, however, FHR variability disappears and one can no longer inhibit late deceleration with autonomic blockade. We therefore know that severe hypoxemia and acidosis are capable of altering CNS responsiveness, and that this is reflected in the FHR pattern. Similarly, it is well established that fetuses with severe nonhypoxic CNS abnormalities may have FHR patterns that differ from those in babies with intact central nervous systems (8–12). Because the ultimate goal is the prevention of fetal CNS damage from intrauterine hypoxia, we must examine what we have learned about FHR patterns associated with CNS dysfunction. Furthermore, recent research on maternal infection with chorioamnionitis and funisitis may result in cytokine-mediated CNS dysfunction and damage (see Chapter 3), and it is my recent experience that FHR patterns found in this condition may also reflect CNS dysfunction without preceding FHR patterns known to be associated with fetal hypoxia.

When the modulatory function of the CNS is impaired, a lack of variability is the most common effect seen in the FHR pattern (10). However, other changes are observed when CNS control is impaired. Many of these changes are also seen in very premature fetuses in which, presumably, the brain is less well developed. They can also occur when the mother has taken drugs that affect the fetal brain (13–18). Interestingly, FHR evidence of CNS dysfunction in anencephalic fetuses varies with the level of the defect, from normal to severely abnormal (8). When the fetus has a complete heart block or when there is a supraventricular fetal tachycardia caused by an ectopic pacemaker not under CNS control, there will also be a complete lack of variability (10).

As more experience is gained with FHR pattern observation in fetuses that subsequently show CNS damage as neonates, it is increasingly clear that the patterns preceding birth are often more characteristic of a lack of CNS control than of ongoing hypoxia. Certainly, these same characteristics are seen in fetuses with CNS dysfunction resulting from acute ongoing hypoxia, and fetuses with chronic oxygen deprivation may also show evidence of CNS dysfunction in the FHR prior to labor. Therefore, while we recognize that preexisting CNS insults or abnormalities may produce changes in the FHR indicating CNS dysfunction, these same changes may accompany FHR patterns indicating ongoing hypoxia (late deceleration or severe variable deceleration); it is not possible to determine the degree of CNS dysfunction that is preexisting and the degree of dysfunction that is due to an ongoing hypoxic process. It should also be pointed out that not all fetuses with CNS abnormalities will have signs of CNS dysfunction on the FHR monitor strip.

The following FHR patterns are evidence of fetal CNS dysfunction:

1. Flat FHR (4,6)
2. Blunted patterns (4,6,19,20)
3. Unstable baseline (1)
4. Overshoot (21)
5. Sinusoidal patterns (1,22)
6. "Checkmark" pattern (23).

FLAT FETAL HEART RATE

When CNS dysfunction is present, there may be virtually no fluctuation in the FHR pattern (Figs. 14.1–14.5). This change does not occur in cycles lasting 20 to 40 minutes, as are observed in cases of fetal state change. We are often restricted to external FHR recordings and, as a result, cannot

(text continues on page 225)

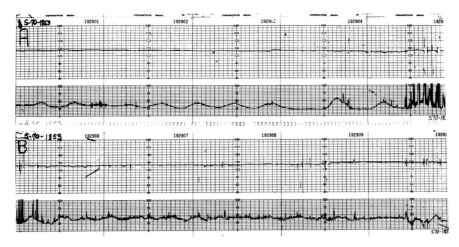

FIGURE 14.1. A flat fetal heart rate pattern with no periodic changes. It could be due to a pre-existing central nervous system (CNS) abnormality, drugs, or, occasionally, a fetus with CNS dysfunction and ongoing hypoxia.

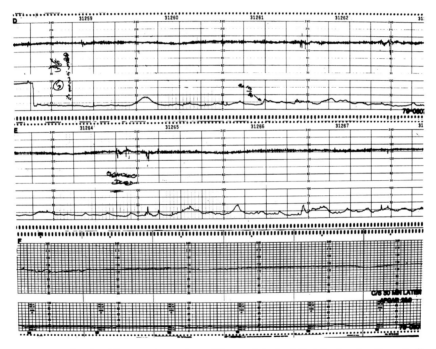

FIGURE 14.2. A flat fetal heart rate tracing with associated subtle late decelerations, indicating the probability of ongoing hypoxia. This fetus was found to have metabolic acidosis, a low Apgar score, neonatal seizures, and subsequent evidence of cerebral palsy.

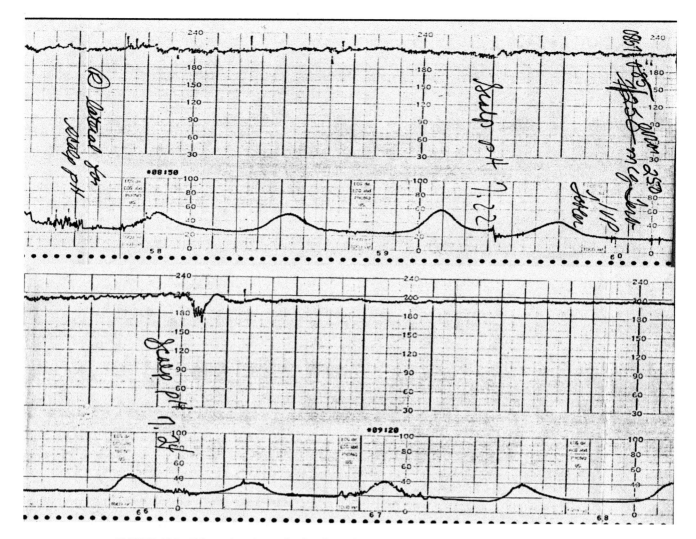

FIGURE 14.3. This tracing shows fetal tachycardia associated with maternal chorioamnionitis. Note the pH of 7.22 and the cord pH was in the same range. The neonate developed encephalopathy and now has cerebral palsy. This may be an example of the fetal inflammatory response to maternal chorioamnionitis mediated by cytokines with neonatal encephalopathy not distinguishable from hypoxic ischemic encephalopathy.

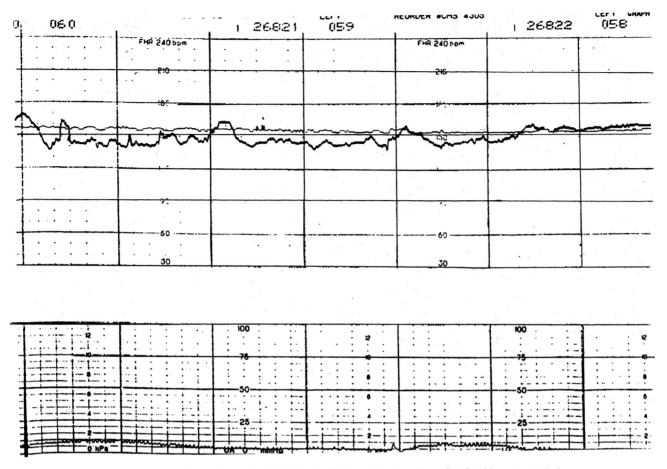

FIGURE 14.4. Twins at 32 weeks. Twin B is the light tracing showing a flat fetal heart rate. Twin A is the dark tracing showing average variability and reactivity. Twin B had a biophysical profile of 2 for fluid and delivered with low Apgar scores and decreased pH. Twin B now has cerebral palsy.

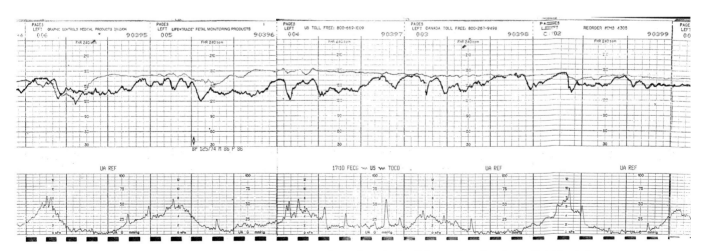

FIGURE 14.5. Twin pregnancy at 35 weeks. Twin A is the light tracing showing a flat blunted fetal heart rate pattern. Twin B is the dark tracing showing normal variability and reactivity. Twin A had a pH of 6.96 and Apgar scores of 0 at 1 minute and 2 at 5 minutes and 4 at 10 minutes. Twin B had a normal pH and Apgar scores. Twin B now has spastic diplegia and magnetic resonance imaging findings of periventricular leukomalacia.

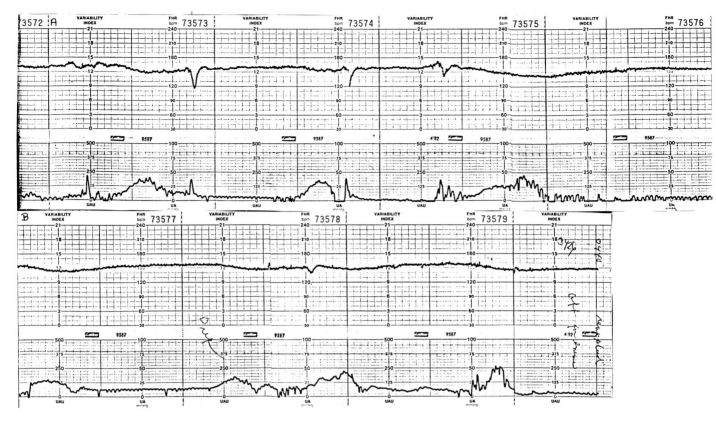

FIGURE 14.6. An example of blunted, rounded variable decelerations associated with a flat fetal heart rate. There is also an unstable baseline. This tracing was observed for several hours before delivery of a neonate with a normal neonatal pH but low Apgar scores. The neonate began convulsing soon after birth and now has cerebral palsy. This represents an example of preexisting central nervous system damage.

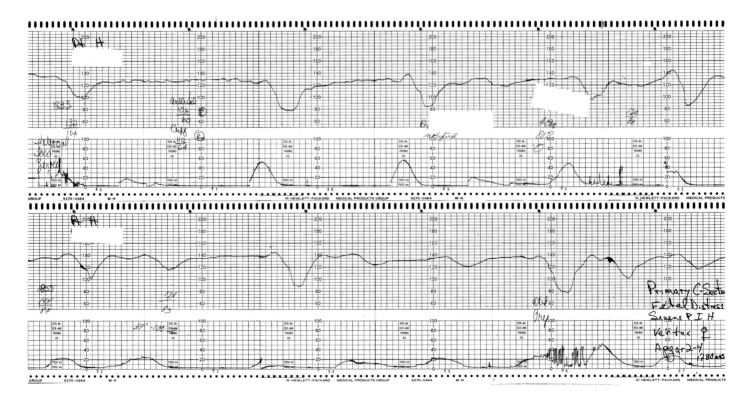

FIGURE 14.7. A flat fetal heart rate pattern and blunted variable decelerations representing central nervous system dysfunction. Note, however, the associated late decelerations indicating ongoing hypoxia. This fetus was born with fetal acidosis and began convulsing soon after birth. The child now has cerebral palsy.

be absolutely sure that short-term variability is absent; however, with the newer autocorrelation method (see Chapter 4) we can get a better idea of short-term variability. Long-term variability (3 to 5 cycles/minute) is reduced or absent, and if present takes on a very smooth shape.

BLUNTED PATTERNS

When periodic changes do occur in patients with fetal CNS dysfunction, the changes are usually smooth and take on a "blunted" characteristic (Figs. 14.6–14.8). This is especially

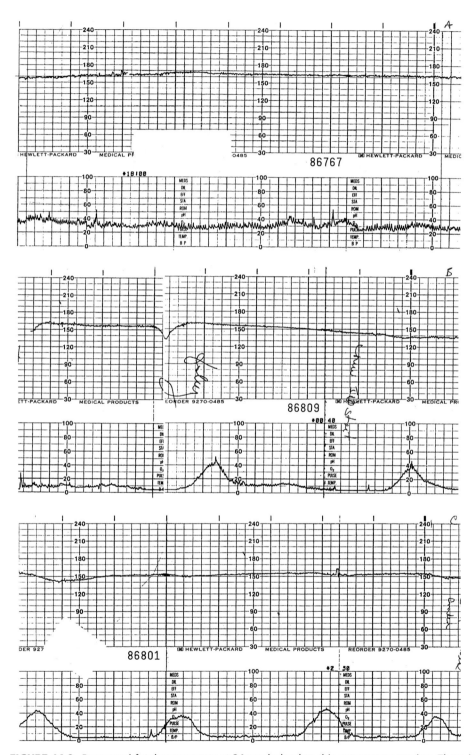

FIGURE 14.8. Decreased fetal movements at 34 weeks lead to this antepartum tracing. There is an unstable baseline associated with blunted variable decelerations. The neonate had a pH of 6.9 and a base deficit of 18. The neonate had seizures and an intraventricular hemorrhage.

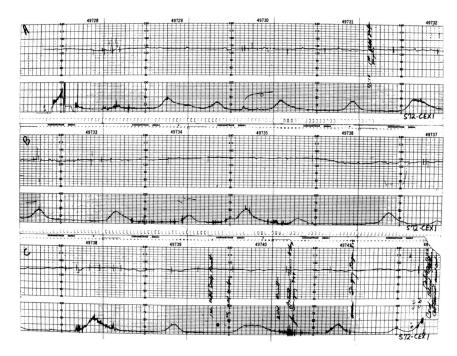

FIGURE 14.9. A flat fetal heart rate pattern with a wandering or unstable baseline. Note there are no late decelerations or other periodic changes suggesting fetal distress. The fetal scalp pH, however, was 7.01, and the neonate was born with low Apgar scores and subsequently died with evidence of central nervous sytem dysfunction.

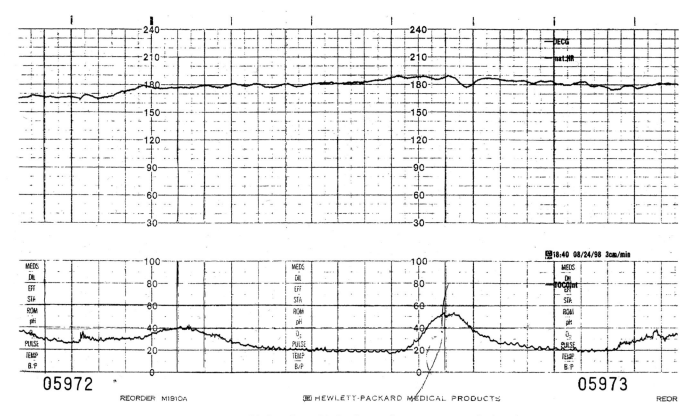

FIGURE 14.10. Unstable baseline with fetal central nervous system dysfunction.

evident with variable decelerations. There is a loss of the angular components of FHR change that are seen with intact fetuses. Blunted variable decelerations may be of low magnitude and, as a result, may not be noticed easily.

UNSTABLE BASELINE

The baseline FHR characteristically remains constant for intact fetuses, although it can change over a long period or in response to maternal fever, acute hypoxia, or certain drugs. However, with the CNS dysfunctional fetus, the baseline may appear to wander, and it may be difficult to establish exactly where the baseline is (Fig. 14.9 and 14.10).

OVERSHOOT

Rarely, in fetuses with CNS dysfunction, a prolonged smooth acceleration occurs following a variable deceleration that may take several minutes to return to baseline. The accelerations that may precede and follow reassuring variable decelerations are often referred to as shoulders and should not be confused with overshoot. The variable deceleration may not be of large magnitude. It is always associated with a smooth baseline FHR. This "overshoot" has the shape of a rapid but rounded rise followed by a very gradual return to baseline (Fig. 14.11 and 14.12).

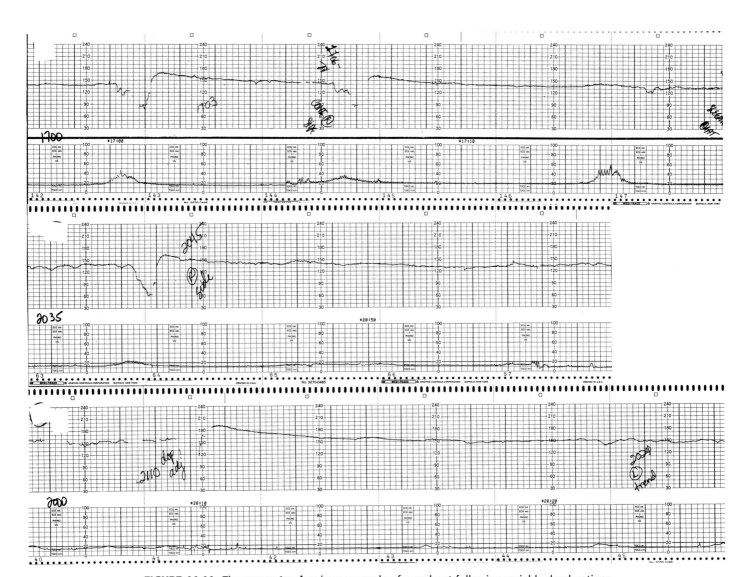

FIGURE 14.11. The **upper tracing** is an example of overshoot following variable decelerations in a fetus who delivered with a subsequent umbilical arterial pH of 7.10. Note the very slow return to baseline and the associated flat fetal heart rate (FHR). The **lower tracing** is from an anencephalic fetus. Note the flat FHR, blunted variable decelerations, and overshoot. This fetus died during labor, and it is not possible to determine whether this FHR change was all due to the central nervous system (CNS) anomaly or was partially related to hypoxic CNS dysfunction.

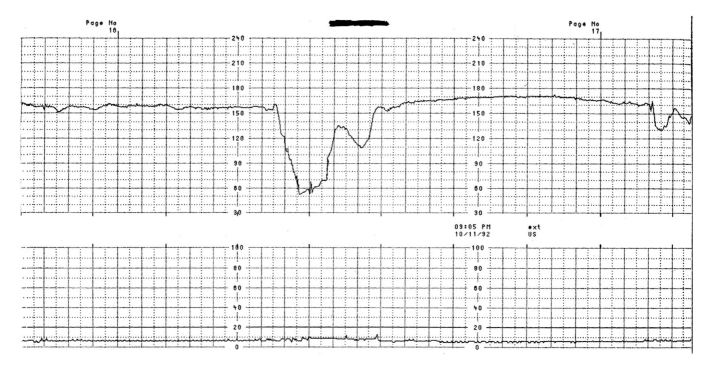

FIGURE 14.12. This tracing shows blunted variable decelerations with overshoot.

SINUSOIDAL PATTERNS

Sinusoidal patterns are described elsewhere in this book. They are very rare and are characterized by a complete lack of reactivity and by a basically smooth FHR, with the exception of the sinusoidal aspect (Fig. 14.13). There is no short-term variability, and the long-term variability is uniform, going above and below the baseline, with a smooth character and a frequency of 3 to 5 cycles/minute with an amplitude that may vary from 10 to 40 beats per minute (BPM). There are often areas of completely flat FHR, and late decelerations may also occur. This pattern has been classically associated with fetal anemia, but it can also occur with fetal hypoxia without fetal anemia (Fig. 14.14A,B.). It does not indicate irreversible damage in all cases.

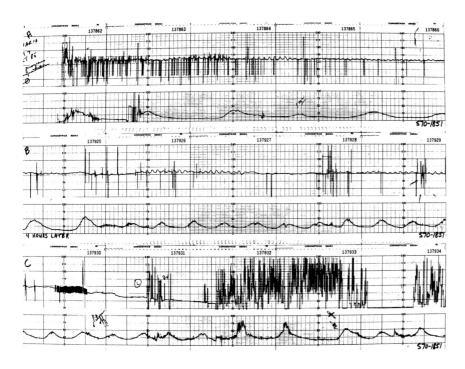

FIGURE 14.13. A flat fetal heart rate (FHR) pattern with intermittent bursts of sinusoidal heart rate. This fetus was severely hypoxic and died during labor. Note that there are no late decelerations or other periodic FHR changes suggesting fetal distress.

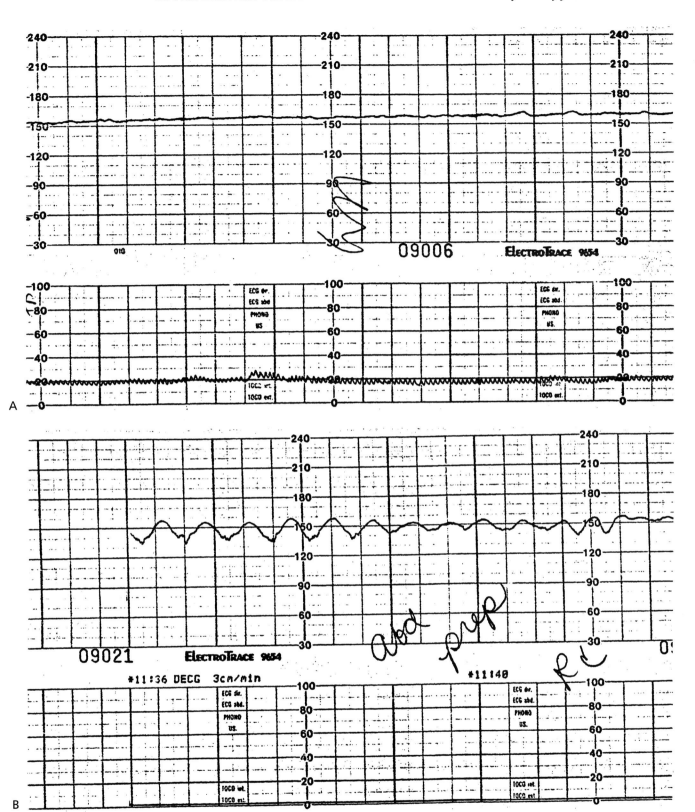

FIGURE 14.14. This tracing was from a patient with gestational diabetes mellitus at term found at the time of a routine nonstress test done at 0830 in **panel A**. The patient was sent to the hospital for a contraction stress test and when first observed at 1200 had the sinusoidal pattern seen in **panel B**. The neonate was delivered by cesarean section and had Apgar scores of 2 at 1 minute and 8 at 5 minutes. The cord arterial pH was 7.06 and the cord hemoglobin was 19.8 gm%. The neonate developed neonatal seizures with cerebral edema seen on a computed tomography scan in the first 24 hours. Now the child has spastic quadriplegia. The sinusoidal pattern appears to be associated with chronic hypoxia without fetal anemia.

"CHECKMARK" PATTERN

This is an extremely rare pattern that was first described by Cruikshank (23) in a case where the mother had had a previous cardiorespiratory arrest. The neonate began convulsing immediately after birth. We have seen this pattern with both normal pH and low fetal pH. Interestingly, there is normal short-term variability, and the checkmark pattern occurs approximately every 20 seconds (Figs. 14.15 and 14.16). The checkmark pattern may represent intrauterine fetal convulsions, because the three cases that we are familiar with all were associated with immediate neonatal convulsions.

It is possible to see some elements of one or all of these patterns in any given fetus with CNS dysfunction. With the exception of the checkmark pattern, FHR variability is characteristically absent. When one sees such a pattern, a

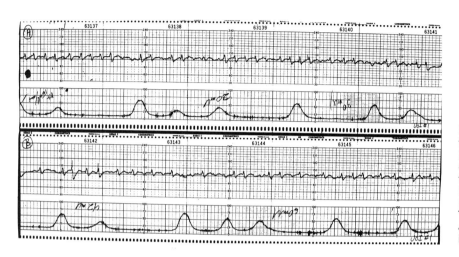

FIGURE 14.15. A pattern with characteristic "checkmark" fetal heart rate changes. Note the normal variability between the checkmark changes. This fetus was born following maternal recovery from a severe hypoxic episode and had an umbilical arterial pH of 7.25 but Apgar scores of 1 and 5. The child never breathed spontaneously and had a flat electroencephalograph until its death on the fifth day of life.

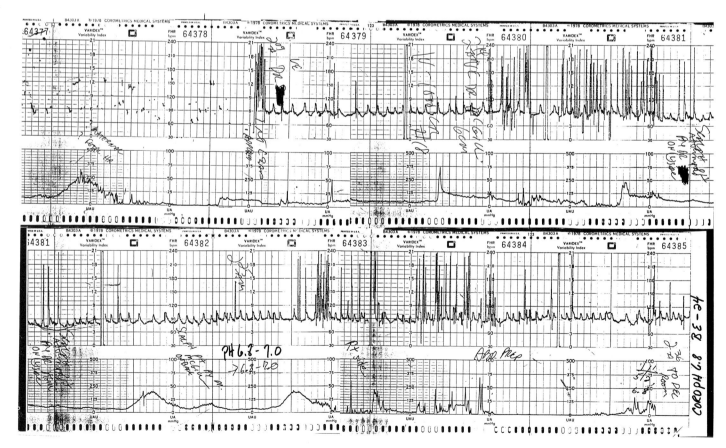

FIGURE 14.16. Checkmark pattern in a fetus with ongoing hypoxia.

fetal scalp blood pH may help to determine whether there is ongoing hypoxia or probable CNS dysfunction without ongoing hypoxia. It is never possible to tell from the FHR pattern whether the CNS dysfunction is reversible or not.

ETIOLOGIES OF FETAL CENTRAL NERVOUS SYSTEM DYSFUNCTION

The following are examples of clinical situations in which CNS abnormalities may be evident on the FHR tracing as a result of a preexisting condition with a hypoxic or nonhypoxic cause:

1. CNS malformation, for example, anencephaly, hydrocephaly (Fig. 14.17)
2. CNS destruction, for example, tumor (Fig. 14.18)
3. CNS infection, for example, rubella, cytomegalovirus, syphilis, and toxoplasmosis (TORCH)
4. Fetal inflammatory response from maternal chorioamnionitis
5. CNS anoxic insult, for example, maternal cardiac arrest (Fig. 14.19)
6. CNS physical trauma, for example, cerebral contusion
7. Toxic fetal encephalopathy, for example, mercury poisoning
8. Fetal cerebral irradiation, with resulting microcephaly
9. Intrauterine fetal CNS hemorrhage
10. Developmental abnormalities, for example, chromosomal (Fig. 14.20)
11. Drugs (Fig. 14.21).

Fetuses with chronic hypoxia preceding labor (nonreactive positive contraction stress test) will usually have reasonably normal umbilical cord blood gas and pH values if they are delivered without the acute stress of labor. When the chronically hypoxic fetus does show metabolic acidosis at birth without having gone through labor, it is probably very near death. When a chronically hypoxic fetus is subjected to labor, it will usually develop metabolic acidosis very rapidly, indicating that the reserve is limited. We believe these observations are explained by the placenta's ability to maintain fetal acid-base balance even when the fetus is utilizing anaerobic metabolism; when labor is superimposed, uterine contractions further interfere with uteroplacental exchange. When a fetus demonstrates evidence of CNS dysfunction on the FHR tracing, possible explanations include the following:

1. A preexisting abnormality of CNS function with no hypoxia at any time
2. A previous hypoxic injury with resolution and no current hypoxia
3. Ongoing chronic hypoxia, but normal acid-base balance because of placental exchange
4. Chronic hypoxia with superimposed acute hypoxia from labor and, therefore, fetal metabolic acidosis
5. No chronic hypoxia and only acute intrapartum fetal hypoxia with metabolic acidosis.

How we attempt to differentiate these situations is important both for patient management and from a medicolegal causation standpoint (Table 14.1).

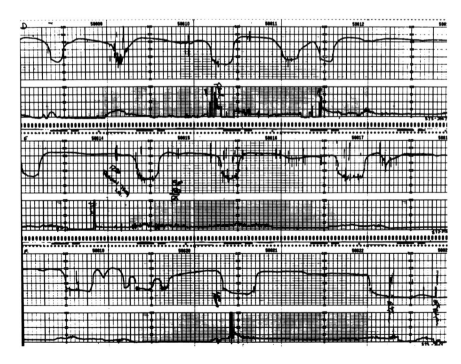

FIGURE 14.17. A tracing from an internal fetal scalp electrode on an anencephalic fetus. Note the blunted character of the variable decelerations and the flat fetal heart rate baseline.

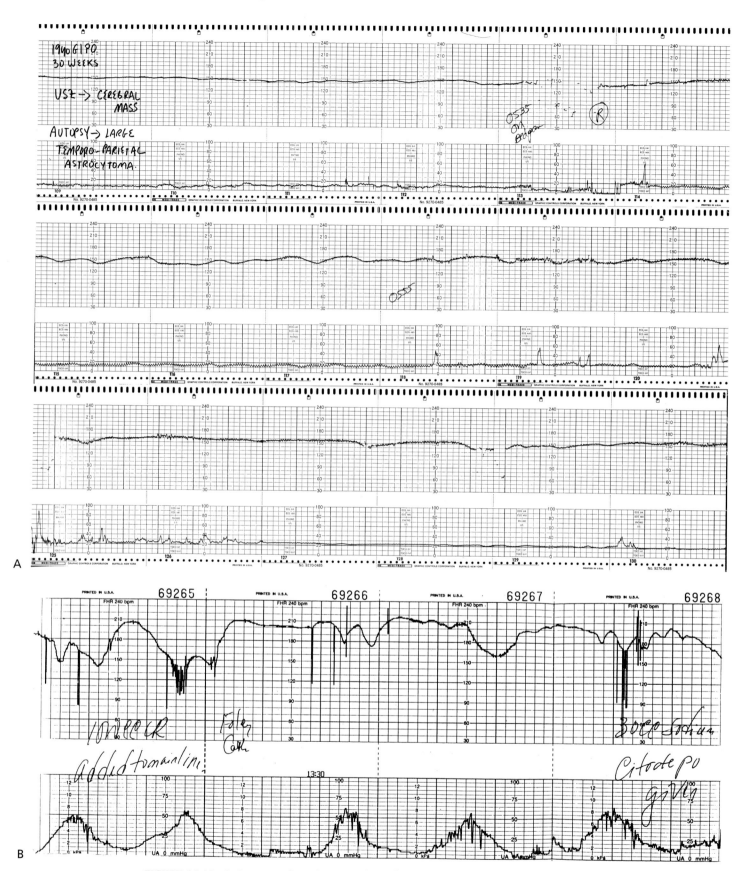

FIGURE 14.18. A: An external monitor recording of a fetus with an intracranial lesion detected on ultrasound that was diagnosed as a parietal astrocytoma in the neonate. Note the flat, blunted character of the pattern. **B:** An internal tracing taken during labor. The outcome was a cesarean section for fetal distress. The fetus had a brain tumor.

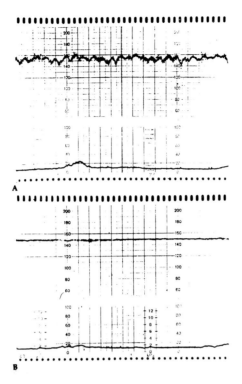

FIGURE 14.19. The **upper tracing** is an example of a 2 cm/minute (20 beats per minute per centimeter vertical scale) external Doppler tracing taken prior to a maternal cardiorespiratory arrest. Note the normal variability. The **lower panel** represents a tracing from the same fetus following resuscitation of the mother with no ongoing hypoxia. Note the flat fetal heart rate that represents central nervous system (CNS) damage from the prior CNS hypoxic insult. (From van der Moer PE, Gerretsen G, Visser GH: Fixed fetal heart rate pattern after intrauterine accidental decerebration. *Obstet Gynecol* 65:125, 1985, with permission.)

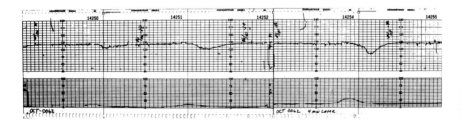

FIGURE 14.20. A tracing from a fetus with trisomy 18.

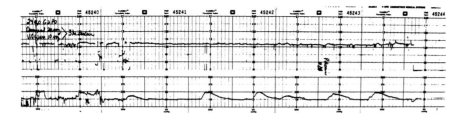

FIGURE 14.21. An external Doppler tracing from a fetus whose mother received meperidine (Demerol) and diazepam (Valium). Note the flat fetal heart rate pattern without any decelerations, representing central nervous depression due to drugs.

If, in a laboring patient, there are no patterns of persistent late deceleration, severe variable deceleration, or prolonged decelerations accompanying signs of CNS dysfunction, it is unlikely that there is no ongoing acute hypoxia. When possible, a normal fetal scalp blood pH value or normal fetal oximetry value can confirm this, and intervention would not be indicated. If, however, there are persistent late decelerations, severe variable decelerations, or prolonged decelerations accompanying signs of CNS dysfunction, ongoing fetal hypoxia can be presumed, and intervention is indicated even without fetal scalp blood pH determination.

Medicolegally, in cases with evidence of CNS dysfunction on the FHR pattern, it would be desirable to be able to assess when CNS dysfunction became irreversible. Unfortunately, the current state of knowledge does not allow us to make this determination. We can only say that the FHR pattern is consistent or not consistent with CNS dysfunction. The observations described in this chapter have usually been made from retrospective analysis of FHR patterns from babies with CNS damage. For this reason, we are unable to determine how often fetuses with evidence of CNS dysfunction on their FHR patterns develop normally, but it certainly does happen. Therefore, we know that these patterns do not always mean that damage has occurred, and an element of reversibility is clearly possible at least in some cases. In addition, we now know that neonates and children demonstrate improvement with time in many instances of initial developmental handicap.

REFERENCES

1. Cetrulo CL, Schifrin B: Fetal heart rate patterns preceding death in utero. *Obstet Gynecol* 48:521, 1976.
2. Emmen L, Huisjes HJ, Aarnoudse JG, et al.: Antepartum diagnosis of the "terminal" fetal state by cardiotocography. *Br J Obstet Gynaecol* 82:353, 1975.
3. Freeman RK, James J: Clinical experience with the oxytocin challenge test. II. An ominous atypical pattern. *Am J Obstet Gynecol* 46:255, 1975.
4. Gaziano EP, Freeman DW: Analysis of heart rate patterns preceding fetal death. *Obstet Gynecol* 50:578, 1977.
5. Hon E, Lee S: Electronic evaluation of the fetal heart rate. VIII. Patterns preceding fetal death in utero. *Am J Obstet Gynecol* 87:814, 1963.
6. Serafini PC, Amisial PA, Murgalo JA, et al.: Unusual fetal heart rate pattern associated with severe neonatal asphyxia and death. *Am J Obstet Gynecol* 140:715, 1981.
7. Martin CB Jr, de Haan J, van der Wildt B, et al.: Mechanisms of late deceleration in the fetal heart rate. A study with autonomic blocking agents in fetal lambs. *Eur J Obstet Gynecol Reprod Biol* 9:361, 1979.
8. Terao T, Kawashima Y, Noto H, et al.: Neurological control of fetal heart rate in 20 cases of anencephalic fetuses. *Am J Obstet Gynecol* 149:201, 1984.
9. Garite TJ, Linzey EM, Freeman RK, et al. W: Fetal heart rate patterns and fetal distress with congenital anomalies. *Obstet Gynecol* 53:716, 1979.
10. Navot D, Mor-Yosef S, Granat M, et al.: Antepartum fetal heart rate pattern associated with major congenital malformations. *Obstet Gynecol* 63:414, 1984.
11. Karp LE, Meis PJ: Trisomy-18 and antepartal fetal distress. *J Reprod Med* 19:345, 1977.
12. Powell Phillips WD, Towell ME: Abnormal fetal heart rate associated with congenital abnormalities. *Br J Obstet Gynaecol* 87:270, 1980.
13. Baxi LV, Gindoff PR, Pregenzer GJ, et al.: Fetal heart rate changes following maternal administration of a nasal decongestant. *Am J Obstet Gynecol* 153:799, 1985.
14. Keegan KA, Paul RH, Broussard PM, et al.: Antepartum fetal heart rate testing. III. The effect of phenobarbital on the nonstress test. *Am J Obstet Gynecol* 138:579, 1979.
15. Rayburn WF, Motley ME, Zuspan FP: Conditions affecting nonstress test results. *Obstet Gynecol* 59:490, 1982.
16. Ayromlooi J, Tobias M, Berg P: The effects of scopolamine and

TABLE 14.1. RELATIONSHIP BETWEEN FETAL HEART RATE CHANGES, HYPOXIA, AND CENTRAL NERVOUS SYSTEM DYSFUNCTION*

	Group 1	Group 2	Group 3
Late deceleration	Yes	No	Yes
Variable deceleration	Yes	Yes	Yes
Decreased variability	No	Yes	Yes
Blunted patterns	No	Yes	Yes
Acidosis	No	No	Yes
Scalp acceleration	Yes	No	No
Unstable baseline	No	Yes	Yes
Sinusoidal patterns	No	Yes	Yes

*Group 1, hypoxia without CNS dysfunction; Group 2, CNS dysfunction without current hypoxia; Group 3, CNS dysfunction with ongoing hypoxia.
CNS, central nervous system.

ancillary analgesics upon the fetal heart recording. *J Reprod Med* 25:323, 1980.

17. Petrie R: How intrapartum drugs affect the FHR. *Contemp Obstet Gynecol* 16:61, 1980.

18. Westgren M, Holmquist P, Svenningsen NW, et al.: Intrapartum fetal monitoring in preterm deliveries: prospective study. *Obstet Gynecol* 60:99, 1982.

19. Baskett TF, Sandy EA: The oxytocin challenge test: an ominous pattern associated with severe fetal growth retardation. *Obstet Gynecol* 54:365, 1979.

20. Krebs HB, Petres RE, Dunn LJ: Intrapartum fetal heart rate monitoring. VIII. Atypical variable decelerations. *Am J Obstet Gynecol* 145:297, 1983.

21. Goodlin RC, Lowe EW: A functional umbilical cord occlusion heart rate pattern: the significance of overshoot. *Obstet Gynecol* 43:22, 1974.

22. Baskett TF, Ko KS: Sinusoidal fetal heart rate pattern: a sign of fetal hypoxia. *Obstet Gynecol* 44:379, 1974.

23. Cruikshank DP: An unusual fetal heart rate pattern. *Am J Obstet Gynecol* 130:101, 1978.

PITFALLS IN ANTEPARTUM AND INTRAPARTUM FETAL MONITORING

Electronic fetal heart rate (FHR) monitoring is a modality that is difficult to learn, difficult to interpret, and probably results in many inappropriate operative interventions. It has become a major factor in obstetric malpractice litigation, in which its inexact nature confuses attorneys and lay juries. Generally, FHR monitoring is at its best in detecting early signs of fetal hypoxia; however, many of the indicators used to identify early hypoxia are nonspecific and easily subject to overinterpretation. At the other end of the spectrum, subtle patterns such as shallow late decelerations are frequently unrecognized or unappreciated. Unusual preterminal or ominous patterns may create difficulty both in interpretation and in deciding on appropriate management. This chapter uses case examples to focus on limitations and common pitfalls. Solutions to many of these FHR monitoring problems are also proposed.

It is not our intent in this chapter to lecture on careful and meticulous clinical management. Examples of all the pitfalls described herein have occurred, sometimes repeatedly. It is our hope that these case examples may prove useful in the learning process and in avoiding such errors.

INTRAPARTUM PROBLEMS

Unrecognized Oxytocin Hyperstimulation

The occurrence of decelerations that result from excessive uterine activity, often caused by oxytocin, is far too common. Shenker (1) suggests that the most frequent cause of late decelerations is oxytocin. Prolonged decelerations and aggravation of existing late or variable deceleration patterns can also occur with excessive oxytocin stimulation. Although it is highly improbable that relatively short periods of hypoxia in a fetus with good reserve will result in any damage, hyperstimulated decelerations create many problems (Fig. 15.1). Frequently, the oxytocin must be discontinued, thwarting efforts to stimulate contractions in the face of a poorly progressing labor curve, or such therapy

as oxygen and repositioning may be instituted, possibly alarming the patient, or unnecessary operative intervention may be initiated. Such decelerations may also create unnecessarily easy foci for plaintiffs' attorneys to concentrate upon when looking for sources of substandard practice, which may or may not be related to any adverse neurological outcome. A review of large awards and settlements from obstetric malpractice cases suggested that problems involving oxytocin were among the most common sources of alleged negligence (2).

There are three main areas on which to concentrate to avoid oxytocin-induced hyperstimulation: adequate contraction monitoring, adequate nursing attention, and lowered dosage. Certain nonreassuring FHR patterns should dictate oxytocin discontinuation.

Inadequate contraction monitoring may allow unrecognized hyperstimulation to occur for prolonged periods (Fig. 15.2) and may postpone recognition of excessive uterine activity, thus delaying the appropriate response to decrease or discontinue oxytocin. One solution is to be meticulous in detecting contractions with patients on oxytocin. If careful external contraction monitoring fails, use internal pressure catheter monitoring whenever feasible. The second and related solution involves adequate nursing attention. Before electronic monitoring, we may have been more careful in our clinical attention to the patient on oxytocin, but the FHR monitor has freed us to other tasks, and we may watch the patient intermittently or on central monitors. If an audit reveals oxytocin hyperstimulation to be a common problem, instituting a policy requiring more direct nursing contact may be of benefit. Finally, work by Seitchik and Castillo (3) has suggested that the most commonly used dosage regimens for oxytocin augmentation may be excessive. They found that frequent decelerations caused by oxytocin-induced hyperstimulation and subsequent discontinuation of the medication were associated with the increase of oxytocin more frequently than every 45 minutes, increments of greater than 0.5 to 1.0 mU/minute, and total doses in excess of

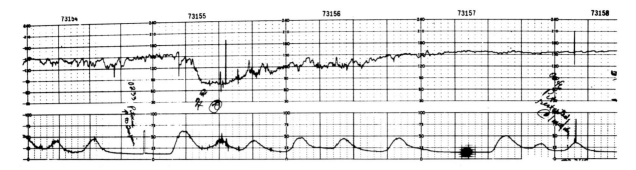

FIGURE 15.1. Contractions have become too frequent in this patient with oxytocin augmentation, allowing insufficient time for adequate intervillous blood flow between contractions. Consequently, a prolonged deceleration ensues and oxytocin must be discontinued, delaying effective efforts at stimulating progressive labor.

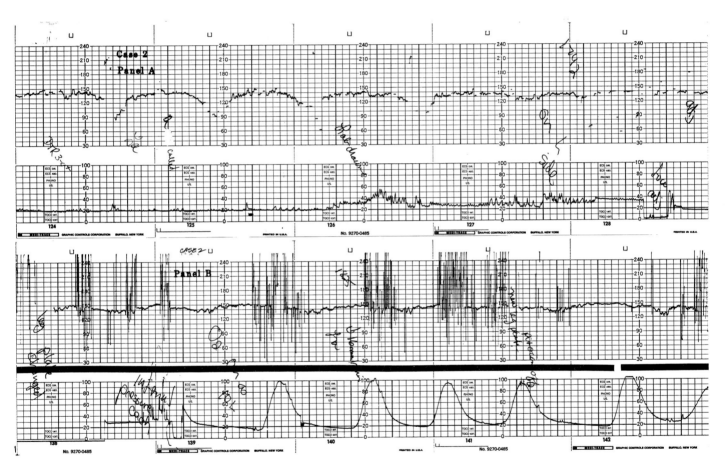

FIGURE 15.2. External monitoring is being used in this patient in the active phase of labor. The fetal heart rate demonstrates frequent symmetric decelerations that cannot be timed because there is inadequate tocodynamometer contraction monitoring. After insertion of internal electrode and pressure catheters **(panel B)**, it is apparent that late decelerations are occurring with frequent contractions of 100 mm intensity and only 1 minute or less recovery time between them. The decelerations are now clearly seen to be late, and the oxytocin must be discontinued.

6.0 to 8.0 mU/minute. The paradoxical end result of higher doses and more frequent increases is slower progress. At the same time, many physicians do not agree with the low-dose regimen and feel that a more rapid increase in oxytocin gives better progress, and thus the controversy continues.

Problems with Auscultation

There have been no substantive data to suggest that electronic FHR monitoring is superior to intensive auscultation for the evaluation of intrapartum fetal well-being in the low-risk patient. However, most studies that have evaluated this question have used as their control auscultation done by a nurse who never leaves the bedside. It is clear that for auscultation to be successful it must be done frequently and well. The American College of Obstetricians and Gynecologists (ACOG) and the American Academy of Pediatrics (AAP), in Guidelines for Perinatal Care (4), suggest that in the active phase of labor, the fetal heart should be auscultated and results recorded every 15 minutes, immediately following a uterine contraction, and in the second stage of labor at 5-minute intervals. Busy labor and delivery units have difficulty predicting staffing needs. Failure to meet requirements for performing and recording auscultative FHR is a common problem.

To identify the occasional low-risk patient with late decelerations not detectable by auscultation, a reasonable option is to run an initial 20- to 30-minute electronic fetal monitoring strip at the time of admission, and if this is reactive and otherwise reassuring, use auscultation for the remainder of the labor.

Electronically Monitoring of High-Risk Patients

Not only is the likelihood of fetal hypoxia greater among high-risk patients, but these patients are also more likely to have late decelerations, especially shallow or subtle ones, which are missed by auscultation (5). For these reasons it is the usual practice, and was formerly recommended by AGOG and AAP, that all patients at high risk for intrapartum asphyxia should have continuous electronic FHR monitoring throughout labor. Because randomized studies have not clearly demonstrated the benefit of electronic fetal monitoring, even in high-risk patients, more recent guidelines have softened the requirement for such monitoring in this group (4). The limitations of auscultation, however, especially in fetuses with shallow late deceleration, should be appreciated, and a judgment of whether to use auscultation made accordingly (Fig. 15.3). Table 15.1 lists a number of high-risk conditions for which continuous electronic FHR monitoring should be strongly considered.

Need for Electronic Monitoring at Labor Check

When evaluating a patient presenting with contractions or other complaints, such as bleeding or suspected premature rupture of the membranes, for possible admission to the labor and delivery unit, it is important to include at least an initial 20- to 30-minute period of continuous electronic FHR monitoring (Fig. 15.4). If the strip is reactive and without significant decelerations, one can be reassured. If the clinical situation does not dictate admission, one can then safely allow the patient to leave. This is particularly important in the patient with any of the high-risk factors listed in Table 15.1.

Discontinuing the Monitor Too Soon

It is important to monitor the fetus until as close to the time of delivery as possible. Frequently, when the patient has to be moved for delivery and there is no monitor in the delivery room, the one from the labor room has to be moved with the patient. Owing to this inconvenience, or because expected imminent delivery does not occur, there may be a prolonged interval without FHR monitoring. Previously reassuring FHR patterns may deteriorate rapidly, especially in the second stage of labor (Fig. 15.5).

For many reasons, it may be valuable to monitor the fetus in the delivery room in the last minutes before delivery. For anticipated vaginal deliveries, a forceps or vacuum delivery may be indicated in the presence of a rapidly deteriorating fetus. If variable decelerations become nonreassuring, the patient can be instructed to push with every other contraction, given oxygen, and repositioned, or other measures can be taken to improve fetal condition (Fig. 15.6). If a conduction anesthetic results in a prolonged deceleration or late decelerations, the patient can be repositioned and given intravenous fluids, and even vasoconstrictors if necessary, and the fetus then allowed to recover (placental resuscitation) before delivery is accomplished (Fig. 15.7). This is true whether anticipating a vaginal or cesarean delivery. The recognition of previously unanticipated fetal hypoxia can facilitate notifying the pediatrician and/or other members of the neonatal resuscitation team. Therefore, a policy that includes electronic or intensive auscultative monitoring of all patients until the time of delivery can allow optimal management. This policy should include anticipated cesarean sections as well as vaginal deliveries.

Commonly Misinterpreted Patterns

Learning FHR monitoring is a process of pattern recognition. Once an individual masters the basics, the vast majority of patterns will be readily recognized. Nonetheless,

(text continues on page 244)

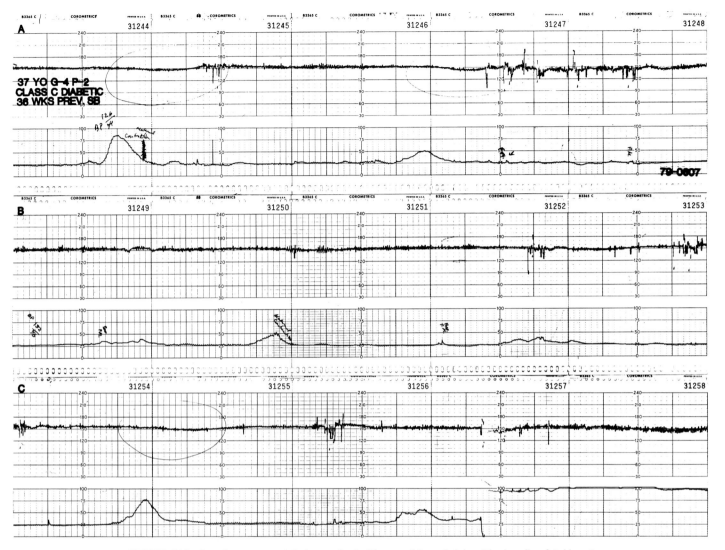

FIGURE 15.3. A patient at term is being evaluated for possible early labor. The baseline fetal heart rate is quite flat, and there are persistent late decelerations. It is unlikely that either the late decelerations or poor variability could be appreciated with auscultation in this high-risk patient.

TABLE 15.1. CONDITIONS THAT IDENTIFY FETUSES AT HIGH RISK FOR ANTEPARTUM AND/OR INTRAPARTUM PERINATAL ASPHYXIA*

Postdate pregnancy	Third trimester bleeding
Chronic hypertension	Maternal anemia
Preeclampsia/pregnancy-induced hypertension	Previous cesarean section
Diabetes	Rh isoimmunization
Intrauterine growth retardation	Multiple gestation
Lupus/collagen vascular disease	Malpresentation
Chronic renal disease	Polyhydramnios
Cyanotic cardiac disease	Meconium-stained amniotic fluid
Premature labor	Abnormal fetal heart rate on auscultation
Preterm premature rupture of membranes	Oligohydramnios

*List is not all-inclusive.

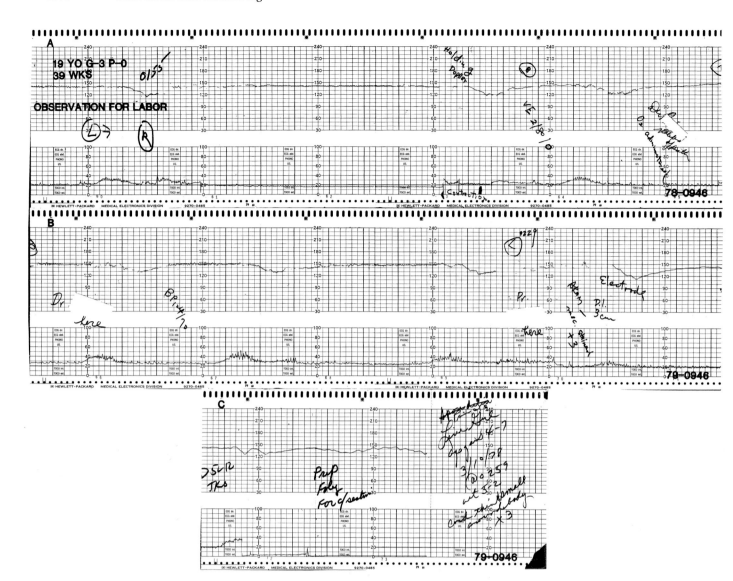

FIGURE 15.4. The patient being evaluated for labor is a low-risk nulliparous woman at term. Her contractions are irregular and her cervix is 80% effaced and dilated only to 2 cm. If these late decelerations were not appreciated, and the patient discharged to return when labor was more active, the fetus may well have been in worse condition or may even have died. An initial fetal monitoring period is important in the evaluation of the patient in early labor.

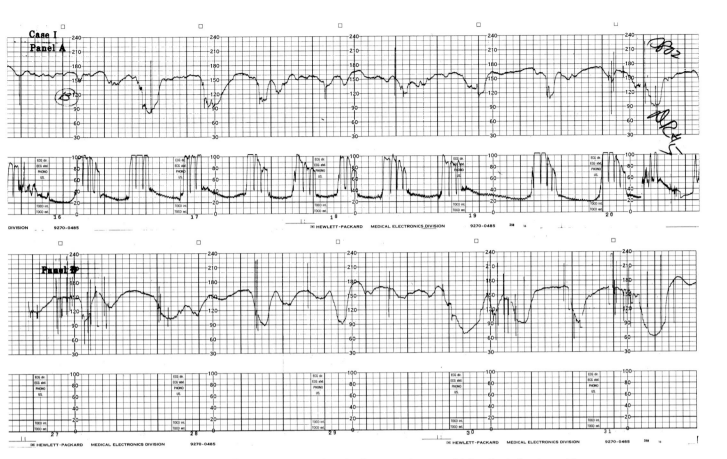

FIGURE 15.5. This nulliparous term patient in the second stage of labor is obviously pushing with her frequent contractions. **Panel A** displays mild-to-moderate variable decelerations accompanied by an upper normal baseline rate and minimum tachycardia. At this point it would be expected that the patient could continue to push and deliver spontaneously. She is brought to the delivery room and the monitor reconnected **(panel B)**. The fetal heart rate (FHR) has now progressed to a clearly nonreassuring one with loss of variability and blunted decelerations, with some of the decelerations demonstrating "overshoot." Intervention to expedite delivery is clearly indicated. If monitoring had not been reinstituted when this patient was taken to the delivery room, the change in the FHR pattern would not have been appreciated, nor would the necessity for expediting delivery.

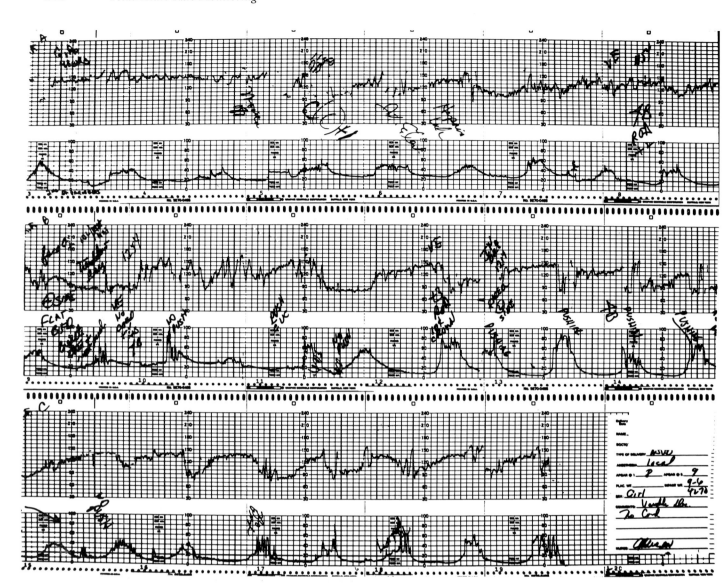

FIGURE 15.6. A primigravida at 41 weeks is in the second stage of an otherwise uneventful labor. In the **middle panel** the variable decelerations are becoming more prolonged. Multiple repositioning attempts and instructions for the patient not to push after the more prolonged decelerations seem to be giving the fetus adequate recovery. When spontaneous delivery occurs, a vigorous newborn arrives. This example again emphasizes the importance of bringing the fetal monitor to the delivery room.

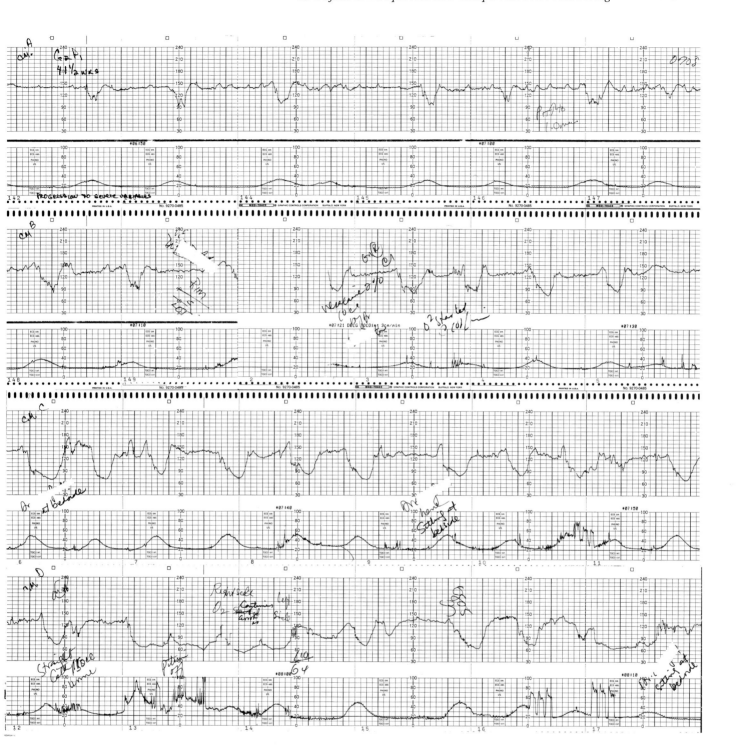

FIGURE 15.7. At nearly complete dilation, this patient on oxytocin was injected with an epidural anesthetic **(middle of panel B)**. Approximately 25 minutes later a prolonged deceleration is seen in association with a prolonged contraction **(panel D)**. Evidence presented by Steiger and Nageotte (6) suggests that the majority of prolonged decelerations associated with epidural anesthetics are correlated with prolonged contractions and not hypotension, and that they occur at an average of 15 minutes following injection. Recognition of this resolvable insult should, in general, allow better timing of delivery, after placental resuscitation has occurred.

subtle patterns, or those that occur only occasionally, are frequently not appreciated or are misinterpreted or missed completely. Such rare patterns as sinusoidal or preterminal heart rates may be missed because they are so infrequent and the individual is not familiar with them.

Unfortunately, the size and depth of decelerations do not always correlate with the degree of fetal asphyxia (Fig. 15.8). Prolonged accelerations or decelerations may create confusion over which part of the pattern is the baseline and

which the periodic change (Fig. 15.9A,B). Poor external monitor signals may mask important patterns. Electrical or other artifacts sometimes mask patterns or cause misinterpretation (Fig. 15.10). Increased FHR variability may similarly mask deceleration patterns (Fig. 15.11). On occasion, fetal arrhythmias are falsely interpreted as patterns indicating hypoxia/asphyxia (Fig. 15.12). (Sinusoidal and preterminal heart rates are demonstrated and described in other chapters.)

(text continues on page 248)

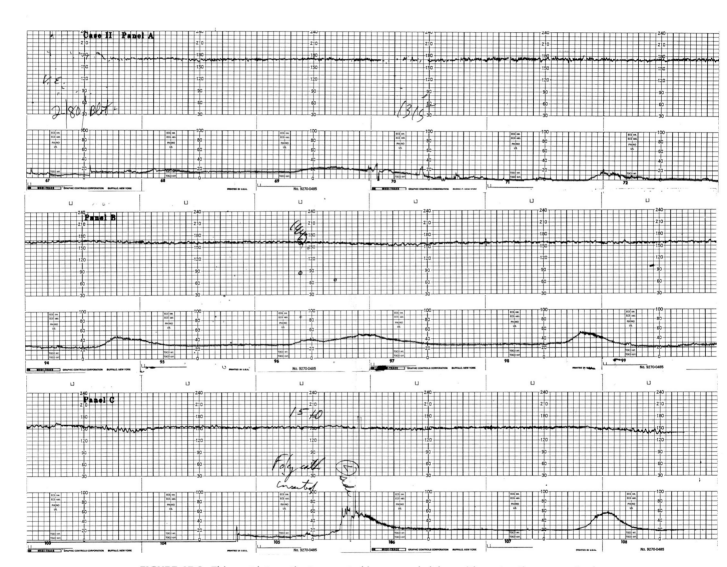

FIGURE 15.8. This postdate patient presented in very early labor with contractions every 7 minutes, cervical dilation 2 cm, and effacement 80%. On external monitor it can be seen that long-term variability is essentially absent, and, on careful scrutiny, late decelerations are seen with all contractions. Late decelerations, particularly in the postmature fetus, can be very shallow and difficult to recognize, especially on an external monitor. In the presence of flat baseline heart rates, take special care to scrutinize the monitor for such shallow late decelerations. Cesarean section in this patient shortly after the end of **panel C** resulted in a postmature-appearing baby with Apgar scores of 5 at 1 minute and 7 at 5 minutes and an umbilical arterial pH of 7.18 showing mild acidosis.

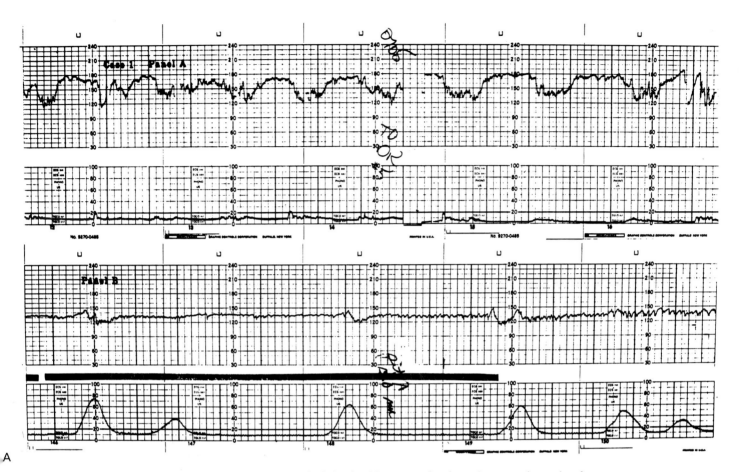

A

FIGURE 15.9. A: The **upper panel** of this fetal heart rate (FHR) monitor record reveals a fetus with heart rate varying between 130 and 180 beats per minute (BPM). The clinician erroneously interpreted the lower heart rate as decelerations below a tachycardiac baseline (180 BPM) and took the patient to cesarean section for a nonreassuring FHR rate pattern. In reality this pattern demonstrates a baseline rate of 130 BPM with frequent and somewhat prolonged accelerations to 180 BPM. The **lower panel** preceded the **upper panel** by some minutes and shows the actual baseline rate of 130 BPM. The absence of contraction monitoring on the **upper panel** makes interpretation of the pattern even more difficult. To avoid this pitfall, review the previous baseline rate and look at the contraction channel to see whether the correlation of timing and contraction makes any sense. In addition, ask the mother if the baby is very active, and see whether the fetal movements coincide with the accelerations. Finally, note that decelerations are rarely flat at their nadir, as is this baseline heart rate of 130 BPM. *(Continued on next page)*

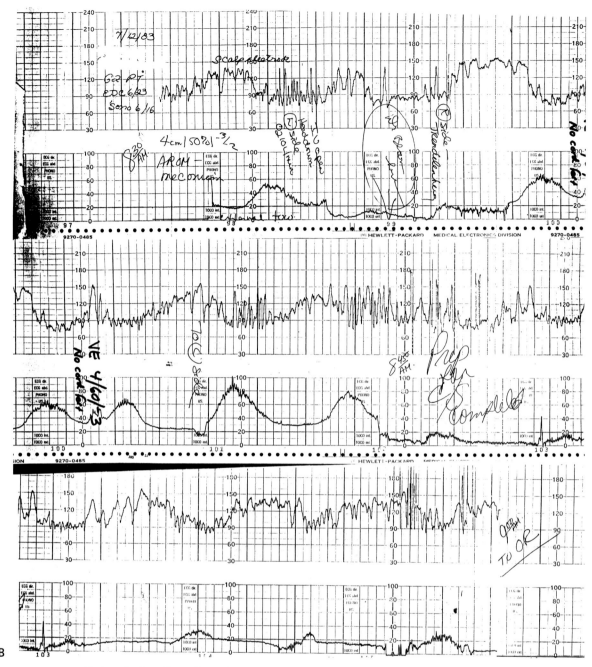

B

FIGURE 15.9. *(continued)* B: The interpretation of this strip is even more difficult than that demonstrated in Fig. 15.9A. The patient was admitted at 43 weeks gestation at 4 cm dilation. Amniotomy was immediately performed, and an internal scalp electrode placed. Meconium was noted. This FHR ranges between 80 to 90 and 150 BPM and shows increased variability. The physician interpreted this strip as demonstrating recurrent prolonged decelerations and, given the clinical information, decided to proceed to cesarean section for presumed fetal hypoxia. The baby had Apgar scores of 8 at 1 minute and 9 at 5 minutes, and umbilical cord pH values were normal. Although there may yet remain some debate over which is the actual baseline rate, the neonatal heart rate throughout its otherwise normal stay in the nursery was 80 to 90 BPM. This case probably represents a benign baseline bradycardia with accelerations to 150 BPM.

FIGURE 15.11. There is fetal heart rate (FHR) variability throughout the portion of the strip shown here. Although this pattern may itself represent very early hypoxia, it is not overly concerning and generally requires only careful observation. The problem is that such increased variability may mask one's ability to appreciate the shallow decelerations that are actually present within the backbone of the increased variability. The clinician can appreciate late decelerations by drawing an imaginary line through the center of the FHR above and below which the heart rate is oscillating *(arrows)*. This baby was delivered somewhat depressed (Apgar scores 5 at 1 minute and 6 at 5 minutes, with a mild metabolic acidosis). The clinicians were surprised to deliver a depressed baby in the presence of what they considered a reassuring pattern.

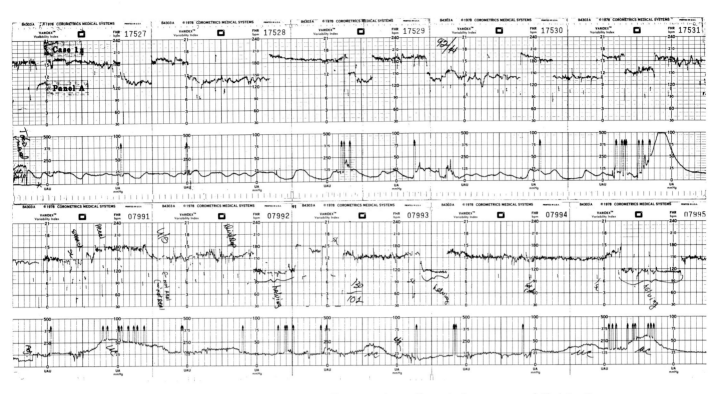

FIGURE 15.10. This fetal monitor strip illustrates the artifactual phenomenon of "halving." Sometimes, on an external Doppler tracing, as the rate goes up to higher levels the monitor logic becomes refractory to the higher rate and halves the interpreted rate. Thus, in this strip, as the fetal heart rate (FHR) accelerates to rates above 180 beats per minute (BPM) (as seen on **panel 07991**), with subsequent accelerations the rate is halved to 110 BPM. These halved FHRs can be easily misinterpreted as some type of concerning deceleration, as opposed to the reassuring accelerations that they actually are.

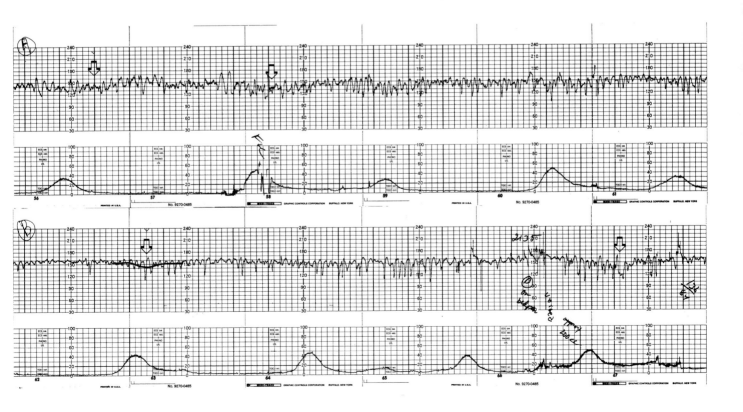

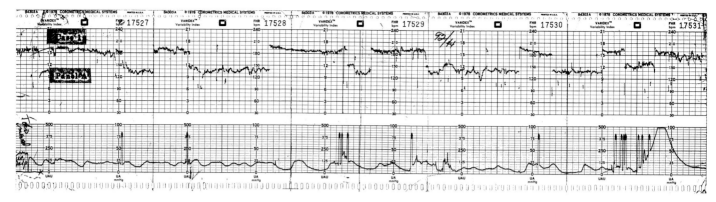

FIGURE 15.12. This pattern could be misinterpreted as tachycardia with prolonged decelerations to 130 beats per minute. In reality, as confirmed by fetal echocardiography, these are real atrial rates, probably representing a benign fetal atrial arrhythmia.

ANTEPARTUM PROBLEMS

Pitfalls in antepartum fetal evaluation may arise from many sources, with false nonreassuring or false reassuring tests consequent to misinterpretation, failing to follow established guidelines for conducting and interpreting tests, failing to test appropriate patients, or failing to respond to abnormal tests appropriately. Because multiple types of

antepartum fetal evaluation modalities have been developed, common pitfalls may vary with the type of test used. These can, nevertheless, be identified and described.

Falsely Nonreassuring Tests

Tests of baseline fetal status, in general, use lack of fetal activity as their endpoints. It should be appreciated that

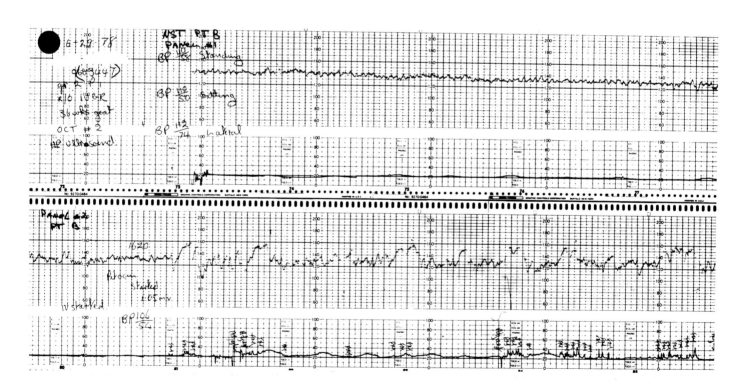

FIGURE 15.13. This nonreactive nonstress test (NST) **(upper panel)** becomes reactive in the **lower panel** as the nurse is preparing to start an intravenous line to perform a backup oxytocin challenge test. A common reason for false nonreassuring (nonreactive NST) tests is the failure to wait an adequate amount of time for sleep cycles to change, with resultant changes in the biophysical parameters used for fetal testing.

fetal sleep-like states may affect the results of nonstress tests (NSTs), fetal movement counting, and fetal respirations. Sufficient time should be allowed before interpreting these tests as nonreassuring. For NSTs and fetal movement counting, up to 60 to 80 minutes may be required before being confident that the absence of fetal reactivity and/or movement may be secondary to a fetal sleep cycle (Fig. 15.13). Depressant drugs will often result in false nonreassuring patterns in tests that depend on central nervous system (CNS) alertness. Drugs such as barbiturates, narcotics, many psychotropics, and, theoretically, beta-adrenergic blockers may precipitate nonreactive nonstress patterns and/or absent fetal movement. Nicotine in cigarettes may decrease fetal respirations. The effect of such drugs on fetal tone has not been well-described but may be similar to the effect on movement, although tone would be less likely to be affected. One may want to weigh whether the use of such depressants is necessary (e.g., phenobarbital in the expectantly managed preeclamptic), because they often make FHR and other test interpretation difficult (Fig. 15.14). Similarly, fetal anomalies may be the origin of abnormal FHR patterns and other tests that appear to be

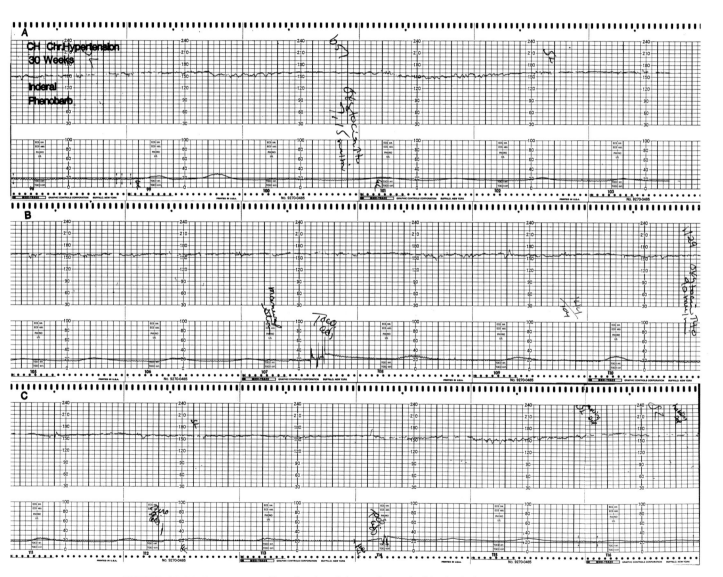

FIGURE 15.14. Drugs may affect fetal activity and certain biophysical parameters. The fetal heart rate in this 30-week fetus is persistently nonreactive; however, both drugs that this patient is taking, phenobarbital and propranolol (Inderal), may diminish reactivity. Phenobarbital reduces fetal movement by central nervous system (CNS) depression. Inderal is a beta-sympathetic blocker that may inhibit the usual cardiac response (accelerations) to CNS stimuli. Hence, in patients taking such medications, it is difficult to tell whether decreased reactivity and/or fetal movement is due to CNS depression secondary to asphyxia or drugs. Similar difficulty may arise when the patient ingests certain illicit drugs.

consistent with CNS depression subsequent to hypoxia and asphyxia. Certainly, such obvious and lethal anomalies as anencephaly can and should be carefully sought and identified before intervening for fetal indications (Fig. 15.15). In the case of the contraction stress test (CST), a number of situations may produce false positive or nonreassuring results. Maternal supine hypotension may decrease uterine perfusion and produce late decelerations. Generally, blood pressure monitoring during testing and care in positioning will aid in the recognition and avoidance of this problem. Unrecognized hyperstimulation may also generate false positive CSTs. Proper positioning of the tocodynamometer and careful administration of oxytocin or nipple stimulation should be ensured (Fig. 15.16).

Falsely Reassuring Tests

The most explicit and definable goal of antepartum fetal evaluation is the prevention of fetal death. Therefore, fetal death within a week (or whatever the usual repeating frequency) of a reassuring test would define a false negative or falsely reassuring test. Although certainly not due to test failure, the most common circumstances associated with antepartum death is the untested patient. As in intrapartum electronic FHR monitoring, careful attention should be paid to maternal risk factors (Table 15.1), because it is usual practice to use some form of antepartum fetal surveillance on all high-risk patients. In theory at least, testing the 15% of patients who are at high risk will result in a 50% reduction in antepartum fetal deaths. The dilemma, of course, is that if this scheme is successful, the majority of stillbirths will then come from low-risk patients or those who are noncompliant or do not seek prenatal care. It is probably appropriate, therefore, to apply some form of antepartum evaluation, such as fetal movement counting, to all patients (Fig. 15.17). As mentioned in Chapter 12, antepartum fetal evaluation is not likely to detect certain causes of fetal deaths, for example, cord accidents, abruptio placentae, anomalies,

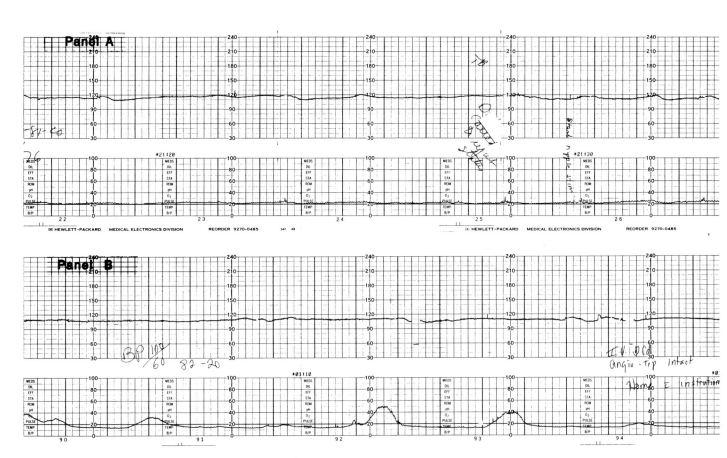

FIGURE 15.15. This is a fetus with holoprosencephaly and structural cardiac defects. Central nervous system (CNS) and cardiac congenital malformations are often associated with abnormal and even bizarre fetal heart rate (FHR) patterns. This FHR is bradycardic (110 beats per minute), shows no accelerations, and has nearly absent long-term variability. When the contractions are induced on the **panel B,** no late decelerations are seen, making it unlikely that asphyxia is the source of the CNS depression producing this alarming pattern. In the presence of nonreactive negative contraction stress tests, the physician should consider drugs and anomalies as possible explanations.

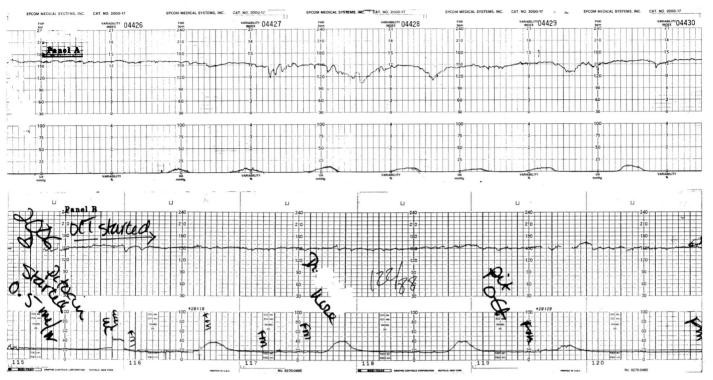

FIGURE 15.16. An oxytocin challenge test (OCT) **(panel A)** was administered to a patient at 33 weeks because of a history of two antepartum stillbirths at approximately this same gestational age. There are obvious persistent late decelerations and no accelerations. This test result was interpreted as nonreactive positive and the patient was transferred to the tertiary center for consideration for possible delivery. On reviewing the tracing, it became apparent that the baseline pressure of the tocodynamometer, set at 0, was too low. It was possible that the actual duration of the contractions was considerably longer than what was printed, and that only the "top of the mountain" was being seen. The test was repeated **(panel B)**, with the clinicians paying careful attention to set the contraction channel baseline at 20 and avoid hyperstimulation. The second test result was negative and reactive. Following subsequent normal antepartum testing, the patient went on to deliver a healthy baby at term. Unrecognized hyperstimulation is an important potential cause of false-positive OCT results and should be carefully avoided.

and sudden deterioration in maternal condition (e.g., preeclampsia). Occasionally, some of these problems can be avoided. Promptly retesting patients with vaginal bleeding or a decrease in fetal movement can sometimes preclude death from sudden causes. In patients with oligohydramnios, those with variable decelerations on previous tests, and those with ultrasonically detected funic presentations may be candidates for more aggressive monitoring and earlier intervention to prevent umbilical cord accidents (Fig. 15.18). A very important additional example of preventing such unexpected fetal deaths in tested patients is in those mothers whose condition significantly changes or deteriorates. A partial list of situations in which immediate fetal testing should be done, regardless of when the previous test was conducted, is provided in Table 15.2. In such situations, fetal retesting may reveal associated deterioration of fetal condition and may lead to either correcting the maternal problem, with resultant improvement in fetal condition or delivery (Fig. 15.19).

Poor quality testing, or failure to follow established guidelines for conducting and interpreting tests, is a dangerous potential pitfall in antepartum FHR testing, especially with the CST (Fig. 15.20). Late decelerations are often subtle, especially on antepartum tests, and can be easily missed in inconsistent or artifactually affected FHR tracings. Meticulous care must be taken and demanded, and a continuous high-quality FHR tracing obtained, to avoid this pitfall. For this reason it is advisable to use the highest quality and latest model monitor available for CST. Published studies on antepartum FHR monitoring and other types of fetal evaluation have reported excellent results, with low stillbirth rates in tested populations. The success of these studies has been attributed to following strict protocols for conducting the tests, test interpretation, and deter-

(text continues on page 254)

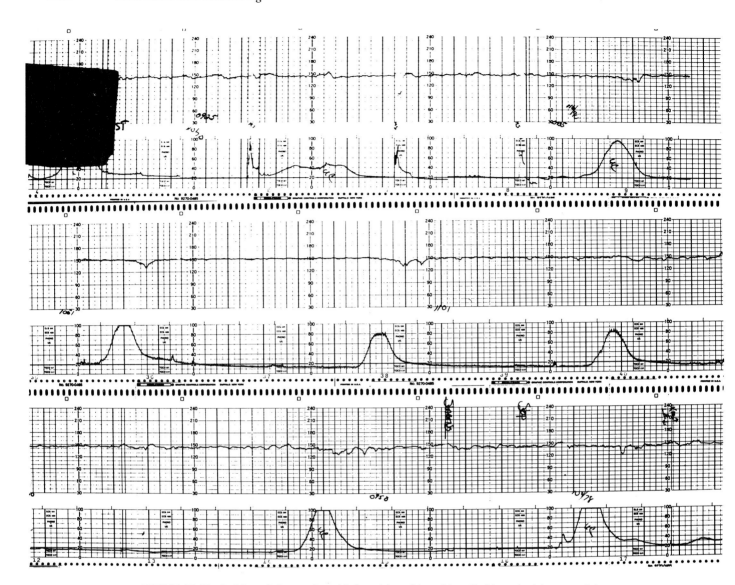

FIGURE 15.17. At 34 weeks' gestation, this low-risk multigravida called her physician complaining of decreased fetal movement over the previous 12 hours. She was told to carefully count movements for 1 hour. She called back, having felt no movements for that hour, and was brought in for an immediate nonstress test. No accelerations were observed, and spontaneous late decelerations occurred with the infrequent contractions. Nipple stimulation produced a contraction stress test with persistent late decelerations. The fetus remained nonreactive. The patient was taken for cesarean section and was delivered of a premature appropriately grown newborn with Apgar scores of 8 at 1 minute and 8 at 5 minutes and a mild metabolic acidosis. No explanation for the nonreassuring antepartum fetal heart rate pattern was apparent. This case illustrates the importance of alerting low-risk patients to observe fetal activity.

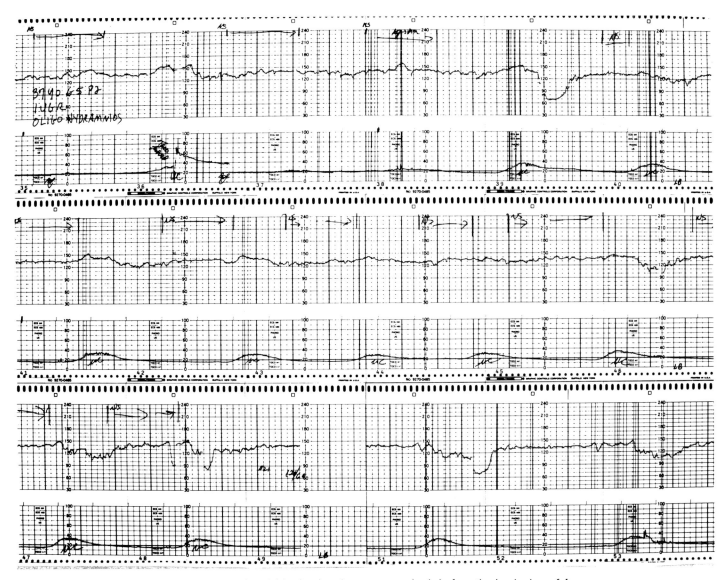

FIGURE 15.18. Several variable decelerations are seen both before the beginning of **(upper panel)** and during **(lower panel)** the oxytocin challenge test in this patient with mild intrauterine growth retardation at 33 weeks and significant oligohydramnios. Such variable decelerations are commonly seen on antepartum fetal heart rate strips in association with oligohydramnios, because the umbilical cord is not afforded the usual protection as with normal fluid volumes.

TABLE 15.2. SITUATIONS REQUIRING IMMEDIATE RETESTING BECAUSE OF A SUDDEN CHANGE IN MATERNAL CONDITION

Worsening preeclampsia
Worsening renal disease
Acute asthmatic episode
Severe maternal dehydration
Acute trauma
Diabetes out of control
Lupus flare

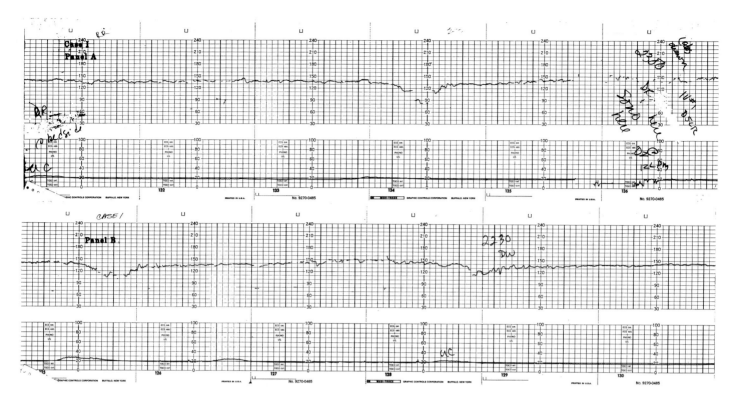

FIGURE 15.19. This patient had been undergoing antepartum testing for mild chronic hypertension and had a normal contraction stress test result 3 days before presenting with scant vaginal bleeding at 32 weeks. There was no associated abdominal pain. The uterus was nontender. For 45 minutes, the strip was persistently nonreactive, with late decelerations occurring with contractions that the patient was not feeling. A portion of the initial strip is shown on **panel A.** An ultrasound was performed, no abruption seen, and the biophysical profile score was only 2 (normal fluid). The patient was taken for cesarean section, delivering an appropriately grown baby with Apgar scores of 4 at 1 minute and 8 at 5 minutes. A 30% abruptio placenta was identified as the cause of the nonreassuring antepartum fetal heart rate pattern. This illustrates the importance of repeat fetal evaluation when any new situation arises, in this case, vaginal bleeding.

mining when to repeat the test. A CST may be quite reactive and may have only one late deceleration among many contractions. Although it is often tempting to ignore the late deceleration and interpret the test as negative, such variances in interpretation guidelines have not yielded good outcome in published studies (Fig. 15.21). Equivocal tests should be strictly interpreted and repeated the next day. NSTs must meet strict criteria for reactivity before discontinuing the test and sending the patient home. Nonreactive NSTs must be followed up with another test such as biophysical profile or CST and not simply repeated the next day (Fig. 15.22). Negative CSTs should be repeated at least weekly and NSTs probably more frequently, although many

still advocate weekly NSTs. As stated previously, immediate retesting should be performed in the presence of a significant change in maternal status that might affect the fetus. As with false-positive test results, misinterpreted NSTs and CSTs may result in false-negative results (unprevented fetal death). Late decelerations are often subtle and easy to miss, even on good quality tracings (Fig. 15.23). Tests should be carefully reviewed by the individual responsible for interpretation. Verbal reports may be incorrect or may not totally convey the seriousness or urgency of the situation. Hospital guidelines providing for an appropriate maximum interval between testing and interpretation may be helpful in avoiding this pitfall (Fig. 15.24).

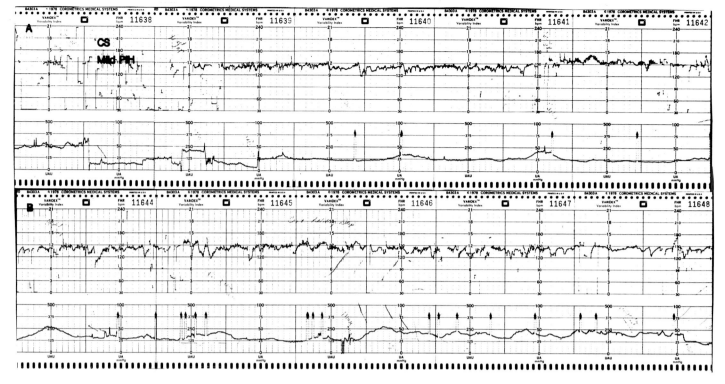

FIGURE 15.20. In this example of an unsatisfactory contraction stress test, the frequent loss of signal, especially on the **lower panel**, could easily lead to missed shallow late decelerations that might be apparent on better quality tracings. (None are seen on this tracing.) For this reason, the quality of the fetal heart rate tracing is especially critical for contraction stress testing.

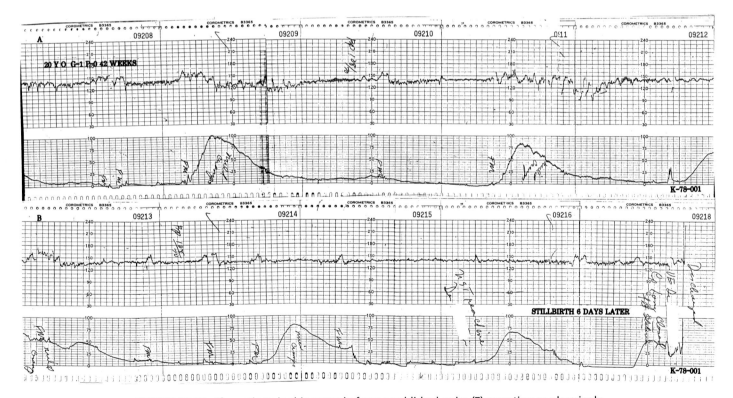

FIGURE 15.21. The patient, in this example from a published series (7) reporting an alarmingly high rate of stillbirths in tested postdate patients, was undergoing a nonstress test for prolonged pregnancy (42 weeks). The test results clearly met the criteria for reactivity, and on that basis a repeat test was rescheduled in 1 week. Six days later, antepartum fetal death was discovered. On **panel A**, there are two late decelerations. While admittedly these are with prolonged contractions (hyperstimulation), this still qualifies as an equivocal test result and requires at least a repeat test in 1 day. (From Miyazaki FS, Miyazaki BA: False reactive nonstress tests in postterm pregnancies. *Am J Obstet Gynecol* 140:269, 1981, with permission.)

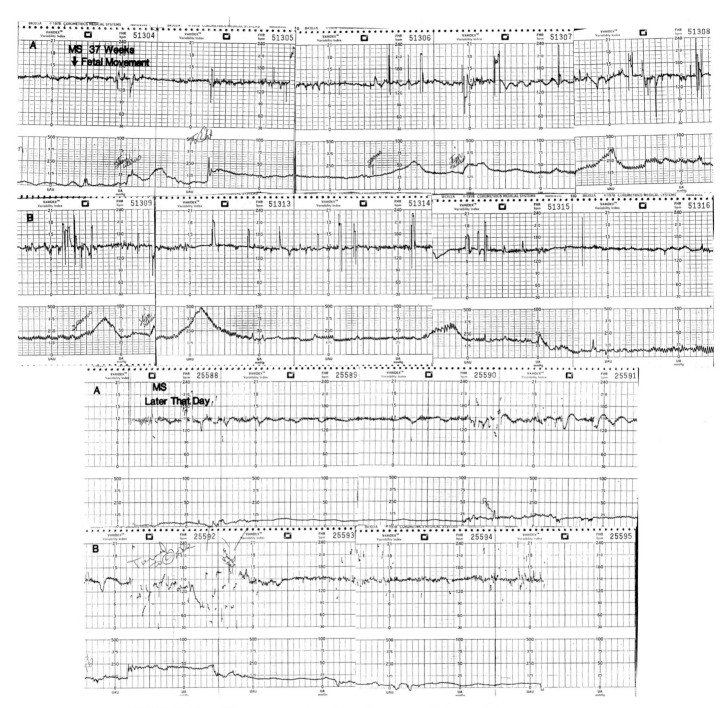

FIGURE 15.22. At 37 weeks' gestation, this patient reported decreased fetal movement. An immediate nonstress test was performed, and on **upper panels A** and **B** it can be seen that this test result does not meet criteria for reactivity. Her contractions were judged of insufficient length, not palpably strong, and not being adequately sensed by the patient to meet criteria for a spontaneous contraction stress test (CST). In accordance with the protocol in this testing unit, the patient was brought back later that day to see if the test would be reactive at that time. On the second test, the fetus remained nonreactive and no contractions were present. Unfortunately, no backup test (CST or biophysical profile) was performed and by the next day the fetus had died.

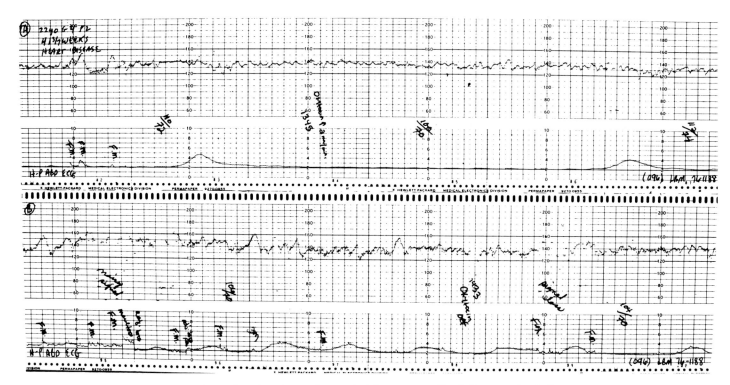

FIGURE 15.23. During the observation period **(upper panel)** of this oxytocin challenge test, two spontaneous contractions occur, both associated with late decelerations. Contractions are then stimulated with oxytocin, and the remainder are without decelerations. The significance of the initial late decelerations should not be ignored and, in this test at least, requires repeating in 1 day. This case also illustrates how carefully one must scrutinize a contraction stress test. Late decelerations, such as those seen here, are easy to overlook.

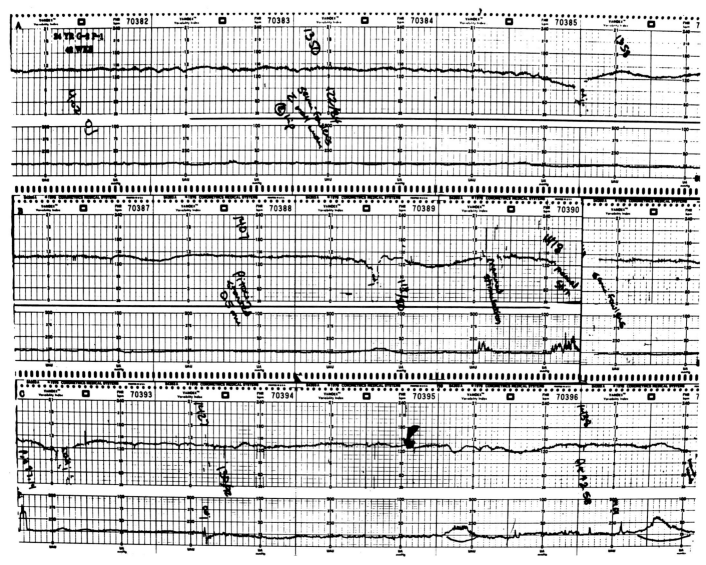

FIGURE 15.24. In this patient being tested because of postdate pregnancy, the test result is non-reactive and positive. It is also clear that the baseline fetal heart rate is quite flat. This is an ominous antepartum tracing. The nurse performing the test informed the physician verbally of the absence of accelerations and presence of late decelerations. The patient was admitted and scheduled for cesarean section later that day, but not monitored continually. Approximately 8 hours later, the patient was seen by the physician in preparation for delivery, but by then the fetus was dead. Verbal reports often fail to convey the urgency of the situation. Abnormal test results should be reviewed promptly.

REFERENCES

1. Shenker L: Clinical experiences with fetal heart rate monitoring of one thousand patients in labor. *Am J Obstet Gynecol* 115:1111, 1973.
2. Gold WR, Levine AM: Pinpointing a major source of Ob malpractice claims. *Contemp Obstet Gynecol* 20:215, 1982.
3. Seitchik J, Castillo M: Oxytocin augmentation of dysfunctional labor. I. Clinical data. *Am J Obstet Gynecol* 144:899, 1982.
4. American College of Obstetricians and Gynecologists, American Academy of Pediatrics: *Guidelines for perinatal care,* 2nd ed. Washington DC, 1988.
5. Miller FC, Pearse KE, Paul RH: Fetal heart rate pattern recognition by the method of auscultation. *Obstet Gynecol* 64:332, 1984.
6. Steiger RM, Nageotte MP: Prolonged decelerations following bupivacaine epidural anesthesia presented at the Society of Perinatal Obstetricians, Houston, TX, February 1990.
7. Miyazaki FS, Miyazaki BA: False reactive nonstress tests in postterm pregnancies. *Am J Obstet Gynecol* 140:269, 1981.

SUBJECT INDEX

Page numbers ending in "*f*" refer to figures. Page numbers ending in "*t*" refer to tables.